REGIONAL PERSPECTIVES IN BIOETHICS

The Annals of Bioethics

Regional Perspectives in Bioethics

Edited by

John F. Peppin
Director
Center for Bioethics, Pain Management & Medicine
Des Moines, Iowa

and

Mark J. Cherry
Department of Philosophy
Saint Edward's University
Austin, Texas

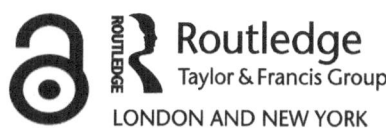 Routledge
Taylor & Francis Group
LONDON AND NEW YORK

Library of Congress Cataloging-in-Publication Data

Applied for

First published 2003 by Swets & Zeitlinger Publishers

Published 2017 by Routledge
2 Park Square, Milton Park, Abingdon, Oxon OX14 4RN
52 Vanderbilt Avenue, New York, NY 10017, USA

First issued in paperback 2014

Routledge is an imprint of the Taylor and Francis Group, an informa business

Copyright © 2003 Swets & Zeitlinger B.V., Lisse, The Netherlands

Although all care is taken to ensure the integrity and quality of this publication and the information herein, no responsibility is assumed by the publishers nor the editors for the publication and/or the information contained herein.

ISBN 13: 978-90-265-1952-9 (hbk)
ISBN 13: 978-1-138-00222-7 (pbk)

Contents

PART III: EUROPE

PART IV: ASIA

Acknowledgements

The development of this volume benefited through the kind efforts of many. In particular we would like to thank Eugene Boisaubin, Joseph Boyle, Ruth Groenhoet, Henk Ten Have, Kazumasa Hoshino, Loretta Kopelman, Anne M. Fagot-Largeault, José Alberto Mainetti, Maurizio Mori, Edmund D. Pellegrino, Ren-Zong Qiu, Michael Rie, Hans-Martin Sass, W. David Solomon, and Griffin Trotter, who were discussion partners that aided in reviewing and focusing the essays. In addition, a number of individuals must be thanked in particular who contributed significant time and energy to the volume: Ana Smith Iltis, Fabrice Jotterand, Lisa Rasmussen, Fr. Allyne Smith, Matthew Lomanno, and Robert Perez. A very special debt is owed to H. Tristram Engelhardt, Jr., who, in addition to having unfailingly and tirelessly supported this project's development, contributed a splendid introduction.

We also wish to recognize the on-going kindness of Saint Edward's University, School of Humanities, the Department of Philosophy, and the Center for Ethics and Leadership, especially Louis T. Brusatti, William J. Zanardi, and Phillip M. Thompson. Each has been instrumental, though in different capacities, to the success of this project.

John F. Peppin and Mark J. Cherry

Preface to a new series

Annals of Bioethics: A Forum of Foundational, Clinical and Emerging Topics

Bioethics has become a truly international phenomenon. Through foundational philosophical, religious, and cultural perspectives, clinical case studies, and legal analysis, the *Annals of Bioethics* documents, reviews, and explores emerging bioethical viewpoints as well as the state-of-the-art of this global endeavor.

In so doing, the *Annals* is, perhaps inadvertently, as much on the nature and depth of our contemporary moral and cultural conflicts as it is on biomedical ethics. Bioethics is grounded in and has implications for the religious, political, and legal elements of cultures. As a field of inquiry, bioethics has coveted an international political forum. Secular Western bioethics in particular lays claim to a universal account of proper moral deportment, including the foundations of law and public policy, as well as the moral authority for national and international institutions to guarantee uniformity of practice, secure basic human rights, and promote social justice. Bioethical expertise is widely sought in the framing of public and institutional policy. Witness, for example, the broad advisory role of the President's Council on Bioethics in the United States, as well as the European Bioethics Convention, which sought not merely to explain or analyze moral issues but to justify political resolutions. Similarly, bioethicists regularly provide testimony as expert witnesses in courts of law. They present themselves as experts of moral rationality and principles of moral probity, including permissible standards of evidence and inference.

Religious and cultural moral diversity runs deep; it strides the divisions that separate regional, religious, and cultural biomedical and moral perspectives. This series illustrates the ways in which the national and international political landscape compasses persons from diverse and often fragmented moral communities with widely varying moral intuitions, premises, evaluations, and commitments. The various volumes explore, document, and critically appreciate diverse moral, cultural, and religious viewpoints representing the various regions of the world, from mainland China and Hong Kong, Taiwan, Japan, India and East Asia more generally, to Europe, the Middle East, Australia and New Zealand, to South America and North America. Moral perspectives range from Orthodox Christianity, Roman Catholicism, and contemporary Protestant Christianity, to Orthodox, Conservative and Reformed Judaism, to Islam, Buddhism, Confucianism, Hinduism, and so forth, to secular liberal egalitarianism. The goal of the series is to document and review the often widely varying bioethical perspectives reflected throughout the international community's regions, religions, laws and policies.

The *Annals of Bioethics* compasses updates in moral theory, normative health care practice, case studies, and public policy. The series begins with three foundational volumes: *Regional Perspectives in Bioethics*; *Religious Perspectives in Bioethics*; and *Legal Perspectives in Bioethics*, which establish an initial framework. Future volumes will document and assess legal, religious and cultural responses to specific aspects of the fast paced developments in health care and medical technology. Future areas to be explored include such contentious issues as abortion, euthanasia, prenatal genetic screening, parental discretion regarding treatment of neonates, genetic engineering, sex reassignment surgery, reproductive technologies, and cloning, as well as the permissible foundations and limits of biomedical ethics and health care policy.

Biomedical policy must be created to span a diverse set of individuals, cultures, and communities. Political struggles regard the structure and content of what will become the prevailing medical, moral, and social ethos. Such discussions concern not merely which policies will best achieve the desired objectives, but which objectives are themselves desirable; that is, which moral understanding should be established (e.g., pro-choice or pro-life; individual versus family or community oriented consent), utilizing which school of practice (traditional Chinese or Western medicine, allopathic, homeopathic, naturopathic, or chiropractic health care, and so forth), at what standard of care (e.g., guaranteed equal access for all, or with regional variation, or varying levels of access depending on insurance coverage). There exists a significant plurality of fundamentally different, incompatible, and often mutually antagonistic moral visions and moral rationalities, within which such complex bioethical issues are addressed. An honest assessment of bioethics requires careful consideration of the various regional, religious, cultural, and legal perspectives on such concerns.

The *Annals of Bioethics* documents and explores such complex concerns while remaining an approachable set of authoritative texts for physicians, nurses and other health care professionals, lawyers, and students, as well as philosophers, theologians, and bioethicists. To that end, guided by the usual scholarly standards of peer review, our international editorial advisory board consists of scholars representing philosophy, law, theology, and medicine. The *Annals* will include clinical case studies as well as foundational philosophical, religious, and cultural positions and critical commentary. As such, the *Annals of Bioethics* documents the diverse moral perspectives within which health care policy must be fashioned.

The series editors welcome proposals from interested scholars for future volumes that further develop and document particular aspects of the ongoing international debates concerning bioethics.

Mark J. Cherry   Ana Iltis
Department of Philosophy   Center for Health Care Ethics
Saint Edward's University   Saint Louis University
3001 S. Congress Avenue   Salus Center
Austin, Texas 78704   3545 Lafayette Avenue
                                                                        St. Louis, Missouri 63104

Introduction: Bioethics as a Global Phenomenon

H. Tristram Engelhardt, Jr.

I. A Global Phenomenon Versus a Global Bioethics

The essays in this volume provide a view of the state of bioethical reflection across the world at the threshold of the 21st century. On the one hand, they amply demonstrate that interest in bioethics spans the globe. On the other hand, the attentive reader will notice differences, often subtle, in moral perspective from country to country. In a number of cases, the differences in moral assumptions underlying the ethics applied by bioethics will be salient and significant. These differences in moral viewpoint underlie an important debate that is now surfacing in the field: is there one or a number of bioethics? This question is in part dependent on a more fundamental issue: do humans share one morality? Or, instead, are humans committed to a cluster of different moralities? In answering these questions, one must bear in mind that overlapping moral interests do not constitute a common morality. It may be the case that humans in general are interested in such cardinal values as liberty, equality, prosperity, and security. However, depending on how persons rank these values, they will live within quite different moral viewpoints and affirm substantively different, settled moral judgments. All moralities, for example, may be concerned with the propriety of killing and lying; however, these moralities may be distinguished in terms of when it is forbidden or praiseworthy to kill or to lie.

This plurality of moral understandings, visions, and narratives can be accounted for in terms of a number of different and competing views regarding the nature of morality, moral knowledge, and the moral life. Somewhat procrusteanly, moral pluralism can be understood as having four major sources:

(1) Moral-metaphysical skepticism. This, the strongest account of moral pluralism, denies the existence of any objective moral truth. Instead, it grounds morality in local custom, convention, and agreement. In this account there is no independent moral truth for all to know.

(2) Moral-epistemological skepticism. This account of moral pluralism does not deny the existence of an independent moral truth. Rather, it denies the ability to know with certainty that one knows this moral truth. Moral pluralism is tolerated by default.

(3) The recognition of special, non-discursive epistemological conditions for knowing moral truth. This account of moral pluralism recognizes a diversity of moral viewpoints, understandings, and narratives to be an undesirable outcome of the failure to pursue

moral knowledge properly. Such accounts, as for example within traditional Christian understandings of epistemology, require a personal, spiritual transformation of the knower in order rightly to know morality.

(4) Limited moral pluralism due to divergent local conditions. In this case, moral pluralism represents only the outcome of applying generally valid moral principles and rules within different contexts.

Of course, moral pluralism may be the result of any one of the first three circumstances for moral divergence plus the fourth. As one looks to the foundations for pluralism in bioethics, one will need to bear in mind at least these fundamental sources of moral difference.

It is also helpful to consider a number of axes along which moral difference in bioethics can be displayed. These axes are offered as heuristics in order to identify the character of moral difference. They are not exclusive and surely can be overlapping.

(1) Traditional versus post-traditional bioethics. Differences among bioethical understandings depend on the extent to which a nation, culture, or religion has become post-traditional. The result will be conflicts, for example, with respect to whether artificial insemination should be restricted only to married couples and their gametes. Here, too, one can locate differences in the plausibility or implausibility of families making medical decisions on behalf of their competent members.

(2) Market versus social-liberal understandings of moral probity. Along this axis, different views will seem plausible regarding the relative importance of market rights versus liberty rights. Those who embrace particular content-rich views of liberty rights may regard a range of market choices as exploitative.

(3) Autonomy interests versus equality interests. Along this axis, different views will seem plausible or implausible as to whether the free choices of individuals may veto the realization of egalitarian goals.

These three axes can surely be supplemented by further ways of attending to the structure of moral controversies and the character of different understandings regarding the proper use of medicine, the allocation of health care resources, and the development of the biomedical sciences.

This dawning recognition of the possibility of conflicting human moralities and bioethics should not come as a surprise to anyone who has become acquainted with the so-called culture wars: the moral-political struggle to define the guiding assumptions that will frame the major institutions of particular countries and of international organizations (Hunter, 1991). After the events of September 11, 2001, it should be clear that there are stark differences in views of right and wrong moral and political conduct. It would be a mistake to regard these differences simply in terms of conflicts among religious views or between secular and religious views. There is an emerging appreciation of differences in bioethical perspective grounded in disparate cultural commitments and moral histories.[1] It may prove to be the case that the world is moving towards being marked by greater moral difference in its bioethical approaches after a period where increasing unanimity seemed to be the rule. As one reads these essays, one might see whether one can scry in them any suggestion of a emerging clash of civilizations (Huntington, 1996). Surely, the markers will not be easy to discern, but may exist nevertheless.

Before us lies the challenge of peaceably coming to terms with moral pluralism. Meeting this challenge will require securing an adequate diagnosis of the philosophical and cultural roots of moral pluralism. One will need to judge as well regarding the extent to which this pluralism inevitably leads to a struggle for the opportunity to impose at law one moral orthodoxy rather than another (Engelhardt, 1996). From a moral perspective, questions regarding political power must be anchored in moral concerns. It is regarding such issues that this volume and this series make such an important contribution. The reader will find in this and the volumes to follow perspectives on bioethics drawn from different cultural, religious, and national contexts. The reader may wish to attend not only to the similarities but to the differences among national and religious approaches to issues in bioethics. As an introduction to using these resources, this essay begins with a focus on the genesis of bioethics in the 1970s and its emergence as an American-made moral movement. The introduction then lays out some general characteristics of the context within which bioethics and bioethicists find themselves. The reader will find essays and authors drawn from five continents and over twenty national perspectives. The richness of its compass is a tribute to the growing maturity of the field.

II. The Creation of Bioethics

In 1972 bioethics emerged seemingly from nowhere. In two important senses, it took shape as a thoroughly American phenomenon. First, it was made in America. Second, its predominant moral commitments reflected a particularly American version of a liberal democratic ethos with its special emphasis on individual autonomy and personal rights. As to the first, bioethics came into existence out of an ingenious cultural diagnosis by André Hellegers, the first director of the Kennedy Institute of Ethics, and by Sargent Shriver, founder of the Peace Corps. They correctly perceived a substantial societal need for a body of moral experts to guide health care and the biomedical sciences. Either jointly or individually, they *de novo* invented the term bioethics, or, according to another account, they insightfully re-applied a term already coined by Van Rensselaer Potter. He had used the term not to identify the current field, but a *Lebensphilosophie* compatible with sustaining the human population in a threatened environment (1970a, 1970b). Despite the controversy regarding the genesis of the term (Reich, 1994),[2] one thing is clear: with the support of the Kennedy family, Eunice and Sargent Shriver in particular, and Georgetown University, the Kennedy Institute of Ethics successfully applied a name to a social phenomenon that by the end of the 20th century had transformed the moral context within which medical and science policy were framed. Although there were other institutions engaged in exploring issues of ethics, medicine, and the humanities prior to the establishment of the Kennedy Institute of Ethics, along with its Center for Bioethics, most especially the Hastings Center (née Institute of Society, Ethics, and the Life Sciences), it was the Kennedy Institute that uniquely associated the name bioethics with an academically established cadre of scholars and a commitment to the training of ethics experts. The result was a cultural turning point: the establishment of a socially recognized body of moral experts in authority to give moral direction regarding moral decision-making and conduct in health care and the biomedical sciences.

The Kennedy Institute of Ethics brought together an academically established body of scholars who generated a literature, taught graduate and undergraduate students, and who conducted total-immersion courses for individuals drawn from a wide range of professional and academic backgrounds. The first two traditional undertakings lent credibility to the last novel undertaking: one-week introductory courses. These one-week intensive courses offered the broader intellectual and professional public acquaintance with the new field. These intensive courses also produced a body of trained bioethicists: after this one-week encounter, some persons considered themselves able "to do" bioethics. The plausibility that such expertise could be so quickly achieved may have come from a distant analogy between these intensive courses and courses designed to train physicians in the use of new procedures and techniques. Courses of four to six weeks were also supported by the National Endowment for the Humanities (NEH). Some individuals after these longer courses came to hold themselves out as able to teach bioethics. This massive production of "ethicists" resulted in the rapid establishment of a field that was at the same time academic as well as practical. In the past, there had surely been numerous departments of philosophy replete with scholars addressing questions of morality. An important *novum* was the creation of a body of moral practitioners recognized as appropriately providing moral guidance for the now major social institution of health care.

Both the academics and the quickly trained practitioners offered services traditionally associated with the roles of moral philosophers and moral theologians. (1) They analyzed concepts, in particular moral concepts, (2) they critically analyzed moral arguments, and (3) they laid out the range of possible positions regarding particular moral and policy issues. Often they did this with a slavish devotion to the Georgetown four principles of Beauchamp and Childress: autonomy, beneficence, non-maleficence, and justice (1979). These four principles conveyed a cultish character to bioethics, especially in the eyes of some academically-based moral philosophers. After less than a decade, a fairly sophisticated literature developed. In addition, the Kennedy Institute gave an academic imprimatur to the field by producing an *Encyclopedia of Bioethics* by the end of the 1970s (Reich, 1978). At the end of the 1970s and during the 1980s, bioethical missionary voyages were undertaken to bring the good news of bioethics to Japan, China, and Europe. These academic missionaries brought with them a view of bioethics framed within the particular context and perspective of America. Remarkably, these attempts were widely influential (though after some initial resistance, given their exotic, American assumptions), no doubt in great measure due to the global influence of the American economy, American science, and American medicine. It seemed plausible to many that if American biomedicine could be so successful, its new ethics should be given a serious hearing.

Although bioethics had many of the trappings of a traditional academic field, there were a number of important and noticeable differences. First, many of those who characterized themselves as ethicists or bioethicists plied their profession not within the usual venues of scholars (e.g., the classroom), but instead increasingly in non-traditional environments, such as hospitals. Second, many of those working in these non-traditional contexts also had non-traditional educational backgrounds, at least from the perspective of philosophers. As already mentioned, some were innocent of advance academic training in the humanities, possessing instead an understanding of the character of moral conflicts in health care derived from personal experience and an autodidact's education, at times supplemented by a one-week intensive course at the Kennedy Institute Center for Bioethics. This state of affairs should not simplistically be considered an indictment of the field for intellectual superficiality or for a failure to provide adequate training for the new cadre of ethicists. Instead, it is an important marker of the considerable perceived societal need for what bioethicists appeared to offer.

The professional roles of analyzing concepts, criticizing arguments, and providing a geography of moral positions were also usually joined to an additional role, (4) that of moral adviser. In this latter role, bioethicists assumed an office to which philosophers had often aspired and which homilists usually possess, namely, that of giving instruction regarding proper deportment. This role was increasingly played in a new context, that of medical education, consultation regarding clinical cases, and service on newly-formed hospital ethics committees. To these roles there came to be added a final and more novel one, (5) that of being a moral expert recognized not simply as an authority but as in authority to pronounce on moral requirements, as when serving as experts recognized by courts (Kipnis, 1997, pp. 325-343). In sum, within less than a third of a century, bioethics was societally recognized and at times legally established as the source of moral guidance for health care and the biomedical sciences.

Numerous plausible accounts can be given of this remarkable phenomenon: the emergence of a group of moral authorities charged with guiding one of society's major institutions. At least this much seems clear: in America, the field of bioethics was the result of a number of significant societal changes. None of these changes was strictly unique to America, but each had a particularly American character: (1) the marginalization of the traditional authority of physicians and of the profession of medicine, (2) the secularization of public life, and (3) the developing emphasis on individual rights and autonomy to the detriment of traditional authority figures. No doubt, there were similar cultural changes occurring in late 20th century Canada, Europe, South America, and the Pacific Rim. Yet, in America these changes came to a focus in one field prior to this happening in other countries.

First, in the mid-20th century through a number of Supreme Court holdings, the American medical profession was recast at law from functioning as a quasi-guild to being constrained to function as a trade. These holdings represented not just a change in the ways in which the medical profession could function economically; they also importantly implied that the norms for medical professional conduct should not collide with the general norms of the society, in this case those that required commerce be unhindered by restraints of trade.[3] An implication of this shift is that medical ethics was not a concern just for physicians. Here it is important to recognize that the medical profession had for a long time understood that its medical ethics were directed not just to the observance of generally endorsed societal norms, but to the protection of the economic interests of physicians. This became clear in the disputes at the end of the 19th century, leading to the establishment of an association of physicians in competition with that of the American Medical Association (AMA). Consider, for example, the address by Francis Delafield, the first president of the Association of American Physicians, who stated at their first meeting in 1886 that they were seeking an association "in which there will be no medical politics and no medical ethics..." (Means, 1961, p. 10). As one entered the mid-20th century, it became plausible not only to criticize medicine for its financially self-serving use of "medical ethics", but also to hold that any parochially professional ethics was not properly an ethics. As a consequence, medical ethics could no longer be considered independently of the dominant culture's moral commitments. This led to a socio-moral need to relocate medical ethics within a broader public understanding of proper deportment. Professional ethics was to be relocated within a general lay ethics. This, indeed, is what bioethics offered.

Second, along with this deprofessionalization of medicine, there was also a dramatic secularization of American society and its public discourse. At the beginning of the 20th century, courts could still without embarrassment recognize America as a Christian nation and affirm Christian moral assumptions (read here, Protestant moral assumptions) as integral to the common-law commitments of the United States.[4] Through a number of Supreme Court holdings, America transformed its legal and public policy expectations from that of a Christian to that of a secular polity.[5] It is difficult to underestimate the profound significance of these changes for moral reflections regarding medicine and the biomedical sciences. Among other things, these secularizing changes made plausible the United States Supreme Court holding in *Roe v. Wade*,[6] which established a constitutional right to abortion. This constitutional development both reflected and enlarged a major cultural cleft in American society. A liberal cosmopolitan secular ethics was emerging. Yet, the traditional commitments of the once-dominant American culture remained. The new bioethics became a counter-ethics to the previously established moral theological ethics that had guided much of American health care decisions into the 20th century. In reaction to this secular bioethics, there has been the redevelopment, especially since the 1990s, of a substantial Christian bioethical literature. This bioethics is set over against the bioethics of the Establishment. The author of this essay should confess that as an Orthodox Christian his recent work is best seen as part of this critical reassessment of the established bioethics born of the 1970s (Engelhardt, 2000). Bioethical debates thus have come to express a larger cultural conflict, a culture war that is not restricted to the United States or the Western world (Hunter, 1991). The dominant understanding of bioethics that emerged came to require that public moral and bioethical debates be conducted in terms of claims justifiable in general, secular terms, or at least claims that can be defended within a notion of public reason that is fundamentally secular. This requirement is itself controversial.

Finally, the rights movements of the 1960s and 1970s brought into question traditional authority figures. The results were multiple, including a progressive abandonment of the professional standard for consent to medical procedures,[7] and the embrace instead of a reasonable-and-prudent-person or objective standard for disclosure,[8] if not in some context a subjective standard for consent.[9] These changes should not be seen simply in terms of the deconstruction of the guild status of medicine and therefore of the authority of physicians to determine what ought prudently to be disclosed to patients in the process of consent. These changes also reflect an independent shift in accent towards individual authority. This shift brought into question the role of the family in determining what should be told to a family member receiving medical care. At stake was a widespread change in who was accepted in the dominant culture as an authority for health care decisions. The authority of physicians, the clergy, the family, and traditional authority figures was displaced by the authority of autonomous, rights-bearing individuals. The result was the disestablishment of those who had traditionally been in authority for giving advice and direction with regard to health care, namely, respected physicians, priests, rabbis, and ministers.

This deconstruction of the traditional sources of authority for guiding medicine and the biomedical sciences occurred just as medicine and the biomedical sciences were becoming (1) more effective, (2) more costly, and (3) more productive of new moral puzzles (e.g., posing questions such as "what moral considerations should guide transplantation and genetic engineering?"). Thus, the culture was confronted by important moral challenges regarding the proper use of medicine and the development of the biomedical sciences, just as it lost taken-for-granted sources for meeting those challenges. In short, the collapse of traditional sources of authority and the growing need for moral direction created a moral leadership vacuum. It was into this moral vacuum that bioethics entered. Again, it must be stressed that it was the creative insight of André Hellegers and Sargent Shriver who understood that an academic and applied field such as bioethics was needed to fill this moral vacuum. Located as they were in a major university in the capital of the United States, they could both convey academic respectability to the field, while providing its members access to influence over public policy at a national level. One might note the role of Tom L. Beauchamp of the Center for Bioethics of the Kennedy Institute in the undertakings of the National Commission for the Protection of Human Subjects of Behavioral and Biomedical Research in its production of what was tantamount to a governmental articulation of fundamental principles to guide the biomedical sciences in their research (1978).

The result of all of these developments was the recognition within less than one decade of the successful role that bioethics had played in creating cadres of scholars, clinically-based practitioners, and individuals involved in the framing of health care policy for the United States. The record was by any measure impressive. This success could be invoked as a model to invite scholars in other countries to do likewise. In particular, it offered those who wished to reform and reconstitute the character of health care ethics in their countries a model for successful intervention. Philosophers and would-be ethicists had at their disposal an approach for refashioning their country's health care ethos. Following the success of American bioethics, while adapting it to the local context, they could redirect social changes already in motion and focus them under the rubric of bioethics. Depending on the circumstances, they could (1) relocate the medical profession and its ethics within a more democratically-based moral context, (2) further secularize their societies, and (3) give greater accent to individual rights over against traditional authority structures.

III. Bioethics and Post-Traditional Cultures

There are a number of accounts that can be and have been given of how this cluster of developments led to the emergence and establishment of bioethics, especially in the United States.[10] This essay gives special accent to changes in the cultural expectations of the dominant culture in the United States and increasingly in the world. This accent is offered in order to locate the emergence of bioethics in terms of a large-scale shift in Western and global culture generally, which occurred in the 20th century, and which called for the redirection of societal moral concerns.[11] It is not that moral interest in medicine did not exist prior to this. It was rather that such concerns were embedded for the most part in the context of professional and religious reflections, disengaged from the interests of professional philosophers and humanists. Philosophy for its part had in the mid-20th century been largely uninvolved in such so-called applied issues. As a result, a further novelty was that philosophy was brought into an engagement with medicine and the biomedical sciences through the founding of the Kennedy Institute and the work of Edmund Pellegrino (1979) and a few others. This remarkable shift of philosophical energies may in part have seemed plausible to Georgetown University, André Hellegers, and Sargent Shriver because of their Roman Catholic faith in reason and its capacity to disclose a common human morality. There was in addition in this Roman Catholic context a faith in an openness to the secular world born of the Second Vatican Council. Under these circumstances, bioethics could only be conceived of as a universal ethics performing the function of the secular equivalent of a liberation theology.

Largely unnoticed in the 1970s was that this enterprise of creating a universal bioethics grounded in a universal morality was undertaken just as the Western Enlightenment faith in reason was being brought into question by post-modernity. That is, just as one hoped to find a universal morality cum global bioethics, it was becoming clearer that it would be impossible to ground discursively the canonical status of a single moral vision, account, or narrative in reason without begging the question, arguing in a circle, or engaging in an infinite regress. Nevertheless, the appeal to rational argument grounded in terms of premises and rules of evidence all persons could affirm, absent any particular historical, religious, or mystical insight, was engaged. This engagement tended to bring into question traditional cultural and religious commitments, even if people were not able to agree regarding these premises or rules of evidence. In this sense, the bioethics born of the 1970s accomplished in part that to which the Enlightenment had aspired: the secularization of public moral discourse.

These changes in moral perspective were profound. They involved a fundamental change in taken-for-granted expectations. They can be summarized under six rubrics:

(1) The partial deprofessionalization of health care. The authority of medicine as a self-governing guild has been brought into question, along with the traditional authority of physicians and physicians' orders (e.g., "doctor's orders"). The result is that physicians have lost a clear sense of professional identity and commitment.

(2) The immanent displacement of theological concerns. Traditional religious concerns regarding such matters as the sanctity of human life and human dignity have been relocated, as far as possible, by bioethics within a fully secular context. As a result, there is often an intense search for a depth of moral meaning that cannot be achieved without a metaphysical anchor (e.g., when God is not recognized as the bestower of human dignity, the dignity of humans is only what humans make of it).

(3) The de-orientation of cosmic and human history. The history of the cosmos and of humanity can no longer be understood as having an ultimate source or direction. In a secular context, it is impossible to determine what directions human evolution should take, now that humans have the capacities to control their own evolutionary development.

(4) The critical deconstruction of traditional moral commitments. For instance, the traditional recognition of abortion as the taking of the life of an unborn child becomes reinterpreted by secular bioethics as a patriarchal enforcement of pregnancy, thus violating the fundamental rights of women. These contrary visions of moral probity depend on conflicting basic moral commitments to either preserving the authenticity of a veridical tradition, or freeing persons from the constraints of such traditions.

(5) The emergence of a liberal cosmopolitan ethics affirming self-determination, equality, self-fulfillment, and a non-moralistic mutual recognition. In terms of this ethos, the quest for moral virtue and character becomes indeterminate.

(6) The affirmation of an Enlightenment expectation that this liberal cosmopolitan ethos should ground a single, canonical, global bioethics despite moral pluralism and post-modernity.

Bioethics cannot innocently be affirmed. Rather, it must be recognized as tied to important controversies regarding the meaning of life, the substance of morality, and the ultimate sense or senselessness of the universe. Traditional Christians, Jews, and Moslems will have good grounds to regard secular bioethics as corruptive of proper moral conduct.

The readers of this first edition of the *Annals* are offered an international perspective on a field that is only recently come to take seriously the place and significance of moral difference. It is very likely that future volumes, which attend to religious, national, and legal responses to issues bioethical, will take their character from the outcomes of the growing and important debates regarding the significance of moral pluralism for the possibilities of a global bioethics. The second volume in this series will confront this issue even more forthrightly in addressing differences in religious perspectives. Bioethics, which was made in America and in the 1970s had a predominantly American cast, is now being reexamined within the context of different national laws and local customs. The field is entering its maturity. This volume makes an important contribution to that maturation.

H. Tristam Engelhardt, Jr.
Department of Philosophy
Rice University

and

Department of Medicine
Baylor College of Medicine
Houston, Texas

Notes

1. See, for example, Kazumasa Hoshino (ed.), *Japanese and Western Bioethics* (1997) and Angeles Tan Alora and Josephine M. Lumitao (eds), *Beyond a Western Bioethics: Voices from the Developing World* (2001).
2. Warren Reich (1994, pp. 319-336). Sargent Shriver described his own role in a letter to the author dated January 26, 2001.
3. *American Medical Association v. United States*, 17 U.S. 529 (1943); *American Medical Association v. Federal Trade Commission*, 638 F.2d 443 (2d Cir. 1980).
4. *Church of the Holy Trinity v. United States*, 143 U.S. 457 (1892), and *United States v. Macintosh*, 283 U.S. 605 (1931).
5. See, for example, *School District of Abington Township v. Edward L. Schempp et al., William J. Murray et al. v. John N. Curlett et al.*, 374 U.S. 203, 10 L ed 2d 844, 83 S Ct 1560 (1963)
6. *Roe v. Wade*, 410 U.S. 113 (1973).
7. *Natanson v. Kline* 350 P.2d 1093 (Kan. 1960).
8. *Canterbury v. Spence*, 464 F.2d 772 (DC Cir. 1972).
9. *Scott v. Bradford*, 606 P.2d 554 (Okla. 1980) and *Spencer v. Seidel*, 742 P.2d 1126 (Okla. 1987).
10. See, for example, Albert R. Jonsen, *The Birth of Bioethics* (1998); David J. Rothman, *Strangers at the Bedside* (1991); and M. L. Tina Stevens, *Bioethics in America: Origins and Cultural Politics* (2000).
11. For a more ample account of how these shifts in moral perspectives that produced bioethics, see Engelhardt, "The ordination of bioethicists as secular moral experts" (2002, pp. 59-82).

Bibliography

Alora, A. Tan & Lumitao, J.M. (eds) 2001. *Beyond a western bioethics: voices from the developing world*. Washington, DC: Georgetown University Press.
American Medical Association v. United States, 17 U.S. 529 (1943).

American Medical Association v. Federal Trade Commission, 638 F.2d 443 (2d Cir. 1980).

Beauchamp, T. & Childress, J.F. 1979. *Principles of biomedical ethics*. New York: Oxford University Press.

Canterbury v. Spence, 464 F.2d 772 (DC Cir. 1972).

Church of the Holy Trinity v. United States, 143 U.S. 457 (1892).

Engelhardt, H.T., Jr. 1996. *The foundations of bioethics (2nd ed.)*. New York: Oxford University Press.

Engelhardt, H.T., Jr. 2000. *The foundations of Christian bioethics*. Lisse: Swets & Zeitlinger.

Engelhardt, H.T., Jr. 2002. The ordination of bioethicists as secular moral experts. *Social Philosophy & Policy* 19(2): 59-82.

Hoshino, K. (ed.) 1997. *Japanese and western bioethics*. Dordrecht: Kluwer Academic Publishers.

Huntington, S.P. 1996. *The clash of civilizations and the remaking of world order*. New York: Touchstone.

Hunter, J.D. 1991. *Culture wars: the struggle to define America*. New York: Basic Books.

Jonsen, A. 1998. *The birth of bioethics*. New York: Oxford University Press.

Kipnis, K. 1997. Confessions of an expert ethics witness. *The Journal of Medicine and Philosophy* 22(4): 325-343.

Means, J.H. 1961. *The Association of American Physicians*. New York: Blakiston.

Natanson v. Kline 350 P.2d 1093 (Kan. 1960).

National Commission for the Protection of Human Subjects of Biomedical and Behavioral Research. 1978. *The Belmont report: ethical principles and guidelines for the protection of human subjects of research*. Washington, D.C.: US Government Printing Office.

Pellegrino, E.D. 1979. *Humanism and the physician*. Knoxville: University of Tennessee Press.

Potter, V.R. 1970a. Bioethics, the science of survival. *Perspectives in Biology and Medicine* 14: 127-153.

Potter, V.R. 1970b. Biocybernetics and survival. *Zygon* 5: 229-246.

Reich, W. (ed.) 1978. *Encyclopedia of bioethics*. New York: Free Press.

Reich, W. 1994. The word "bioethics": its birth and the legacies of those who shaped its meaning. *Kennedy Institute of Ethics Journal* 4: 319-336.

Roe v. Wade, 410 U.S. 113 (1973).

Rothman, D.J. 1991. *Strangers at the bedside*. New York: Basic Books.

School District of Abington Township v. Edward L. Schempp et al., William J. Murray et al. v. John N. Curlett et al., 374 U.S. 203, 10 L ed 2d 844, 83 S Ct 1560 (1963).

Scott v. Bradford, 606 P.2d 554 (Okla. 1980).

Spencer v. Seidel, 742 P.2d 1126 (Okla. 1987).

Stevens, M.L.T. 2000. *Bioethics in America: origins and cultural politics*. Baltimore: Johns Hopkins University Press.

United States v. Macintosh, 283 U.S. 605 (1931).

Part I: North America

1 Bioethics in Canada

Nuala Kenny

I. Introduction

Bioethics was firmly entrenched in academic, clinical, and health policy discussions and debates as Canada entered the twenty-first century. This chapter presents an overview of important and distinctive features of bioethics in Canada. As the largest country in the Americas with a relatively small population, bordering and profoundly affected by medical and social developments in the United States, Canada revels in its unique identity. The distinctive nature of Canadian bioethics is rooted in these realities. This reflection begins by sketching the early development of bioethics and then moving to a more detailed review of Canadian bioethics during the period of 1990-2002.

Canada's bioethics has developed with contributions from many sources: ethics education for health professionals, professional codes of ethics, difficult clinical cases, federal and provincial legislation, court decisions, commission and committee reports, and working papers. Here, selections from each of these sources will be presented to provide a flavor of the vitality of Canadian bioethics and the challenges it faces.

The Canadian health care system is the particular context in which these developments occurred. The system is understood by Canadians to be a manifestation of the values of justice, fairness, and compassion. This macro-ethical framework is central to Canadian bioethics.

II. History

The early history of ethics in Canada can be divided into the "traditional" period before 1960 and the period of modern bioethics from 1960s to the present. There is no authoritative early history of bioethics in Canada (Roy & Williams, 1995). However, Canada and the Canadian Medical Association (CMA) were both founded in 1867. In 1868, the CMA adopted a Code of Ethics patterned on that of the American Medical Association. The Canadian Nurses Association was established in 1908 and adopted a Code of Ethics prepared by the International Council of Nurses in 1854. These two important professional organizations contributed no specific "Canadian content" to the codes they adopted.

The Roman Catholic Church played an important role in Canadian health care and in early deliberations regarding moral and ethical issues in health care. The Catholic

Hospital Association of the United States and Canada (CHAUSC), founded in 1915, adopted a Code of Ethics in 1921. The Catholic Hospital Association of Canada became independent in 1954 and adopted its own moral code in 1955. This Code was most recently revised in 2000. By the 1940s, one notes Canadian publications in medical-morals and medical ethics (LaRochelle & Fink, 1943). As was the case in the United States, theological writing focused on emerging ethical issues in health care before the entrance of philosophers.

There were few formal contributions to medical ethics until the 1940s. Medical ethics was a hybrid of etiquette and adherence to general codal precepts. The renowned Canadian physician William Osler (1849-1919) taught about medical practice and the virtues of equanimity, imperturbability, and detachment (Bliss, 1999). These indicate clearly the tone of medical ethics of the time. By the mid-1960s, medical ethics was transformed by scientific and technological advances and social change. While influenced by developments in the United States, Canadian bioethics advanced through the work of some prominent pioneers in Canadian bioethics and professional health care associations, academic institutions, and public commissions.

Ethics education is a required component of health professional education in Canada. Under the leadership of Dr. Vincent Sweeney and Alistair Browne, meetings were held in the late 1980s to explore the programs that had been developed for undergraduate ethics education in the sixteen Canadian medical schools; the goal was to learn from the best programs and to develop some consistency among them. This was voluntary until the Medical Council of Canada (MCC) issued its policy "Considerations of the Legal, Ethical and Organizational Aspects of the Practice of Medicine (CLEO)" (Kenny & Baylis, 1998) which requires the formal inclusion of ethics and health law in the licensing examinations for new physicians. Specific ethics learning objectives include confidentiality, consent to investigation or treatment, truth telling, resource allocation, research ethics, physicians and industry, the doctor-patient relationship, personal and professional conduct, and controversial and evolving ethical issues in practice (e.g., euthanasia, maternal-fetal conflict, genetic testing, and so forth).

The Royal College of Physicians and Surgeons of Canada (RCPSC), the accreditation body for all specialty training programs in Canada, has mandated ethics in postgraduate training. The College's Bioethics Committee, under the leadership of Peter Singer, developed the Bioethics Education Project, an ethics curricula for residency programs, which is mounted on the RCPSC website. The Pediatrics Ethics Network (PedEthNet), led by Abbyann Lynch, developed a full ethics curriculum for use in Canadian pediatrics residency programs (1996). This project, begun prior to the Bioethics Education Project, was incorporated as the pediatric component.

In 1996, continuing education for practicing physicians was improved through a regular series in the Canadian Medical Association Journal (CMAJ) entitled "Bioethics for Clinicians" (Singer, 1996, pp. 189-190) and subsequently published as a text (Singer, 1999). The series has become a regular feature in the journal. Philip Hebert (1996) and Michael Yeo (1996) contributed to ethics education by providing texts for use in Canadian educational programs. Virtually all health professional groups have developed educational guidelines. The Alberta Provincial Health Ethics Network (PHEN) has been a pioneer in educational programming for clinical and research ethics boards as well as health care administrators.

Royal Commissions and Commissions of Inquiry are used to address social and policy issues. Between 1970 and 1989, there were more than thirty commission inquiries into a wide range of bioethical issues (Williams, 1989, pp. 425-444). In the absence of a formal federal mechanism, commissions are still the dominant approach to achieve public and professional input into pressing policy issues with social and ethical implications.

The 1867 Constitution Act was amended in 1982 by the Canadian Charter of Rights and Freedoms. This obliges government agencies not to violate fundamental rights, such as life, liberty, and security of the person, freedom of conscience, thought, belief, and expression, and freedom from discrimination. Democratic support for legislation that violates the Charter does not compel the courts to support the legislation, since the Charter protects fundamental rights.

As the selected case law dramatically demonstrates, the Charter has had a profound effect on the interpretation of ethical and legal obligations in the context of health care and medical decision-making. A comprehensive discussion of the interaction between bioethics and law in Canada has been the subject of study over the last decade in particular (Roy, Williams, & Dickens, 1994; Downie & Caulfield, 1999). Some selected examples from case law relevant to bioethics will demonstrate this relationship. The landmark 1980 decision in *Reibel v. Hughes* (1980) moved the standard for patient consent from the "reasonable practitioner" standard (i.e., what would the reasonable clinician have disclosed), to a reasonable patient standard (i.e., what would the reasonable patient need to know in order to make a decision). The 1983 *Stephen Dawson* decision emphasized the ethical significance of accurate medical information in life and death decisions. The 1986 case of *Eve* followed mid-1970s through 1980s debates and position papers on contraceptive sterilization for some mentally disabled persons. For some, this procedure could be truly beneficial because it would allow these persons to enjoy sexual fulfillment without the responsibility of bearing and rearing children. Sensitive to the history of involuntary sterilization of mentally disabled persons for other, more ignoble, reasons, the majority of Canadians supported sterilization. Controversy ensued over by whom and how the decisions should be made. The *Eve* decision declared categorically that sterilization should never be authorized for non-therapeutic reasons. In the absence of a person's consent, the Court believed it impossible to determine that the procedure was for the person's benefit. The decision continues to be the focus for discussion and debate about the dilemma posed when what appears to be ethically correct is judged to be illegal.

The Canadian national health insurance system, as defined in the Hospital Insurance Act of 1957, was affirmed in the 1984 Canada Health Act (CHA). The principles of the CHA and provincial jurisdiction over health are distinctive features of Canadian health care (Taylor, 1987). The principles are comprehensiveness, universality, accessibility, portability – across all Canadian provinces – and public administration. They ground a single-tier, not-for-profit system. The federal government contributes a substantial component of the funding; provincial governments, in return, incorporate these principles into their operation of the system. For Canadians, this health care system is a strong manifestation of equality of both opportunity and outcome. It has been said that in Canada equality before the health care system is as strong as equality before the law (Evans, 1998, pp. 155-189). The sustainability of the health care system has been the object of serious discussion and debate at both the provincial and federal levels over the past decade. In November of 2002, a federally appointed Commission on the Future of Health Care in Canada, a major exercise in public, expert, and advocate consultation, reported to the Prime Minister affirming the fundamental principles of the CHA and suggesting areas for modernization and change. These included expansion of coverage to home care, palliative care and out of hospital drugs; a reform of primary care; improved information access; the formation of an oversight National Health Council and the development of a new Health Covenant between citizens and the government.

III. Topics

A. Bioethics in General

Academic institutions have had a major role in the development of Canadian bioethics. Courses developed widely in philosophy and health professional education. Advanced work in bioethics was facilitated by the creation of some key centers and institutes. In 1976, the Center for Bioethics of the Clinical Research Institute of Montreal, Quebec, was the first such institute in Canada. Some, like the Westminster Institute for Ethics and Human Values founded in London, Ontario, focused on bioethics while others, like the McGill Center for Health, Law and Ethics, incorporated both the legal and ethical components of research and academic work. By 2000, more than twenty-five established research centers and institutes in Canada were dedicated to health law and bioethics.

Further definition of the field occurred in 1988 with the creation of the Canadian Bioethics Society, an amalgamation of the Canadian Society of Bioethics (CSB) and the Canadian Society for Medical Bioethics (CSMB). The CSB had been established by a group of philosophers, theologians, lawyers, nurses, and physicians to facilitate discussion and debate about bioethical issues. The CSMB was founded in response to the heightened physician sensitivity to bioethical issues by the Canadian Medical Association, the College of Family Physicians, the Association of Canadian Medical Colleges, the Medical Research Council, and the Royal College of Physicians and Surgeons of Canada. It soon became clear that a single multidisciplinary society would enrich discussions and debate, so both groups united to form the new Canadian Bioethics Society (CBS). Edward W. (Ted) Keyserlingk became the first president of the CBS. Pioneers in this formation were Abbyann Lynch, Michael Burgess, Benjamin Freedman, John Dossetor, Robert Green, George Webster, Sydney Segal, Douglas Kinsella, Michael Coughlin, Marcel Melancon, Bruno Leclerc, Judith Miller, and John Williams. The CBS has flourished and by the 2002 Annual meeting, membership had grown to over six hundred persons representing the diversity and enthusiasm its founders envisioned.

Canada's proximity to the United States and the cross-border fertilization of academic activity means that theoretical perspectives on bioethics have closely paralleled U.S. thought. Case-based and principle-based reasoning dominated early bioethics. However, there is a distinct stream of Canadian thought on many issues. It has been enriched by Francophone philosophers and ethicists deeply rooted in the traditions of continental philosophy. Canadian thinkers have provided critique of what is seen as a U.S. autonomy-dominated bioethics and have contributed to development of a more distinctive Canadian literature. Baylis, Downie, Freedman, et al., "Health Care Ethics in Canada" (1995) and Keatings and Smith (1995), "Ethics and legal issues in Canadian Nursing" are examples.

Susan Sherwin's (1992) contribution to feminist theory is recognized internationally. The Feminist Health Ethics Network, including Sherwin, Baylis, Downie, and Purdy, has been the source of rich conceptual work.

B. Professionalism

Professional codes of ethics have been central to the patient-professional relationship. These codes underwent remarkable expansion in every field of health care in the 1990s (Baylis, Downie, & Dewhurst, 1999). In 1996, after four years of discussion and debate, the CMA adopted a new Code of Ethics for the medical profession (CMA, 1996, pp. 1176A-1176B). Two years later, the CMA ratified a "Charter for Physicians" to clarify that Canadian physicians must achieve the goal of providing the best health care possible. This "Charter" has been identified as a departure from the ethical tradition of professional codes and its impact is yet to be seen (Kenny, Weijer, & Baylis, 1999, pp. 3999-4000). The Canadian Nurses Association (CNA) released a new "Code of Ethics for Registered Nurses" (1997) containing sections on health and well-being, choice, dignity, fairness, confidentiality, accountability and practice environments conducive to safe, competent, and ethical care. The CMA approved policies on the management of physicians who test positive for hepatitis B (CMA, 1998, pp. 71-73) and HIV (CMA, 1993, pp. 1800A-1800D). The CMA position is that neither health care professionals nor patients have a right to know each other's HIV status. The CMA and the Canadian Dental Association (CDA) oppose the mandatory testing of health care workers and recommend a voluntary system instead. A statement on resolving ethical conflicts was released in June 1999 (Joint Statement on Resuscitation Inventions, 1994, pp. 1176A-1176C) by the Canadian Healthcare Association (CHA), the CMA, the CAN, and the Catholic Health Association of Canada (CHAC). It received attention in the bioethics community for its apparent conferral upon physicians of authority to make decisions regarding futile treatments.

C. Decision-Making, Consent, and Privacy

Medical decision-making has been a major area of work focused on clarity regarding disclosure, the determination of capacity to make decisions, and appropriate use of advance directives and third-party decision-making. Each of the provinces has a Health Care Consent Act containing practical advice on obtaining consent from patients or substitute decision-makers, definitions of essential terms, such as personal directives (including who can make a directive, other requirements, revocation, and so forth), agents (i.e., proxy decision-makers), duties of service providers, liability and protection. Generally, when a health care provider has determined that an adult is incapable of giving or refusing consent in accordance with the established criteria, the health care provider is required to obtain a health care decision from a substitute decision-maker, except in cases of urgent or emergency care or a preliminary examination.

In December 2000, Ontario amended the Ontario Mental Health Act and the Health Care Consent Act (2000), setting a new standard for the involuntary commitment and treatment of the mentally ill. Previously, individuals were involuntarily committed only if they posed an "imminent" risk of serious bodily harm to themselves or others. The new law removed the "imminent" requirement and introduced "community treatment orders"

(CTO) for individuals with a cyclical history of multiple hospital admissions for mental illness. Under a CTO, a person may be required to take treatment outside the hospital setting. Ontario's law is in keeping with similar legislation already enacted in British Columbia, Manitoba, and Saskatchewan.

A few selected court cases serve to illustrate the importance of balancing respect for autonomy with care. In May 1986, Carole Arndt became infected by chicken pox in the 12th week of pregnancy. She consulted Dr. Margaret Smith, who informed her about some, but not all, of the risks to a fetus. The child was born with varicella syndrome and serious medical complications. Ms. Arndt sued Dr. Smith for damages. The judge found that Dr. Smith's failure to disclose all material risks amounted to medical negligence, but concluded that there was no causative link between this negligence and the decision not to abort. On appeal, the Supreme Court reaffirmed the "modified objective test" of informed consent set out in its 1980 *Reibl v. Hughes* judgment, which requires that the court consider what the "reasonable patient" in the plaintiff's circumstances would have done in the situation had she been fully informed. It concluded that "it is appropriate to infer ... that a reasonable person in the plaintiff's position would not have decided to terminate her pregnancy in the face of the very small increased risk to the fetus" (Crow, 1998, pp. 3-13).

A 1991 Ontario Court of Appeal decision in *Malette v. Shulman* demonstrates the influence of ethics on case law. Malette, a Jehovah's Witness, was taken to the hospital unconscious and bleeding after an accident. The attending physician was informed she carried a signed card refusing blood products. He transfused her to prevent death from hemorrhage. The patient survived and successfully sued the physician for battery. The trial judge declared that the transfusion may have saved her life but the ethical principle of respect for autonomous persons prevailed over beneficence and non-malevolence.

In 1992, *Norberg v. Wynrib* involved a male physician who supplied his female patient with free drugs in return for sexual favors. In its judgment for the plaintiff, the Court explained the requirements for consent, including the lack of coercion in a relationship where there exists a "power relationship".

The withdrawal of a previously given consent was also the focus of legal action (*Ciarlariello v. Schacter*, 1993). A patient experienced discomfort during an angiogram for which she had given consent. She told the doctor to stop the test; he informed her it would take only a few minutes more and continued. As the dye was injected, she suffered an immediate reaction, which caused quadriplegia. The Court reaffirmed the "reasonable patient" standard and confirmed that if consent is withdrawn during a procedure, it must be respected unless cessation poses an immediate or serious threat to the patient.

A highly controversial case regarding surrogate decision-making and futility evoked much discussion from the bioethics community in 1998. Helene Sawatzky, wife of Andrew Sawatzky, a 79 year-old man with severe Parkinson's Disease, obtained an injunction lifting a do-not-resuscitate order placed on her husband's chart. The Court ordered medical assessments to determine Mr. Sawatzky's competence and found him unable to make informed decisions. They concluded that a do-not-resuscitate order was appropriate. Mrs. Sawatzky rejected the findings and filed suit to have the public trustee removed as Mr. Sawatzky's official guardian. The defendant argued that the Court does not have the authority to impose an order that would result in a doctor providing medical treatment that he or she thinks is not in the patient's best interests. The Court responded that "in the case of non-consensual medical decisions, be they decisions to provide, withdraw or refuse care or treatment, there is a role for the courts to play in making factual determinations and advising of the legality or illegality of disputed decisions before the patient is dead." The Court granted the injunction (Sawatzky, 1998).

Obligations to infants and children present particular challenges to health professionals. Richard and Beena B., a Jehovah's Witness couple, refused consent for a blood transfusion for their infant daughter, Sheena B. (*R. B. v. Children's Aid*, 1992). The Children's Aid Society of Metropolitan Toronto applied for and received wardship of the infant who received the transfusion. The parents subsequently appealed the wardship orders on the grounds that the Ontario Child Welfare Act infringed two sections of the Canadian Charter of Rights and Freedoms: section 2, which guarantees freedom of religion, and section 7, which states that "Everyone has the right to life, liberty and security of the person and the right not to be deprived thereof except in accordance with the principles of fundamental justice." The Supreme Court upheld the judgments of the lower courts that the parents had no right to refuse the transfusion.

In November 1997, a 3 month-old infant admitted to the hospital with severe brain damage resulting from a beating was apprehended by Child and Family Services of Central Manitoba. Physicians determined that the infant was in a persistent vegetative state and recommended a DNR order. The parents refused and Child and Family Services applied for and received a court order authorizing the order. The parents appealed this decision. The Court did not overturn the DNR order. Mr. Justice Twaddle stated that "philosophical arguments apart, it is in no one's interest to artificially maintain the life of a terminally-ill patient who is in an irreversible vegetative state." He was unable to find a Canadian precedent dealing with the authority of a physician making a DNR order but stated:

> neither consent nor a court order in lieu is required for a medical doctor to issue a non-resuscitation direction where, in his or her judgment, the patient is in an irreversible vegetative state. Whether or not such a direction should be issued is a judgment call for the doctor to make having regard to the patient's history and condition and the doctor's evaluation of the hopelessness of the case (p. 12).

This decision evoked much debate regarding qualitative and quantitative futility and physician authority. In fact, as of this time, Canadians have not conferred upon physicians the authority to make unilateral decisions regarding futile treatment.

The Minister of Social Services had the authority to consent to the care and treatment of 13 year-old Tyrell Dueck, who was diagnosed with osteosarcoma (T.T.D., 1999). Midway through the chemotherapy, Tyrell refused any more treatments. The court was asked to determine whether Tyrell was a mature minor and thus able to make decisions on his own behalf. It determined that Tyrell was unable to appreciate or understand the medical treatment he required. However, the disease had progressed and Tyrell died soon after.

The CMA issued a policy affirming that medical records are confidential documents and are the property of the physician or health care organization that compiled them (CMA, 1992, p. 1860A). It clearly recognizes the right of the patient to the information contained therein and recommends that physicians should assist patients in understanding their records. Third party disclosure of information requires explicit patient authorization.

The duty to warn others regarding patients who threaten seriously to harm another member of the public became a concern after an unusual case was dealt with by both the Nova Scotia Court of Appeal and the College of Physicians and Surgeons of Nova Scotia (CPSNS). In June 1992, Kenneth Ross was convicted of having sexually assaulted a 29 year-old woman (R. v. Ross, 1993). Hearing media accounts of the trial, Dr. Hansen, a psychiatrist who had treated the woman, feared a miscarriage of justice, since the woman's testimony may have been mistaken, even though she believed it to be true. He consulted legal counsel and the Provincial Medical Board (the predecessor of the CPSNS) and advised his solicitor to bring his concerns to the Crown prosecutor. The Nova Scotia Supreme Court ordered an in-camera examination of Dr. Hansen, stating that "The public interest in avoiding a miscarriage overrides any claim of privilege that might be advanced in these circumstances respecting the patient/physician communications" (p. 255). The Court held that Dr. Hansen's evidence was admissible and ordered a new trial, where Mr. Ross entered a guilty plea.

In peer review, the CPSNS concluded that Dr. Hansen's breach of patient confidentiality was not justified. He had not assessed the facts, and he had not provided his patient with sufficient information to allow her to make an informed decision regarding the release of her confidential medical information to a third party. He was judged him guilty of professional misconduct, and had his medical license suspended.

In another case, the accused, charged with aggravated sexual assault, was convinced by his lawyer to undergo a psychiatric evaluation and was assured that the medical report would be protected by solicitor-client privilege. The psychiatrist judged the accused dangerous and likely to repeat the offence. The accused was convicted. The psychiatrist learned that the sentencing judge would not be provided with his report and sought a judicial declaration entitling him to disclose the information on the basis of the public safety exception to the solicitor-client privilege. The Supreme Court held that the solicitor-client privilege attaching to the report should be set aside "by implication, if a public safety exception applies to solicitor-client privilege, it applies to all classifications of privileges and duties of confidentiality" (Smith v. Jones, 1999).

While there is a professional consensus that physicians should be protected from liability when they break confidentiality because of a threat to harm another person, these recent decisions have made physicians uneasy.

The privacy of medical information has become the object of considerable attention as information technology is increasingly used in health decisions and systems management. A number of professional groups have addressed issues regarding the regulation, development, testing (including pilot projects), implementation and application of emerging technologies, smart cards and biometric identification systems that have a potential to infringe on the privacy of personal information. Ethical and legal concerns have focused on the need to deal with privacy, protection from discrimination, and inappropriate use of health information in the workplace and insurance coverage.

In 1998, the CMA adopted a "Health Information Privacy Code" (CMA, 1998), which articulates the principles of precedence to patient privacy, the confidentiality of health information, and trust between provider and patient within the therapeutic context. Provincial medical associations have also addressed the issue of privacy in the particular context of the physician's office.

The most significant privacy legislation to date is the January 2001 "Personal Information Protection and Electronic Documents Act", which applies to organizations that collect, use, or disclose personal information in the course of commercial activity and in connection with a federal work, undertaking, or business. In Canada, the health care sector involves actors and activities in both the private and public sectors that intersect across the entire continuum of care (e.g., private practitioners' offices, hospitals, long-term care residences, home care, rehabilitation centers, and so forth). Health researchers, especially those in health services and population health, require data from a variety of sources to conduct important research (e.g., clinical records, hospital records, health care utilization data, billing data, vital statistics, employee information, and so forth). Some of the data custodians are engaged in commercial activity, while others are not. The ethical requirement for informed consent is a fundamental principle. However, a strict reading of the new Act could require that formal consent be obtained every time an organization seeks to collect, use, or disclose personal health information.

D. Reproductive and Genetic Technologies

While issues of abortion dominated reproductive ethics in the decades immediately preceding the 1990s (and have not disappeared), the focus of ethical concern has shifted to an array of complex technical interventions into human genetics and reproduction. The Canadian Fertility and Andrology Society (CFAS) and Society of Obstetricians and Gynaecologists of Canada (SOGC) published their reflections, "Ethical Issues in Assisted Reproduction" (Martin, et al., 1999, pp. 369-371).

The Report of the Royal Commission on the New Reproductive Technologies (RCNRT) "Proceed with Care", released in November 1993, dominated the agenda for most of the decade. This highly visible and controversial Royal Commission attempted to elicit public input into the policy decisions being made in this sensitive area. In response, the federal government called for a voluntary moratorium on nine reproductive and genetic technologies and practices: (1) sex selection for non-medical purposes, (2) commercial pre-conception ("surrogacy") arrangements, (3) buying and selling of eggs, sperm, and embryos, (4) egg donation in exchange for *in vitro* fertilization services, (5) germ-line genetic alteration, (6) ectogenesis (creation of an artificial womb), (7) the cloning of human embryos, (8) formation of animal-human hybrids by combining animal and human gametes, (9) and the retrieval of eggs from cadavers and fetuses for donation, fertilization, or research.

The SOGC also published a policy statement on "Preconception Arrangements", which reviews types of preconception arrangements, Canadian and international experience and moral issues. Their principal conclusion is that commercial and non-commercial preconception arrangements are morally unacceptable.

Federal Bill C-47, "An Act respecting human reproductive technologies and commercial transactions relating to human reproduction", was introduced to provide for the long-awaited regulation in this area. Simultaneously with the introduction of Bill C-47 was the release of a document (Health Canada, 1996) that proposed a regulatory structure to develop national standards for the uses of reproductive materials in medical research and practice, issue licenses and enforce compliance with the legislation for issues, such as *in vitro* fertilization, donor insemination, use of fetal tissue, storage and donation of human eggs, sperm, embryos, and embryo research, including pre-implantation diagnosis.

Bill C-47 died when Parliament was dissolved in April 1997. In May 2001, the federal government tabled draft legislation governing assisted human reproduction with the hope that implementation would occur in 2002. In 2002, Bill C-13, the Assisted Human Reproduction Act, proposed the formation of an Assisted Reproduction Agency of Canada to provide oversight in this rapidly developing area of science. It prohits human cloning, the creation of embryos except for assisted reproduction, the creation of chimeras, payment for surrogate motherhood among other things. It recommends a high degree of regulation in this area of human science. Calls for stem cell research approval in Canada have highlighted the need for more formal, clear, and consistent advice into policy development in these emerging areas. The newly constituted Canadian Institutes for Health Research (CIHR) initiated a Working Group to advise the new Council regarding the funding of stem cell research. Both the Canadian Biotechnology Advisory Committee (CBAC) and Health Canada are addressing the need for ethically sound public policy in this area. CIHR has taken the lead on providing guidelines for CIHR-funded research on human pluripotent stem cells. It has provided a needed forum for education and debate in this area through its website (www.cihr-irsc.gc.ca).

In October 1997, the Supreme Court of Canada upheld a highly controversial decision not to allow a pregnant woman who was addicted to sniffing solvent to be placed in the custody of the Director of Child and Family Services and detained in a health center for treatment until the birth of her child (Feasby & Chambers, 1998, pp. 707-809). It reiterated that the law of Canada does not recognize the unborn child as a legal person possessing rights and, therefore, there is no legal person in whose interests a court order could be made. Moreover, courts do not have *parens patriae* jurisdiction over unborn children, and so they have no power to order the detention and treatment of a pregnant woman for the purpose of preventing harm to the unborn child. It is up to the legislature, not the courts, to make changes to such laws.

In 1992, the Privacy Commission of Canada issued a policy statement on issues in genetic testing (1992). The privacy of individual genetic information was seen as fundamental to respect and integrity. Canadians have been active in this area, notably Bartha Knoppers (1994, pp. 2035-2036) and Marcel Melancon (1994). Knoppers has developed "humgen" – a web site that provides access to a wide range of information and policy statements on topics related to human genetics around the world.

E. *Death and Dying*
Care of the dying has generated professional and governmental position papers and has been the object of a number of legal case decisions. Withdrawal/withholding of care was highlighted in the 1992 case of Nancy B. (1992), a 25 year-old women with Guillain-Barre Syndrome. She petitioned to have her respirator disconnected. Respecting her autonomous decision to refuse treatment the petition was accepted; she died soon after discontinuation of ventilator support.

The CMA issued a position against euthanasia and assisted suicide, which can be accessed on the CMA web site (CMA Website). "Of Life and Death", the report of the Special Senate Committee on Euthanasia and Assisted Suicide (Senate of Canada, 1995), contained recommendations including: the need to make palliative care a priority in the restructuring of the health care system, the need for national guidelines and standards, increased training of health care professionals in palliative care, integrated delivery of care and increased research funding, especially in pain control and symptom relief. It further recommended that the Criminal Code be amended to:

- Clarify the practice of providing treatment (for the purpose of alleviating suffering that may shorten life) and standards for the practice of the total sedation of patients.
- Clarify the circumstances in which the withholding and withdrawal of life-sustaining treatment is legally acceptable.
- Inform the public of their rights with respect to the refusal of life-sustaining treatment.
- Require provinces and territories to advance directive legislation.

The Committee recommended that counseling for suicide, involuntary euthanasia, non-voluntary and voluntary euthanasia remain criminal offences but the Criminal Code be amended to provide for a less severe penalty in cases where there is the essential element of compassion or mercy.

The Standing Senate Committee on Social Affairs, Science and Technology issued an update, "Quality End-of-Life Care: The Right of Every Canadian" (Report of the Special Senate Committee, 2000). This recent study, led by Senator Sharon Carstairs, identifies the urgent need for a national strategy for end-of-life care; reports on progress achieved on the recommendations made in 1995 and urges implementation of the 1995 recommendations for improving end-of-life care in Canada. The urgency of clarification is seen in selected court decisions.

Sue Rodriguez (1993), who was affected with amyotrophic lateral sclerosis, wanted assistance in ending her life at a time of her choosing through revision of the criminal code.

In January 2001, the Supreme Court of Canada dismissed Robert Latimer's appeal against his conviction for second degree murder for the 'mercy killing' of his severely disabled daughter, Tracy (R. v. Latimer, 2001). The Court upheld the ruling that the defense of necessity was not available to Mr. Latimer. The three components of the defense – imminent peril, no reasonable legal alternative, and proportionality (that is, that the harm avoided was proportionate to the harm inflicted) – could not, on any reasonable interpretation of the facts, be met in this case. Mr. Latimer also appealed a constitutional exemption from his sentence on the basis that it amounted to cruel and unusual punishment. The Court rejected this argument, finding that the gravity of the offence, the aggravating circumstances (such as Mr. Latimer's lack of remorse), his position of trust, and Tracy's extreme vulnerability did not outweigh his "laudable perseverance as a caring and involved parent." Consequently, the Court concluded that there was no violation of Mr. Latimer's constitutional rights and denied the appeal.

In another case, Mr. Mills was dying, and family and physicians agreed that Mr. Mills be taken off life support. When life support was removed, he showed signs of distress and the intravenous pain medication he was receiving appeared ineffective (subsequent evidence suggested there was inappropriate intravenous line placement). The prosecution alleged that Dr. Morrison injected Mr. Mills with nitroglycerin and later potassium chloride. Mr. Mills died within a minute after the potassium chloride injection. A preliminary inquiry judge discharged Dr. Morrison (R. v. Morrison, 1998). On appeal of the discharge, the Court disagreed with the inquiry judge's finding that there was not sufficient evidence to proceed to trial but ruled that the inquiry judge had not exceeded his jurisdiction in

making the decision to discharge Dr. Morrison. The case presented confusing and conflicted direction regarding appropriate end of life care.

In another case, Dr. Maurice Genereux pleaded guilty to assisted suicide in connection
with the suicide attempts of two of his AIDS patients (*R. v. Genereux*, 1999). His sentence
of two years less a day was appealed, but the Crown stated "more particularly, in the context of doctor-assisted suicide, the criminal sanction imposed will resonate throughout the
medical profession, whose members are precisely the type of people who will be influenced
by the threat of severe criminal penalties" (p. 12).

Canada has been a leader in palliative care with hospice and hospital based programs
across the country. Dr. Neil MacDonald has pioneered physician specialty education in
palliative care. Another of the original leaders in Canadian ethics, David Roy, established
The Journal Of Palliative Care (Roy), which serves as an important source of clinical and
bioethical thought.

F. Access to Health Care

Equitable access to health care within a universal single-tier health care system is the subject
of much bioethical discussion and debate, including the work of Somerville (1999), Stingl
(1996), and others. For specialized medical services, traditionally understood as "medically
necessary", Canadian citizens and permanent residents receive care based on need, not ability to pay. The College of Family Physicians of Canada (CFPC) undertook a study of the ethical implications of health care reform for family physicians (Yeo, 1997). A number of
organizations have focused on justice and health reform (CHAC, 1997). The CMA's "Core
and Comprehensive Health Care Services: A Framework for Decision-Making" addressed
which health services should be publicly funded (Sawyer & Williams, 1995, pp. 1409-1411)
and suggested a framework which requires consideration of quality of care, ethical, and economic factors. Ethical factors include substantive (fairness, age, lifestyle, the identifiable
versus the statistical patient, and futility) and procedural (the role of the public, the role of
physicians, and accountability) criteria for decision-making.

The National Forum on Health was established in 1994 by the Prime Minister to assist
in developing solutions and strategies to improve the health of Canadians and ensure the
sustainability of the Canadian health system. The Forum focused on four themes: determinants of health, evidence-based decision-making, values, and striking a balance. The
Values Working Group sought a better understanding of how values affect the development of the principles and policies governing health and health care in Canada. The
Forum's final report included the Working Group's conclusions (Kenny et al., 1997).
Canadians support the fundamental principles of the CHA, which embody values of fairness and equality, and do not want to see a health system in which the rich are treated differently from the poor. They have affirmed the shared risk inherent in a universal health
care system in the Commission on the Future of Health Care (2002). Despite increasing
pressures to "privatize" covered services, health policy experts in Canada see no evidence
of increased efficiency or improved outcomes from increasing the market's role in health
care. Thus Canada remains the only country with a universal health care system without
some formal incorporation of a parallel private system.

Because not all potentially "medically necessary" services are covered, legal challenges
regarding access are emerging. A childless couple underwent fertility treatments not

covered in the provincial plan (IVF and ICSI) and sued the Nova Scotia government for the costs they incurred in obtaining the treatment. The Supreme Court of Canada upheld the Nova Scotia decision that these procedures could qualify as being "medically necessary" but that the judgment should be left to the administrators of the health care system (Cameron, 1999).

G. Research Ethics

Canadians have contributed much to research ethics. Benjamin Freedman (1951-1997), one of Canada's leading thinkers in bioethics, is best known for the concept of "clinical equipoise" (Freedman, 1987), which affirms the position that offering clinical trial enrollment is consistent with a physician's duty of care if there exists genuine uncertainty in the community of expert clinicians regarding the preferred treatment. The concept is widely regarded as central to the ethics of clinical trials. In 1990, Freedman and Abraham Fuks established McGill University's Clinical Trials Research Group (CTRG), the first such think tank on research ethics.

The CTRG has provided critical analysis on the use of placebo control trials, particularly in psychiatry. This work continues in Charles Weijer's conceptual work on of research risk: putting clinical equipoise into the broader framework of risk analysis and raising the issue of protection for communities in research (Weijer & Emanuel, 2000). This work has been adopted by the U.S. National Bioethics Advisory Commission (NBAC) in its recommendations for regulatory change in the United States (Weijer, 2000).

Other contributions to research ethics include Keyserlink and Glass's work involving persons with dementia in clinical research (Keyserlingk et al., 1995), genetics research by Knoppers (1998), research involving children by Lynch (1992) and Baylis, Kenny, and Downie (1999), and research involving women.

In 1987, an International Summit Conference on Bioethics, held in Ottawa, recommended the establishment of "appropriate fora devoted to the issues arising in research with human subjects". This recommendation, coupled with the need to revise existing research guidelines, led to the collaborative effort of the Medical Research Council (MRC), The Royal College of Physicians and Surgeons of Canada, and Health Canada to establish the National Council on Bioethics in Human Research (NCBHR) in 1989. This Council was charged with assisting REBs in the protection of human subjects through education, site visits, and with fostering high ethical standards through work with other ethics committees of various professional and funding bodies in Canada. NCBHR's work focused on the REBs and reported on its first round of site visits in the 16 Canadian medical schools (NCBHR, 1995).

In 1994, the Canadian Medical Research, Natural Sciences and Engineering, and Social Sciences and Humanities Research Councils established a Working Group (WG) to revise existing guidelines for research. Initially led by Dr. Frederick Lowy and subsequently by Dr. Jean Joly, the WG was to establish a single set of guidelines for all research in Canada involving human subjects. This proved to be more difficult than anticipated. Numerous drafts were circulated for discussion and comment by the academic community. The document was further revised by an editorial board of the three national research Councils and published in 1997 (Tri-Council, 1998). However, there is ongoing dissatisfaction with these guidelines, including their internal inconsistencies and inability to respond to the differing cultures of research represented by the three Councils.

NCBHR's mandate was then expanded beyond biomedical research and changed its name to the National Council on Ethics in Human Research (NCEHR) to reflect the broadened mandate including the social and natural sciences.

With the development of a Tri-Council Advisory Group (TCAG) to continue to work on completing and updating the policy statement and the establishment of the new Canadian Institutes for Health Research (CIHR), roles and responsibilities in regards to human participant protection have become less distinct. In late 2000, the Law Commission of Canada (LCC) had released its report on "The Governance of Health Research Involving Human Subjects" (2000). The report led by Michael MacDonald, a former member of the Tri-Council Working Group, addressed how health research involving human subjects is governed and how effective governance relationships are in consistently achieving effective governance of ethical research. The report concludes that much improvement is needed regarding the coordination and quality of research oversight in Canada. It identifies many gaps in accountability and effectiveness of governance for health research and calls for greater involvement from major parties, more independence in research oversight, monitoring and standard-setting, and more research into the effects of research on human subjects. Current regulation of research in Canada is inadequate, as all research participants are not protected by a single set of over-arching ethical standards, REBs are not accredited, and there is no mandatory certification for human subjects investigators.

A very public issue of research integrity has emphasized the importance of protections for research subjects and researchers. Dr. Nancy Oliveri, who signed a contract with Apotex for support of a randomized clinical trial, became concerned first regarding the drug's efficacy and then with potential risks to participants. She submitted concerns to her REB over objections from the sponsor. The REB Chair indicated that the REB responds to the Principal Investigator to fulfill its mandate to protect research subjects. The REB advised changes to the information and consent forms and to the disclosure of the study findings to all relevant bodies.

For almost five years there was ongoing discussion and controversy over the involvement of researchers, the sponsor, the hospital, medical schools, and proposed external reviewers. In 1999, Oliveri was dismissed from her position at HSC. The Canadian Association of University Teachers (CAUT) called the investigator's treatment "classic bully behaviour" and completed its own report in December (Thompson, Baird, & Downie, 2001). It is highly critical of institutional policies and practices and enunciated clearly that the highest priority is the safety of research subjects in clinical trials and the integrity of research over and above corporate interests.

H. Other Issues

Ethical issues in risk and public policy have become concerns, starting in the late 1970s with HIV and Hepatitis C contaminated blood, continuing with the SARS epidemic in Toronto and the occurence of BSE ("mad cow") disease. The Krever Report on the blood supply set the precautionary principle as the standard for risk management in Canada (Commission of Inquiry, 1997). However, ethical analysis of risk at this macro level is not yet well developed. The Bayer Advisory Council on Bioethics, a private forum, has published two ethical reflections on risk and policy decisions regarding blood, "Creutzfeldt-Jakob Disease, Blood and Blood Products: A Bioethics Framework" (Bayer, 1998) and "Plasma Product Supply in Canada: A Bioethical Analysis" (Bayer, 2000).

In 1999, Federal Industry Minister John Manley established the Canadian Biotechnology Advisory Committee (CBAC) to provide independent advice on the ethical, social, regulatory, economic, environmental, and health aspects of biotechnology, as well as to raise public awareness and engage Canadians in an informed discussion on biotechnology. It reports to the federal Biotechnology Ministerial Coordinating Committee, including the ministers of agriculture and agri-food, environment, fisheries and oceans, foreign affairs and international trade, health, industry and natural resources. CBAC has released several commissioned papers that deal with ethical issues in biotechnology and they are available on their CBAC website.

The Trial Division of the Federal Court of Canada upheld a decision of the Commissioner of Patents not to allow the patenting of transgenic mammals, specifically mice (*President and Fellows of Harvard College v. Canada*, 2000). The Commissioner has stated, "On the plain and ordinary meaning of the words ... I do not find that a non-human mammal like a mouse falls within the definition of "invention". The inventors do not have full control over all the characteristics of the resulting mouse since the intervention of man ensures that reproducibility extends only as far as the cancer forming gene" (p. 37). The court agreed. Although the essential feature of the transgenic mouse is the transgene, which is what makes these mice useful for the testing of carcinogens, and so forth, and although the transgene would not be present without human intervention, the appellant cannot claim a patent over every descendant mouse which possesses that gene. Justice Nadon concluded, "In my view, the mouse is not truly reproducible as that term is understood in the Patent Act because too much is left to luck and chance" (p. 31).

Xenotransplantation, too, presents new issues. Xenografts are therapeutic products and subject to the requirements of Canada's Food and Drugs Act. Therefore, clinical trials involving xenografts must first be approved by the Therapeutic Products Directorate (TPP) of Health Canada. TPP's consultative efforts include a National Forum on Xenotransplantation, a website, development and distribution for comment of a Proposed Canadian Standard for Xenotransplantation, and a national survey of Canadian opinion on xenotransplantation.

IV. Conclusions

Inevitably, some major contributors to Canadian bioethics have been omitted from this overview. Most topics have been presented in too brief a fashion to do the complex issues justice. However, Canadian bioethics is very much in development, and these persons and issues will be the focus of future work. A particular challenge for Canada is the development of the ethical and legal capacity to address the important and complex questions that will be posed in the twenty-first century.

Bibliography

Bayer Advisory Council on Bioethics (BACB). 1998. Creutzfeldt-Jacob disease, blood and blood products: a bioethical analysis. [On-line] Available: <www.bayer-bioethics.org>.

Bayer Advisory Council on Bioethics (BACB). 2000. Plasma product supply in Canada: A bioethi-
   cal analysis working paper. [On-line] Available: <www.bayer-bioethics.org>.
Baylis, F. (ed.) 1994. *The health care ethics consultant.* Ottawa: Humana Press.
Baylis, F., Downie, J., Freedman, B., et al. 1995. *Health care ethics in Canada.* Toronto: Harcourt
   Brace.
Baylis, F., Downie, J. & Dewhurst, K. (eds) 1999. *Codes of ethics: Ethics codes, standards, and
   guidelines for professionals working in a health care setting in Canada (2nd ed.).* Toronto:
   Department of Bioethics, Hospital for Sick Children.
Baylis, F., Downie, J. & Kenny, N.P. 1999. Children and decision-making in health research. *IRB:
   A Review of Human Subjects Research* 21(4): 5-10.
Bliss, M. 1999. *William Osler: a life in medicine.* Toronto: University of Toronto Press.
Cameron v. Nova Scotia (Attorney General), (1999) N.S.J. No. 297 (C.A.).
Canadian Biotechnology Advisory Committee. [On-line] Available: <http://cbac.gc.ca>.
Canadian Medical Association. 1992. The medical record: confidentiality, access and disclosure.
   Canadian Medical Association Journal 147: 1860A.
Canadian Medical Association. 1993. HIV infection in the workplace. *Canadian Medical Associa-
   tion Journal* 148: 1800A-1800D.
Canadian Medical Association. 1994. Joint statement on resuscitation inventions. *Canadian
   Medical Association Journal* 151: 1176A-1176C.
Canadian Medical Association. 1996. Code of ethics. *Canadian Medical Association Journal* 155:
   1176A-1176B.
Canadian Medical Association. 1998. Prevention of Transmission of Hepatitis B. *Canadian Medical
   Association Journal* 159: 71-73.
Canadian Medical Association. 1998. *CMA health information privacy.* Ottawa: Canadian Medical
   Association.
Canadian Medical Association. [On-line] Available: <http://www.cma.ca/inside/policybase/
   index.htm>.
Canadian Nurses Association. 1997. *Code of ethics for registered nurses.* Ottawa: Canadian Nurses
   Association
Catholic Health Association of Canada. 1997. *Justice in the workplace: principles and guidelines for
   health care organizations in times of restructuring.* Ottawa: Catholic Health Association of Canada.
Child and Family Services of Central Manitoba v. Lavallee 75 A.C.W.S. (3rd), 1997.
Ciarlariello v. Schacter, 2 S.C.R. 199 (1993).
Commission of Inquiry on the Blood System in Canada. 1997. *The Krever Report.* Ottawa:
   Canadian Government Publishing – PWGSC.
Commission on the Future of Health Care in Canada, Building on Values: *The Future of Health
   Care in Canada – Final Report.* 2002. Commissioner Roy Romanow.
Crow, M. 1998. Confusion over causation: A journey through *Arndt v. Smith. Health Law Review*
   7: 3-13.
Downie, J. & Caulfield, T. (eds) 1999. *Canadian health law and policy.* Toronto: Butterworths.
Evans, R. 1998. We'll take care of it for you: health care in the Canadian community. *Daedalus*
   117(4): 155-189.
Feasby, C. & Chambers, S. (eds) 1998. Case comments and notes on *Winnipeg Child and Family
   Services (Northwest Area) v. G. (D. F.). Alberta Law Review* 36: 707-809.
Freedman, B. 1987. Equipoise and the ethics of clinical research. *New England Journal of Medicine*
   317: 141-145.
Health Canada. 1996. *New reproductive and genetic technologies. Setting boundaries, enhancing
   health.* Ottawa: Health Canada.
Hebert, P.C. 1996. *Doing right: A practical guide to ethics for physicians and medical trainees.*
   Toronto: Oxford University Press.

Humgen Website. [On-line] Available: <www.humgen.umontreal.ca>.

In re *Eve v. Mrs. E.* 31 D.L.R. (4th) 1 (1986).

In *re Superintendent of Family and Children Service and Dawson et al.; re Russell et al.* and *Superintendent of Children and Family Service et al.* 145 D.L.R. (3rd) 610 (1983).

Keatings, M. & Smith, O.B. 1995. *Ethics and legal issues in Canadian nursing.* Toronto: W.B. Saunder.

Kenny, N.P. & Baylis, F. 1998. Critical reflection and competent care: the ethics of practice. *Echo Newsletter, The Medical Council of Canada* 9 (supplement): 2.

Kenny, N.P., Dickson, R. & Dion Stout, M. et al. 1997. *Values working group: synthesis report, Canadian health action: building on the legacy, Vol. II, national forum on health.* Ottawa: Minister of Public Works and Government Services.

Kenny, N.P., Weijer, C.W. & Baylis, F. 1999. Voting ourselves rights: a critique of the Canadian medical association charter for physicians. *Canadian Medical Association Journal* 16 (4): 3999-4000.

Keyserlingk, E.W., Glass, K. & Kogan, S. et al. 1995. Proposed guidelines for the participation of persons with dementia as research subjects. *Perspectives in Biology and Medicine* 38: 319-362.

Knoppers, B.M. & Chadwick, R. 1994. The human genome project: under an international ethical microscope. *Science* 265: 2035-2036.

Knoppers, B.M. (ed.) 1998. *Socio-ethical issues in human genetics.* Cowansville: Les Editions Yvon-Blais Inc.

LaRochelle, S.A. & Fink, C.T. 1943. *Precis der morale medicale pour infumieres, medicins et pretres.* Quebec: L'Action catholique. English translation: M.E. Poupore, A. Carter, & R. Power: *Handbook of medical ethics for nurses, physicians and priests.* Montreal: Catholic Truth Society.

Lynch, A. (ed.) 1992. *Report on research involving children.* Ottawa: National Council on Bioethics in Human Research.

Lynch, A. (ed.) 1996. *The good pediatrician: an ethics curriculum for use in Canadian pediatric residency programs.* Toronto: The Pediatric Ethics Network Project, Hospital for Sick Children.

Malette v. Shulman (1990). 67 D.L.R. (4th) 321; 71 O.R. (2nd) 417; 20 A.C.W.S. (ed) 301.

Martin, R., Nisker, J., Daya, S., Miron, P. & Parrish, B. 1999. Policy statement: ethical issues in assisted reproduction. Joint Canadian fertility and andrology society/society of obstetrics and gynecology report. *Journal of Society of Obstetricians and Gynaecologists of Canada* 21(4): 369-371.

McDonald, M. 2000. *The governance of health research involving human subjects.* Ottawa: Law Commission of Canada.

Melancon, M. J. (ed.) 1994. *Bioethique et genetique: unreflexion.* Quebec: Editions JCL.

Nancy B. v. Hotel-Dieu de Quebec (1992). 86 D.L.R. (4th) 385; 69 C.C.C. (3d) 450; 31 A. C.W.S. (3rd) 160.

National Council on Bioethics in Human Research (NCBHR). 1995. *Communiqué 1995* 6: 3-32.

Norberg v. Wynrib, 2 S.C.R. 224 (1992).

Ontario Mental Health Legislative Reform, S.O. 2000, C9.

Personal Information Protection and Electronic Documents Act. S.C. 2000, c.5.

Preconception Arrangements. 1997. *Journal of Society of Obstetricians and Gynaecologists of Canada* 19: 393-399.

President and Fellows of Harvard College v. Canada (Commissioner of Patents) (2000) F.C.J. No. 1213 (F.C.A.).

Privacy Commissioner of Canada. 1992. *Genetic testing and privacy.* Ottawa: Minister of Supply and Services.

R. B. v. Children's Aid Society of Metropolitan Toronto (1992). 10 O.R. (3d) 321 (C.A.).

R. v. Genereux (1999). O.J. No. 1387 (Ont. CA).

R. v. Latimer (2001). SCC1.

R. v. Morrison (1998). N.S.J. No. 441 (N.S.S.C).

R. v. Ross (1993). 121 N.S.R. (2d) 242 (C.A.).

Reibel v. Hughes (1980). 114 D.L.R. (3d) 1 (S.C.C.).

Report of the Special Senate Committee on Euthanasia and Assisted Suicide. 1995. *Of life and death*. Ottawa: Minister of Supply and Services Canada.

Report of the Special Senate Committee on Euthanasia and Assisted Suicide. 2000. *Quality end of life care: the right of every Canadian*. Ottawa: Minister of Supply and Services Canada.

Rodriguez v. British Columbia (Attorney General) 3 S.C.R. 519 (1993).

Roy, D.A. (ed.). *Journal of Palliative Care*. Montreal: Center for Bioethics, Clinical Research Institute of Montreal.

Roy, D. Williams, J. & Dickens, B. 1994. *Bioethics in Canada*. Scarborough, Ontario: Prentice Hall.

Roy, D.J. & Williams, J.R. 1995. Canada. In: W.T. Reich (ed.), *Encyclopedia of bioethics* (pp. 1632-1639), New York: MacMillan.

Royal College of Physicians and Surgeons of Canada [On-line] Available: <http://rcpsc.rcpsc. medical.org/rcpsc/public/bioeth.htm>.

Royal Commission on New Reproductive Technologies (1993). *Proceed with care* (Vol. 2, Final Report). Ottawa: Canada Communication Group.

Sawatzky v. Riverview Health Centre Inc. (1998). M.J. No. 506 (Q.B.).

Sawyer, D.M. & Williams, J.R. 1995. Core and comprehensive health care services: 3. Ethical issues. *Canadian Medical Association Journal* 152: 1409-1411.

Sherwin, S. 1992. *No longer patient: feminist ethics and health care*. Philadelphia: Temple University Press.

Singer, P.A. 1996. Bioethics for clinicians. *Canadian Medical Journal Association* 155: 189-190.

Singer, P.A. (ed.) 1999. *Bioethics at the bedside: a clinician's guide*. Ottawa: Canadian Medical Association.

Smith v. Jones, 1999, 169 D.L.R. (4th) 385 S.C.C.

Somerville, M.A. (ed.) 1999. *Do we care? Reviewing Canada's commitment to health*. Montreal: McGill Queens University Press.

Stingl, M. & Wilson, D. (eds) 1996. *Efficiency vs. equality: health reform in Canada*. Halifax: Fernwood Publishing.

T.T.D. (Re). 1999. S.J. No. 144 (Sask Q.B.).

Taylor, M.G. 1987. *Health insurance and Canadian public policy: the seven decisions that created the Canadian health insurance system*. Montreal: McGill-Queen's University Press.

Thompson, J., Baird, P. & Downie, J. 2001. *Report of the committee of inquiry on the case involving Dr. Nancy Olivieri, the Hospital for Sick Children, the University of Toronto, and Apotex Inc*. Toronto: Canadian Association of University Teachers.

Tri-Council. 1998. *Tri-council policy statement on the ethical conduct of research involving humans*. Ottawa: Tri-Council.

Weijer, C. 2000. The ethical analysis of risk. *The Journal of Law, Medicine & Ethics* 28 (4): 344-361.

Weijer, C. & Emanuel, E.J. 2000. Protecting communities in biomedical research. *Science* 289: 1142-1144.

Williams, J.R. 1989. Commissions and biomedical ethics: the Canadian experience. *The Journal of Medicine and Philosophy* 14 (4): 425-444.

Yeo, M. & Moorhouse, A. (eds) 1996. *Concepts and cases in nursing ethics (2nd ed.)*. Ontario: Broadview Press.

Yeo, M. 1997. *Ethical implications of health reform for family medicine*. Toronto: College of Family Physicians of Canada.

2 United States Perspectives on Assisted Reproductive Technologies

Scott B. Rae

In the United States, the use of assisted reproductive technologies (ART) has continued to develop and its popularity as a treatment for infertility has continued to grow. More frequently, insurance plans now cover at least part of the cost of such treatments. There are now hundreds of ART clinics that are members of the Society for Assisted Reproductive Technology, the umbrella organization that provides voluntary guidelines and loose oversight to the infertility industry. In the last twenty years, medicine has made some remarkable accomplishments in the field of reproductive technology. When used successfully, these technologies provide the miracle of life for couples, who have often spent years trying to have a child and have exhausted all other avenues for conceiving a child of their own. But these techniques raise significant moral questions and can create thorny legal dilemmas that must be resolved in court.

I. Overview of Major Assisted Reproductive Technologies

There are a variety of technologies that constitute the mainstream treatments for infertility. New technologies are also arising that are more expensive, more novel, and possibly more invasive that "push the envelope" of assisted reproduction. Mainstream technologies include the following:

Fertility drugs, which attempt to stimulate multiple ovulation or make ovulation more regular and thus predictable.

Intrauterine insemination (IUI) is the procedure in which the husband's sperm is collected through masturbation and then is given a simple and technologically unsophisticated "push" into his wife's body. Usually, the sperm is treated in the lab and then inserted into the woman's body using a syringe without the needle attached. Sperm can come from the woman's husband (formerly known as artificial insemination by husband, or AIH) or from a donor (formerly known as artificial insemination by donor, or AID). Increasingly, IUI is done in conjunction with fertility drugs, which enable multiple ovulation and thereby increase the prospects of achieving pregnancy. When sperm comes from a donor, the procedure is known as donor insemination (DI). In DI, either a single donor is used, or multiple donors are employed. In this latter case, the sperm of multiple donors is mixed to help insure donor anonymity. Normally, when the donors donate their sperm, they also sign a waiver of parental rights, indicating that they give up any parental claims to the child produced with their sperm and they will not attempt to establish any contact with a child born through use of their sperm. Thus the husband of the woman who actually bears the child is assumed to be the child's legal father. In some clinics, couples can choose the traits of their donor(s) and thus increase the chances for a child bearing traits desired by the parents.

Egg donation is the female equivalent of DI, in which a woman, sometimes anonymous and sometimes not, contributes one or more eggs to an infertile couple. Usually the eggs are fertilized with the sperm of the husband in the infertile couple in a lab, and the fertilized eggs, or embryos, are inserted into the uterus of the infertile wife, who will gestate and give birth to the child.

Gamete intrafallopian transfer (GIFT) is a process by which the wife's eggs are removed surgically and reinserted with sperm in the fallopian tubes where fertilization can occur naturally. This is usually proceeded with hormone treatments to stimulate maximum production of eggs in the woman's cycle.

In vitro fertilization (IVF), the first well-publicized reproductive technology, is a process in which fertilization takes place "in vitro" or in glass, outside of the body. Here also the woman's body is stimulated hormonally to produce a number of eggs which are surgically removed, fertilized in a petri dish and then surgically reinserted in the woman's uterus.

Zygote intrafallopian transfer (ZIFT) is a process much like IVF. The only difference is that the embryos are reinserted into the woman's fallopian tubes, where they have a better chance of implanting. This technique is also more expensive than IVF.

Surrogate motherhood is probably the most controversial of all the reproductive advances made recently. However, to call surrogacy a new reproductive technology is a bit misleading, since it is neither new nor does it normally involve much technology. It dates back to Biblical times (Genesis 16, 30). Some distinctions in the kinds of surrogate motherhood are helpful. (a) *Genetic surrogacy*: the surrogate mother contributes the egg and uterus; i.e., she is artificially inseminated by the husband of the infertile couple and actually gives birth to the child, then turning him or her over to the couple shortly after birth, similar to adoption. Only IUI is used in achieving the pregnancy in these types of cases. (b) *Gestational surrogacy*: The surrogate contributes only the gestational environment with the egg coming from the wife of the infertile couple. The wife's eggs are fertilized by her husband's sperm by means of *in vitro* fertilization, then implanted in the surrogate mother who will carry the child during pregnancy and give birth. This is usually done when the wife of the infertile couple can produce eggs but for some reason cannot carry a child to term. Both of these types of surrogacy can be done for a fee, in addition to expenses. This is referred to as *commercial surrogacy*. By contrast, *altruistic surrogacy* occurs when the surrogate does not charge a fee to the couple. Generally, the couple only pays for the expenses incurred during the pregnancy. This is often done by a close friend or family member. In just over half of surrogacy arrangements, the surrogate is a genetic surrogate who does it for the money. When done commercially, the couple who contracts with the surrogate usually employs a surrogacy broker, who recruits and screens the surrogate, drafts the contract, and monitors the process until the child is turned over to the contracting couple, the point at which the surrogate's work is complete.

Prenatal genetic testing is also on the leading edge of new reproductive technology. These procedures, such as ultrasound imaging and amniocentesis, can help an infertile couple know the genetic makeup of the child, whom the woman is carrying. Infertility clinics can also do some genetic screening of embryos prior to implantation.

Intracytoplasmic sperm injection (ICSI) is a technology often used as a last resort when other less expensive and less sophisticated technologies have failed to achieve a pregnancy. Here an opening is made in the woman's egg, enabling the sperm more easily to penetrate and fertilize it. However, this procedure does bypass the normal process of natural selection of the sperm as they travel toward the egg, raising concerns that this procedure will increase the incidence of genetic abnormalities.

The following technologies are not yet mainstream, but may be in the future.

Cloning has recently been accomplished with human embryos. This has been done with animals for some time, but, in 1993, was done for the first time with human embryos. It was done by infertility researchers who were trying to help infertile couples keep the cost of IVF down. Instead of removing a number of the woman's eggs and fertilizing them in the lab, they removed one or two, fertilized them and essentially copied them, creating more embryos that could later be implanted in the woman's body should they be necessary. For the most part, scientists duplicated in the lab what the body does when identical twins are produced. This technology is very new and very controversial, but promises to be helpful to infertile couples in the future.

More well known is *somatic cell nuclear transfer*, what most people commonly refer to as cloning. Here DNA is obtained from a cell of a mature adult and is placed in an egg which has had its nucleus removed; it is then treated and placed in the uterus to develop and grow. This process produces a twin identical to the donor, though separated by an age span determined by the age of the donor. At present, this has only been successful with animals, though there are researchers who are preparing to do this with human beings.

Fetal egg donation is a possibility that may come to fruition if public policy permits it. Here the eggs from aborted fetuses are used as donor eggs, rather than obtaining them from adult donors.

Post-menopausal pregnancies are now possible through the use of an egg donor and treatments to restore the vitality of the uterine wall.

Artificial wombs are being used to gestate some animals successfully and researchers are optimistic about developing this technology for use in human beings.

One group of these techniques involves primarily medical intervention into natural reproductive processes using the genetic materials of husband and wife (fertility drugs, IUI, GIFT, ZIFT, IVF, and ICSI). A second group of these technologies goes further and requires participation of another person in order to achieve conception and birth (DI, egg donation, and surrogate motherhood).[1] In some cases, the genetic material of the third-party is required and in others, such as gestational surrogacy, it is not.

II. Tradition of Procreative Liberty

In the United States, public policy concerning ARTs has not played a major role in regulating the industry, which is still largely self-regulated. In the aftermath of some well-publicized scandals, there have been increasing calls for further regulation of the industry. ARTs in the United States still largely operate under the broad umbrella doctrine of procreative liberty. It is difficult to understand the American perspective on these technologies without grasping the longstanding tradition of procreative liberty established by the United States Supreme Court.

With the exception of commercial surrogate motherhood, which has gained neither widespread legislative nor judicial support, the tradition of procreative liberty gives couples the legal right to use virtually any reproductive technique to have a child. Though the United States Supreme Court has not specifically addressed any particular reproductive technology including surrogate motherhood,[2] states in general have refused to write laws that would interfere with a couple's or a single person's liberty to have a child.

Procreative liberty as a legal right is a strongly held tradition, tied closely to the right to privacy. This tradition has strongly affected the way society views most reproductive technology. Since procreative liberty is considered to fall within the realm of privacy, there are few legal limits on their use. This is why, with the exception of surrogate motherhood, there are few restrictions on infertility clinics. Many couples expect that procreative decisions will be theirs alone, since these are private decisions that affect the most intimate areas of life. This tradition makes it more difficult for any religious tradition to suggest moral limits on the use of reproductive interventions, especially if a particular tradition, such as Roman Catholicism, desires to see its moral stand on such technology become law.[3] Because the discussion of reproductive technology is set against the backdrop of a long-standing legal tradition of procreative liberty in the United States, any public policy on reproductive technology that does not take this tradition into account will face significant obstacles in the process of being enacted into law and withstanding Constitutional challenge once enacted.

As the legal precedent for procreative liberty developed, the focus of the cases shifted from general concerns about family life to a more narrow concentration on contraception. Cases that dealt with contraception were based on the reasoning that came out of the earlier, more general cases. Though the earlier cases may not appear at first glance to apply to reproductive technologies, they are important in that they lay the foundation upon which the edifice of procreative liberty is built. Of course, the abortion cases, such as *Roe v. Wade* (1973), take procreative liberty to the extent of allowing women to end pregnancies that they do not want to keep or are not prepared to keep. Those built the foundations for the cases that followed.

A. *Meyer v. Nebraska (1923)*

In the first of the cases in which the United States Supreme Court established the tradition of procreative liberty, the Court continued to broaden the scope of the liberties protected by the Fourteenth Amendment. Though the Constitution does not specifically recognize the right to privacy, the Court has continually expanded the notion of liberty to include various zones of privacy inherent in the due process clause.

In *Meyer v. Nebraska*, the Court affirmed that the protected Constitutional liberties include the freedom for an individual "to marry, establish a home and bring up children" (*Meyer v. Nebraska*. 262 U.S. 390, [1923], at 399). The state cannot interfere with one's decision to establish a family. Though non-coital means of reproduction were not addressed in this case, some have argued that the freedom for coital reproduction extends by implication to methods that use some of the new reproductive technologies, such as IVF and DI.[4] However, the decision here clearly confined procreative liberty to married couples, and the Court appeared to assume that children (conceived by normal means) are to be brought up in a home occupied by a heterosexual married couple.

B. Pierce v. Society of Sisters (1925)

Though this case did not deal with conception, the decision affirmed the liberty of parents to raise their children in the manner in which they see fit. It clearly limited the power of the state to interfere in the realm of family matters. This is a foundational decision that was later applied more specifically to privacy relating to contraception and abortion. Though it does not address procreative liberty per se, this decision was instrumental in beginning to define the zones of privacy that were later specified to include procreation as chief among them.

Here the Court made the phrase in the Meyer decision more precise, that an individual has the freedom to "bring up children." Assuming that the way in which that is done does not harm the child in a way in which the state could readily prevent, the state does not have the authority to mandate how parents should raise their children. "It is an unreasonable interference with the liberty of parents and guardians to direct to upbringing of the children, and in that respect violates the Fourteenth Amendment" (Pierce v. Society of Sisters. 268 U.S. 510 [1925], at 534). The state of Oregon in this case was prevented from mandating that parents send their children to public schools until the age of sixteen.

C. Skinner v. Oklahoma (1942)

The Court in this case struck down a mandatory sterilization law for habitual criminals. In addition, the Court ruled that the law denied an essential civil liberty, and the language suggested that the right to procreate was so basic as to be inalienable. "We are dealing here with legislation which involves one of the basic civil rights of man. Marriage and procreation are fundamental to the very existence and survival of the race. [When sterilized] he is forever deprived of a basic liberty" (Skinner v. Oklahoma. 316 U.S. 535 [1942]). Thus, the right to marry and start a family established in Meyer cannot be forfeited by any criminal behavior.

D. Griswold v. Connecticut (1965)

In this landmark case, the Court struck down a Connecticut law forbidding the use of contraceptives, and in doing so, affirmed the right of marital privacy. Though the Constitution does not specifically mention many of the rights that are now clearly recognized as consistent with it, the Court recognized that the right of privacy in marriage is within the penumbra of specific guarantees made by the Bill of Rights. Clearly the Court placed the decision not to procreate within the zones of privacy, consistent with earlier decisions that affirmed the freedom to procreate (Griswold v. Connecticut. 381 U.S. 479 [1965]).

E. Eisenstadt v. Baird (1972)

This case broadened the right to use contraception recognized by Griswold to include unmarried individuals as well as married couples. The Massachusetts law in question made it a felony for anyone except a licensed physician or pharmacist, at a physician's direction, to distribute contraceptives. The law provided that they could only distribute them to married couples. It was struck down by the appeals court as a violation of the equal protection clause of the Fourteenth Amendment, and that decision was affirmed by the Supreme Court. The Court affirmed the direction set in Griswold that keeps the government from intruding into the private realm of the bedroom (Griswold v. Connecticut. 381 U.S. at

485-486; *Eisenstadt v. Baird*. 405 U.S. 438 [1972]).[5] In the majority opinion, Justice Brennan clarified the right to procreative privacy. If under *Griswold* the distribution of contraceptives to married persons cannot be prohibited, a ban on distribution to unmarried persons would be equally impermissible. It is true that in *Griswold* the right to privacy in question inhered in the marital relationship. Yet the marital couple is not an independent entity with a mind and heart of its own, but an association of two individuals each with a separate intellectual and emotional makeup. If the right of privacy means anything, it is the right of the individual, married or single, to be free from unwarranted governmental intrusion into matters so fundamentally affecting a person as the decision whether to bear or beget a child (*Griswold v. Connecticut*. 381 U.S. at 453).

The Court affirmed a fundamental privacy right in decisions to prevent conception. These decisions are so fundamental to an individual's goals, aims, and happiness in life that decisions in this area are to be left to the individual, assuming that no harm comes to the parties to the decision or others affected by it. This case thus marked an important shift in the way procreative privacy rights are recognized. The *Griswold* decision assumed that marriage constituted a separate entity that should not be subject to intervention by the state. It only protected married couples from such intervention. *Eisenstadt*, however, affirmed the individuality of the people within the marriage relationship. Thus, the right of privacy was extended beyond the marital couple as a unit to the individuals that make it up. In this way, *Griswold* now applies to individuals irrespective of their marital status.

F. Stanley v. Illinois (1972)

In a case that has important implications not only for procreative liberty but also for parental rights, the Court reversed a decision by the Illinois Supreme Court that denied Stanley a hearing to determine his fitness as a parent prior to the state placing his children for adoption. The Illinois law in question held that upon the death of a single mother, the children were to be declared wards of the state and placed in guardianship, irrespective of the unwed father's claim to parental rights. Stanley was thus denied a hearing to determine his parental fitness, and he charged that he was being denied his rights under the Due Process Clause of the Fourteenth Amendment. The Court recognized a fundamental right of parents to associate with and raise their children. The private interest here, that of a man in the children he has sired and raised, undeniably warrants deference and, absent a powerful countervailing interest, protection. It is plain that the interest of a parent in the companionship, care and custody of his children comes to this Court with a momentum for respect lacking when appeal is made to liberties which derive merely from shifting economic arrangements (*Stanley v. Illinois*. 405 U.S. 645 [1972], at 651).

G. Moore v. City of East Cleveland (1977)

This case reversed an appeals court decision that upheld a city housing ordinance that limited occupancy of single family homes to nuclear families. In this case, that definition excluded a family in which a grandmother chose to live with her son and two grandsons. The law was struck down as an arbitrary limit on the due process clause.

Two important points were made in the concurring opinion of Justice Marshall. First, the city cannot define a family in the way it did, restricting it to the nuclear family. This definition effectively excluded the notion of the extended family living together under the same roof which, the Court recognized, has a long history and plays an important role when the nuclear family faces economic hardship or loss of one of the parents. Second, classifying families in this way "unconstitutionally abridges the freedom of personal choice in matters of family life [that] is one of the liberties protected by the Due Process Clause of the Fourteenth Amendment" (*Moore v. City of East Cleveland.* 431 U.S. 494 [1977]).[6] The family and family-related decisions, such as marriage, having children, and the manner in which they are raised, are within a zone of privacy protected by the penumbra of rights guaranteed by the Constitution. This is an example of the Court's tendency to defend a narrow privacy right with broad language about the overriding right to privacy. Though the Court has yet to hear a case dealing with a specific reproductive technology, one could argue that the reasoning in this case surely supports procreative decisions that involve different definitions of family and non-coital means of reproduction that involve third-party participants.

H. Carey v. Population Services International (1977)

The Court affirmed a lower court decision that struck down a New York law that (1) restricted the sale of contraceptives to minors, (2) only allowed contraceptives to be purchased from a licensed pharmacist, and (3) prohibited anyone from advertising contraceptives. The language of the decision goes beyond the narrow issue of contraception and the right to prevent conception. It explicitly protects the right to achieve pregnancy. After the Court cited the long precedent for privacy in family matters,[7] it applied the *Griswold* decision to this case. "The decision to bear or beget a child is at the very heart of this cluster of constitutionally protected choices. That decision holds a particularly important place in the history of the right to privacy. Decisions *whether to accomplish or prevent conception* are among the most private and sensitive" (*Carey v. Population Services International.* 431 U.S. 678 [1977], at 685, emphasis added). The Court summarized by stating, "Read in light of its progeny, the teaching of *Griswold* is that the Constitution protects individual decisions in matters of *childbearing* from unjustified intrusion by the State" (at 687, emphasis added).

III. Religious Views on Assisted Reproductive Technologies

In the United States, much of the criticism of the broad tradition of procreative liberty and its application to ARTs has come from the religious communities. The religiously based opposition to abortion is well-documented, though clearly opposition to abortion has grounds other than simply one's religious views. But the most stringent limits on procreative liberty, particularly as applied to ARTs, have come from official Roman Catholic teaching. Less restrictive views tend to be found in Protestant and evangelical Christian communities, as well as conservative and Reform Judaism.

A. Roman Catholicism

1. *Humanae Vitae (1968).* Roman Catholic theologians have provided the vast majority of the religiously-based discussion of reproductive technologies. Contemporary Catholic

teaching on procreation comes out in two official Vatican documents. The first of these is called *Humanae Vitae (On the Regulation of Birth)* (1968). This work is considered the foundational modern philosophical and theological contribution to Catholic reproductive ethics. The general tenor of the encyclical is that "Marriage and conjugal love are *by their nature* ordained toward the begetting and educating of children. Children are really the supreme gift of marriage and contribute very substantially to the welfare of the parents" (emphasis added) (Paul VI, 1968, p. 486). That is, God ordained marriage for the procreation of children, to the benefit of the parents.

The crux of the argument is the notion of the essential unity of sexual relations in marriage. Every individual "marriage act," that is, sexual encounter in marriage, must be open to the possibility of creating new life. The reason for this, in Catholic teaching, is that when God designed sexual relations, He invested the action with two inseparable meanings, the unitive and the procreative. These are both parts of the essential structure of the action, neither of which can be separated from the other. The encyclical put it this way:

> That teaching [that every sexual act must be open to procreation], is founded upon the inseparable connection, willed by God and unable to be broken by man on his own initiative, between the two meanings of the conjugal act: the unitive meaning and the procreative meaning. Indeed, by its intimate structure, the conjugal act, while most closely uniting husband and wife, capacitates them for the generation of new lives, according to laws inscribed in the very being of man and of woman. By safeguarding both these essential aspects, the unitive and the procreative, the conjugal act preserves in its fullness the sense of true mutual love and its ordination towards man's most high calling to parenthood (Paul VI, 1968, p. 488).

This statement is foundational to official Catholic teaching on reproduction. These two elements, the unitive and procreative, are rooted in the nature of human beings and ultimately in the will of God who placed that nature in them. The Pope states, "To use this divine gift [of sex in marriage] destroying, if only partially, its meaning and purpose [by separating the unitive and procreative] is to contradict the nature of both man and woman and of their most intimate relationship, and therefore it is to contradict the plan of God and His will" (Paul VI, p. 489). Contraception, sterilization, and elective abortion are all prohibited by the teaching of this encyclical, though a rhythm method of birth control is considered acceptable.

2. *Donum Vitae (1987)*. This document addresses assisted reproductive technology and attempts to apply Catholic teaching on procreation to the various new reproductive technologies. The instruction is a further application of the spirit of *Humanae Vitae* to a set of new questions. The instruction acknowledges that science and technology are a significant expression of the dominion that God originally entrusted to mankind at creation, of which medicine in general is a significant part. But that does not mean that technology can be exempt from moral assessment; that is, moral principles from natural law serve to limit technology appropriately (Paul VI, 1968, pp. 699-700). The fundamental values that limit the application of reproductive technology are twofold: "the life of the human being called into existence and the special nature of the transmission of human life in marriage"

(Paul VI, 1968, p. 700). The first of these values deals with the moral status of the embryo (and fetus, by extension) and the concern to protect embryos from the moment of conception. *Donum Vitae* goes into great depth in discussing the embryonic right to life from conception until death and dealing with questions about prenatal diagnosis, research and experimentation on embryos, and use of embryos in reproductive technologies such as *in vitro* fertilization. In general, reproductive methods that involve intentional destruction of embryonic life are not morally allowed.

The second fundamental value related to assisted reproduction is "the special nature of the transmission of human life in marriage." Here *Donum Vitae* reaffirms the essential teaching of *Humanae Vitae*, that all human procreation must take place in marriage and be connected to a specific sex act. *Donum Vitae* states that:

> from the moral point of view a truly responsible procreation vis-à-vis the unborn child must be the fruit of marriage ... The fidelity of the spouses in the unity of marriage involves reciprocal respect of their right to become a father and a mother only through each other ... in marriage and in its indissoluble unity [is] the only setting worthy of truly responsible procreation (1987, pp. 704-705).

Therefore, any reproductive interventions that involve third-party genetic or gestational contributors would not be allowed. *Donum Vitae* insists that these interventions violate the reciprocal commitment between the spouses in marriage, violates the right of the child, can hinder developing personal identity, and potentially damages the stability of the family for society (1987, p. 705). The only reproductive technologies that are possible for faithful Catholic couples are those that use the genetic material of husband and wife. IUI, egg donation, and surrogate motherhood are not consistent with Catholic teaching.

In keeping with *Humanae Vitae*, *Donum Vitae* goes further and evaluates reproductive technologies that do not involve third-party contributors. In answer to the question, "What connection is required from the moral point of view between procreation and the conjugal act?", *Donum Vitae* quotes the central point of *Humanae Vitae*, which inseparably links the unitive and procreative meanings of sex in marriage (1987, p. 705). But it specifies further and clarifies this central tenet of Catholic teaching. It states that "The same doctrine concerning the link between the meanings of the conjugal act and between the goods of marriage throws light on the moral problem of homologous artificial fertilization, since it is never permitted to separate these different aspects to such a degree as positively to exclude either the procreative intention or the conjugal act" (1987, p. 706). Thus, the only morally legitimate way for fertilization to occur is between husband and wife in marriage and as a result of a specific act of intercourse. The intrinsic nature of the act of sex is rendered incomplete by separating sexual relations from procreation. *Donum Vitae* puts it this way:

> From the moral point of view, procreation is deprived of its proper perfection when it is not desired as the fruit of the conjugal act, that is to say, of the specific act of the spouses' union... The moral relevance of the link between the meaning of the conjugal act and the goods of marriage as well as the unity of the human being and the dignity of his origin, demand that

the procreation of a human person be brought about as the fruit of the conjugal act specific to the love between spouses (1987, p. 706).

Morally legitimate procreation must occur as the result of a specific sexual union in marriage. Concerning *in vitro* fertilization, for example, *Donum Vitae* states that:

the generation of the human person is objectively deprived of its proper perfection: namely that of being the result and fruit of a conjugal act in which
the spouses can become cooperators with God for giving life to a new person.
The act of conjugal love is considered in the teaching of the Church as the
only setting worthy of human procreation (1987, p. 707).

Therefore, IVF, ZIFT, and most forms of IUI are all considered morally impermissible.

Catholic teaching does make an important distinction between a technology that
assists normal intercourse and one that *replaces* it in the process of trying to conceive a
child. Anything that assists intercourse is considered a part of God's wisdom that can be
utilized in reproduction (1987, p. 707). For example, fertilization must always occur
inside the body and masturbation may not be used as a substitute for sex in order to collect sperm outside the body to be reinserted back into the woman. A technology such as
GIFT could be permissible within Catholic teaching, as long as sperm is obtained through
normal sexual relations.

B. *Other Religious Views of ARTs*

Less restrictive views of ARTs are found in non-Catholic religious traditions. Though
there is wide variety among Protestants and evangelicals, there tends to be greater openness to technological interventions to treat infertility, similar to conservative and reform
Judaism. Orthodox Judaism and Islam tend to be more restrictive, sanctioning fewer
interventions. These traditions are particularly skeptical about those which involve third-
party contributors, either of gametes or gestational environment. Further, some are hesitant about technology that achieves conception outside the body, thus substituting
technology for normal sexual relations. However, it is difficult to generalize about views
in these other traditions that operate without anything like the teaching hierarchy of
Catholicism.

For Protestants and evangelicals, there is fairly broad consensus that reproductive
technologies that utilize the genetic materials of husband and wife are acceptable. This
would mean that in principle, IUI, GIFT, IVF, ZIFT and ICSI would fall into the range of
appropriate technologies, though some are uncomfortable with even these interventions
(see, e.g., Cameron, 2000; Meilander, 2000). However, for those with pro-life leanings,
for whom personhood begins at conception, the status and disposition of embryos created
through the use of these technologies raises problems. Specifically, the standard of practice in GIFT, ZIFT and IVF is to harvest as many eggs as possible and attempt to create as
many embryos as feasible in the lab, implanting 3-4 embryos per attempt to achieve a
pregnancy. Should there be leftover embryos, this creates a moral dilemma for those who
hold that embryos have moral status and, thus, consider disposing of them the moral equivalent to abortion. The standard way of dealing with leftover embryos in most infertility

clinics is to keep them in storage until it is clear that they are no longer necessary, then discard them. For those with pro-life leanings, the acceptable options would seem to be implantation of embryos with the couple who created them taking responsibility for them, or donation of the embryos to another infertile couple or couples. Embryo adoption agencies are being formed to meet this need in some major metropolitan areas in the United States.

A further moral tension is raised with the standard practice of offering selective reduction in the number of pregnancies if the woman is carrying multiple fetuses. In some cases, this is necessary for the mother's safety and to safeguard the lives of the remaining fetuses. But in some cases it is offered when there do not seem to be any medical indications, but it is the preference of the couple. Protestants with pro-life leanings view these kinds of abortions as particularly problematic, since they can be easily avoided, simply by limiting the number of embryos implanted to the number the couple is willing to raise or the woman can safely carry to term. It seems especially callous intentionally to create life and then terminate it because the outcome is not what the couple desired.

There is more debate in Protestant, evangelical, and some Jewish circles about the morality of using third-party contributors to procreation. Some hold that using third-party donors is an acceptable way to create a family, though they would have problems with single women, gays, lesbians, and post-menopausal women using donors to bring children into "no-dad" families. Some would also have no trouble with gestational surrogacy, viewing the surrogate as a form of prenatal baby-sitter for another couple's child. These are probably not majority views within these circles, but they do indicate that they are areas of ongoing debate and discussion.

IV. Surrogate Motherhood

Undoubtedly, surrogate motherhood is among the most controversial of the new reproductive technologies and has generated the most public debate. What follows is an attempt to capture the essence of that debate in U.S. courts and public policy arenas.

A. Arguments In Favor of Surrogate Motherhood

1. *Surrogacy as consistent with the constitutional tradition of procreative liberty.* There is a long tradition in the Western world that gives couples the freedom to make their own decisions about childbearing and childrearing. The family has historically been a place in which the right to privacy has reigned and thus family decisions have for the most part been beyond the scrutiny and intervention of the government. Laws have been crafted to insure as much freedom as possible for parents to make choices concerning their children.[8]

In response to this argument, opponents of surrogacy hold that the tradition of procreative liberty only opens the door to *altruistic* surrogacy, in which a woman performs the role of surrogate out of a charitable motive and only receives reimbursement for reasonable expenses incurred during the pregnancy. This is very different from the way in which surrogacy is usually done. Normally, the surrogate is paid at least $10,000 for her services, and another $10,000-25,000 is paid to a surrogacy broker for his services in recruiting the surrogate and drawing up the contract that will govern the arrangement. Whether procreative liberty allows for *commercial* surrogacy is another matter, since most states have laws that forbid the exchange of money for the transfer of parental rights to a child.[9]

2. *The fee paid to the surrogate is for services rendered, not the sale of a child.* Surrogacy proponents are sensitive to the charge that paying a surrogate a large amount of money for bearing a child for another couple is baby-selling. Therefore, the argument is that the fee only pays for gestational services rendered and is not the sale of a child. Proponents insist that it is only fair for a woman to be compensated for her time, risk, and the sacrifice that pregnancy entails. People have a right to be compensated appropriately for services rendered. Just as it is legitimate to pay surrogate *childrearers* in a day care setting, proponents insist that it should be legitimate to pay surrogate *childbearers*.

Opponents of surrogacy respond that this argument fails to take into account that the fee is for much more than childbirth services rendered. The service provided in bearing the child is clearly not the intended end product of the arrangement. What really counts in a surrogacy arrangement is not only the successful birth of the child, but also the transfer of parental rights from the surrogate to the infertile wife, who must adopt the child for the "deal to be done." In most surrogacy cases, in which the surrogate supplies both the egg and the womb, she is the legal mother of the child.[10] Should she so desire, she may keep the child and share custody with the natural father. Thus, for any surrogacy arrangement to be completed, she must turn over parental rights to the contracting couple. Opponents of surrogacy insist that the fee also pays for this transfer of parental rights and is thus baby-selling.

For example, in the well-known Baby M case, only in the event of the surrogate's delivering a healthy baby to the contracting couple and turning over parental rights would she be paid the full $10,000 fee. If she miscarried prior to the fifth month of pregnancy, she would receive nothing. If she miscarried after the fifth month or gave birth to a stillborn child, she would receive only $1,000. The contract was clearly oriented to the delivery of the end product, not the gestational process. To be consistent, if the fee paid to the surrogate is only for gestational services rendered, the surrogate would be paid the same amount whether or not she turned over the child to the contracting couple. If the fee only pays for childbirth services, it is hard to see how a couple could take the surrogate to court to get the child, since the surrogate would have fulfilled her part of the contract once the child was born. In addition, if she miscarried at some point in the pregnancy, her fee should be prorated over the number of months that she performed a gestational service. Proponents of surrogacy respond that the natural father cannot buy back what is already his, and thus surrogacy cannot be baby-selling. But the child is not *all* his. At best, he can only claim the equivalent of joint tenancy in a piece of property, in which he "buys out" his partner, the surrogate, and thus is still baby-selling.[11]

3. *Surrogacy is very different from black market adoptions.* Some proponents of surrogacy will admit that children are being sold, but that the circumstances are so different from black market adoptions that it does no harm to exchange parental rights for money. The laws that prevent payment to birth mothers were designed to prevent black market adoptions, in which birth mothers were exploited based on their financial need and in which the well-being of the children was not considered the highest priority. Surrogacy is a completely different situation. Here the natural father is also the adopting father, and surrogacy results from a planned and wanted pregnancy as opposed to an unwanted pregnancy. Thus the child is not going to a stranger but to a genetic relative, and the surrogate is not coerced into making a decision she will later regret.

Opponents of surrogacy respond that the differences between black market adoptions and surrogacy are overstated. For example, there is little screening of the contracting couple done in order to insure that they are fit parents and that the best interests of the child are being maintained. In addition, the element of coercion is not entirely absent from a surrogacy arrangement, since it is quite possible that the surrogate could end up being coerced by the contract into giving up a child, whom she may end up wanting to keep. Further, given the desperation of the contracting couple to have a child, since they usually do not resort to surrogacy until all other means have been exhausted, it leaves them open to exploitation by the surrogacy brokers. Thus, to say that the environment surrounding surrogacy is free from coercion may not be accurate.

Even if the child is treated well and the arrangement comes off without coercion, the problem of baby selling remains. Even if something like slavery during the Civil War era had cases in which slaves were treated well and considered like family members, the fact remained that they had been bought and sold and had become objects of barter. The circumstances in which such barter takes place is irrelevant according to opponents of surrogacy.

4. *Restriction on the fee means restriction on the practice of surrogacy.* Proponents of commercial surrogacy hold that it is inconsistent to affirm procreative liberty and forbid the fee to the surrogate. If the fee is prohibited, then the number of available surrogates will dramatically decrease and, in all likelihood, curtail the practice. The right to procreate in this way would thereby become an empty right, since the state would have interfered to prevent people from exercising it.

The precedent for this argument is the *Carey v. Population Services* Supreme Court case (431 U.S. 678 [1977]). In this case, the Court struck down a New York law that put burdens on people who wanted to purchase contraceptives, saying that such restrictions infringed on a protected right. This reasoning has been applied to commercial surrogacy by suggesting that a restriction on the fee is tantamount to a restriction on a protected procreative liberty.

However, one should recognize that there is a significant difference between the issue in *Carey* and that in surrogacy. In *Carey*, what is at stake is the sale of *contraceptives*. In surrogacy, what is at stake is the sale of *children*. Though one has a fundamental right to procreate, nowhere does one have a right to sell the "product" of procreation. Any restriction on the sale of children is legitimate and, according to opponents of surrogacy, the argument from the Carey decision does not apply to surrogacy.

B. Arguments against Surrogate Motherhood

1. *Surrogacy involves the sale of children.* Certainly the most serious objection to commercial surrogacy is that it reduces children to objects of barter by putting a price on them. Most of the arguments in favor of surrogacy are attempts to avoid this problem. Opponents of surrogacy insist that any attempt to deny or minimize the charge of baby-selling fails, and thus surrogacy involves the sale of children. This violates the thirteenth amendment, which outlawed slavery because it constituted the sale of human beings. It violates commonly and widely held moral principles which safeguard human rights and the dignity of human persons, namely that human beings are made in God's image and are His unique creations. Persons are not fundamentally things that can be purchased and sold for a price. The fact that proponents of surrogacy try so hard to get around the charge of baby-selling indicates their acceptance of these moral principles as well. The debate is not whether human beings should be bought and sold. Rather it is over whether commercial surrogacy constitutes such a sale of children. If it does, most would agree that the case against surrogacy is quite strong.

As the New Jersey Supreme Court put it in the Baby M case, "There are, in a civilized society, some things that money cannot buy... There are values... that society deems more important than granting to wealth whatever it can buy, be it labor, love or life" (*In re Baby M.* 537 A. 2d, 1249 [1988]). The sale of children, which normally results from a surrogacy transaction (the only exception being cases of altruistic surrogacy), is inherently problematic, irrespective of the other good consequences that the arrangement produces, in the same way that slavery is inherently troubling, because human beings are not objects for sale.

2. *Surrogacy involves potential for exploitation of the surrogate*. Most agree about the potential for commercial surrogacy to be exploitive. The combination of desperate infertile couples, low-income surrogates, and surrogacy brokers with varying degrees of moral scruples raises the prospect that the entire commercial enterprise can be exploitative. The fee alone should not be considered exploitation but an inducement to do something that the surrogate would not otherwise do. But money functions as an inducement to do many things that people would not normally do without being exploitive.

However, this does not mean that the potential for exploitation should not be taken seriously. Should surrogacy become more socially acceptable and states pass laws making it legal, it is not difficult to imagine the various ways in which surrogacy brokers would attempt to hold costs down in order to maximize profit. One of the most attractive ways in which this could be done would be to recruit surrogate mothers more actively from among the poor in this country and particularly from the third world. For example, some are suggesting that those with financial need actually make the best candidates for surrogates since they are the least inclined to keep the child produced by the arrangement.[12] Others are making plans actively to recruit women from the third world to be brought to the United States to serve as surrogates. The advantage to using these women is that it dramatically reduces the cost involved in a surrogacy arrangement. It is not difficult to see the potential for exploitation of poor women in desperate circumstances, a potential that is already being seriously considered by brokers in the industry.

3. *Surrogacy involves detachment from the child in utero*. One of the most serious objections to surrogacy applies to both commercial and altruistic surrogacy. In screening women to select the most ideal surrogates, one looks for the woman's ability to give up easily the child she is carrying. Normally, the less attached the woman is to the child, the easier it is to complete the arrangement. But this is hardly an ideal setting for a pregnancy. Surrogacy sanctions female detachment from the child in the womb, a situation in any other pregnancy that one would never want. This detachment is something that would be strongly discouraged in a traditional pregnancy, but is strongly encouraged in surrogacy. Should surrogacy be widely practiced, bioethicist Daniel Callahan of the Hastings Center describes what one of the results would be. He states:

> We will be forced to cultivate the services of women with the hardly desirable trait of being willing to gestate and then give up their own children, especially if paid enough to do so... There would still be the need to find women with the capacity to dissociate and distance themselves from their own child. This is not a psychological trait we should want to foster, even in the name of altruism (Callahan, 1987, p. B21).

Surrogacy actually turns a vice, the ability to detach from the child in utero, into a virtue.

4. *Surrogacy violates the right of mothers to associate with their children.* Another serious problem with commercial surrogacy might also apply to altruistic surrogacy. In most surrogacy contracts, whether for a fee or not, the surrogate agrees to relinquish any parental rights to the child she is carrying to the couple who contracted her services. In the Baby M case, the police actually had to break into a home to return Baby M to the contracting couple.[13] A surrogacy contract forces a woman to give up the child she has borne to the couple who has paid her to do so. Should she have second thoughts and desire to keep the child, under the contract she would be forced to give up her child.

Of course, this assumes the traditional definition of a mother. A mother is defined as the woman who gives birth to the child. Society has never had carefully to define motherhood, because medicine has previously not been able to separate the genetic and gestational aspects of motherhood. It is a new phenomenon to have one woman be the genetic contributor and a different woman be the one who carries the child. There is debate over whether genetics or gestation should determine motherhood, but in the majority of cases of surrogacy, the surrogate provides both the genetic material and the womb. By any definition, she is the mother of the child, which courts have generally recognized. To force her to give up her child under the terms of a surrogacy contract violates her fundamental right to associate with and raise her child. This does not mean that she has exclusive right to the child. That must be shared with the natural father, similar to a custody arrangement in a divorce proceeding. But the right of one parent (the natural father) to associate with his child cannot be enforced at the expense of the right of the other (the surrogate).

As a result of this fundamental right, some states that allow a fee to be paid to the surrogate do not allow the contract to be enforced if the surrogate wants to keep the child. Any contract that requires a woman to agree to give up the child she bears prior to birth is not considered a valid contract. This is similar to the way that most states deal with adoptions. Any agreement prior to birth to give up one's child is not binding and can be revoked if the birth mother changes her mind and wants to keep the child. Many states that have passed laws on surrogacy have chosen to use the model of adoption law rather than contract law that essentially says that "a deal's a deal."

V. Conclusion

With technological innovations continuing at a remarkable pace, assisted reproductive technologies will continue to pose great opportunities for infertile couples as well as ethical challenges for those who utilize these technologies and those who reflect on their use. Many of the techniques discussed in this article have become mainstream in the infertility industry in the developed countries. In the rest of the world, access to these expensive technological options is similar to access to other types of advanced medical technologies. While assisted reproductive technologies are not life-sustaining treatments, they provide infertile couples with the means to achieve long-held dreams of having children. For many couples, this is a very important component of their flourishing as human beings.

Ethical issues that remain on the table for discussion revolve around these issues of access. It could be argued that assisted reproductive technologies are unnecessary in parts of the world where overpopulation is a serious problem and other forms of basic medical care are the highest priorities for governments and communities. Other ethical issues include the more novel technologies that are still in experimental stages, such as artificial wombs and procreative human cloning. As new reproductive technologies evolve, the likelihood is high that they will involve ethical issues that need public reflection and resolution.

Notes

1. To be exact, GIFT, ZIFT, and IVF normally involve the genetic materials of husband and wife only, though they can be used with donor genetic materials too. For egg donation to work, one of the above techniques must also be employed.
2. A number of state Supreme Courts have addressed surrogacy, including California (*Johnson v. Calvert*. 114 S. Ct. 206 [1993]) and New Jersey in the well-publicized Baby M case (*In re Baby M*. 537 A. 2d 1227, N.J. [1988]). To date, 14 states have passed laws prohibiting commercial surrogacy and making the contracts void. For a detailed discussion of these state laws and the state of the law internationally, see Scott B. Rae (1994, pp. 146-158).
3. The Vatican's *Instruction on Respect for Human Life in Its Origin and on the Dignity of Procreation (Donum Vitae)* makes it clear that the ideal is that Catholic moral teaching in this area become the law. See Part III, entitled, "Moral and Civil Law: The Values and Moral Obligations that Civil Legislation Must Respect and Sanction In This Matter."
4. See for instance, John Robertson's statement about this and other Supreme Court decisions. He states, "In dicta, however, the Supreme Court on numerous occasions has recognized a married couple's right to procreate in language broad enough to encompass coital and most non-coital forms of reproduction." He then cites the Meyer case as one example (1986, p. 958).
5. Justice Douglas used a graphic illustration in *Griswold* to make this point. "Would we allow the police to search the sacred precincts of marital bedrooms for telltale signs of the use of contraception? The very idea is repulsive to the notions of privacy surrounding the marriage relationship" (*Griswold v. Connecticut*. 381 U.S., at 485-486).
6. Justice Marshall was citing *Cleveland Board of Education v. LaFleur*. 414 U.S. 632 (1974), at 639-640.
7. "It is clear that among the decisions that an individual may make without unjustified government interference are personal decisions relating to marriage (*Loving v. Virginia*. 388 U.S. 1, 12, [1967]), procreation (*Skinner v. Oklahoma*. 316 U.S. 535, 541-542, [1942]), contraception (*Eisenstadt v. Baird*. 405 U.S. 453-454, 460, 463-465), family relationships (*Prince v. Massachusetts*. 321 U.S. 158, 166, [1944]), and child rearing and education (*Pierce v. Society of Sisters*. 268 U.S. 510, 535, [1925]; *Meyer v. Nebraska*. 262 U.S. 390, 399, [1923], *Cary v. Population Services International*. 431 U.S. at 685).
8. This freedom assumes, of course, that parents are acting in the best interests of their children and that no harm comes to children in the exercise of freedom on the part of the parents.
9. This normally applies to adoption. In 25 states it is against the law to pay birth mothers a fee beyond expenses to give up her child for adoption. The state rightly wants to protect birth mothers from being exploited and children from being objects of barter.
10. In cases in which the surrogate does not supply the egg, there is debate over who is actually the mother, the woman who bears the child (the traditional definition), or the genetic contributor. Good arguments can be made for both genetics and gestation being the determinant of motherhood. For further detail on this see Scott B. Rae (1994).
11. This real estate analogy is taken from Alexander M. Capron (1987).
12. Statement of staff psychologist Howard Adelman of Surrogate Mothering Ltd. in Philadelphia, cited in Gena Corea (1985, p. 229).
13. This sounds worse than it may be, since Mary Beth Whitehead had left the area with the child because she wanted so badly to keep her. The police were obeying the dictates of a lower court

decision, which awarded sole custody of the child to the contracting couple. But in any case, they still took the child from the woman who bore her by force. That struck most people as unfortunate if not barbaric.

Bibliography

Callahan, D. 1987. Surrogate motherhood: a bad idea. *New York Times*, 20 January, B21.

Cameron, N.M. De S. 2000. Separating sex and reproduction: the ambiguous triumphs of technology. In: J.F. Kilner, et al. (eds), *The reproduction revolution: a Christian appraisal of sexuality, reproductive technologies and the family* (pp. 27-35). Grand Rapids: Eerdmans.

Capron, A.M. 1987. Surrogate contracts: a danger zone. *Los Angeles Times*, 7 April, B5.

Carey v. Population Services International. 431 U.S. 678 (1977).

Cleveland Board of Education v. LaFleur. 414 U.S. 632 (1974).

Corea, G. 1985. *The mother machine*. New York: Harper and Row.

Eisenstadt v. Baird. 405 U.S. 438 (1972).

Griswold v. Connecticut. 381 U.S. 453 (1965).

In re Baby M. 537 A. 2d 1227, N.J. (1988).

Johnson v. Calvert. 114 S. Ct. 206 (1993).

Loving v. Virginia. 388 U.S. 1 (1967).

Meilander, G. 2000. A child of one's own: at what price? In: J.F. Kilner, et al. (eds), *The reproduction revolution: a Christian appraisal of sexuality, reproductive technologies and the family* (pp. 36-45). Grand Rapids: Eerdmans.

Meyer v. Nebraska. 262 U.S. 390 (1923).

Moore v. City of East Cleveland. 431 U.S. 494 (1977).

Paul VI 1968. *Humanae Vitae*. A.A.S. IX, 481-518 [On-line]. Available: <www.nccbuscc.org/prolife/tdoes/humanaevitae.htm>.

Pierce v. Society of Sisters. 268 U.S. 510 (1925).

Prince v. Massachusetts. 321 U.S. 158 (1944).

Robertson, J. 1986. Embryos, families, and procreative liberty: the legal structure of the new reproduction. *Southern California Law Review* 59(5): 958.

Rae, S. 1994. *The ethics of commercial motherhood: brave new families?* Westport: Praeger Publishing.

Sacred Congregation for the Doctrine of the Faith. 1987. *Donum Vitae* [On-line]. Available: <www.nccbuscc.org/prolife/tdocs/donumvitae.htm>.

Skinner v. Oklahoma. 316 U.S. 535 (1942).

Stanley v. Illinois. 405 U.S. 645 (1972).

3 Conceptual, Normative, and Policy Issues in United States Health Care Allocation

B. Andrew Lustig

I. Introduction[1]

Issues of access to health care, general concerns regarding allocation of health care resources, and more recently, specific arguments about the legitimacy and efficacy of health care rationing have been items central to policy debates during the last fifteen years. Yet, for nearly three decades, in discussions among health care theorists and policy analysts, the basic terms of the debate have remained subject to controversy (Fried, 1975, 1976; Lewis, Fein, & Mechanic, 1976; Outka, 1974). To speak of allocating health care resources, for example, assumes that we can establish priorities among various levels of health care needs; yet, such priorities themselves require and incorporate assumptions about the meaning of health as a general concept. According to the World Health Organization, health should be understood as "a state of complete physical, mental, and social well-being" (Callahan, 1973). If we are inclined to be generous in our judgment, we will interpret that definition as idealistic rather than realistic. That is to say, it expresses our aspirations and may, though only if refined and operationalized, illuminate our policy choices in some general way. But the WHO definition does not apply to the current reality of health care delivery in the United States, or in any other nation for that matter. Moreover, such breadth of definition may well "over-medicalize" some needs which are better addressed, as objects of policy choice, in other than "medical" terms. Obviously, adequate housing and proper nutrition are basic needs, and providing them to all citizens would dramatically influence health outcomes for the better. But for reasons of conceptual clarity and of effective legislative division of labor, we quite properly view housing and nutrition as spheres which are linked with, though separate from, the sphere of "health care" needs, as usually understood.

Some commentators stress that any notion of health defined in terms of normal function or physiological regularities overlooks the social context within which we define illness and disease (Engelhardt, 1981; Kass, 1985). While we tend to think about health and disease in objective terms, these concepts are inevitably value-laden. Therefore, how we describe health and health care *ab initio* sets the terms for policy discussion. For that reason, establishing working definitions for disease, illness, health, or well-being will always be, in crucial ways, a philosophical task; the definitions we offer will be stipulative as well as pejorative. They will indicate not only how people generally use such terms, but also how such terms should be employed.

Nonetheless, for all the lack of conceptual clarity which persist in our understanding of health and disease, and despite the changes in modern medicine, many commentators define medicine as a social practice according to identifiable and traditional objectives – to relieve pain and suffering, to heal from disease when possible, and to restore the individual to some semblance of normal function (Kass, 1985, pp. 157-86). Even those who disagree about how to establish spending priorities within medicine (for example, the priority of preventive over tertiary care) do so from a broadly shared understanding: viz., that certain states or chronic conditions are dysfunctional or ultimately life-threatening (Daniels, 1994, p. 426).

There is something perverse in judging a prosperous society as even minimally decent, much less good, if it shows systematic indifference to the serious medical needs of its citizens. To be sure, ours would not appear to be such a society. Yet, few commentators are happy with the status quo. Consider for example, the usual litany of disturbing facts, as set forth in recent statistics reported by the Health Care Financing Administration. As of 1998, more than 43 million Americans lack health insurance of any kind, with more than a third of the uninsured being children. The uninsured population includes 33% of Hispanics, 21% of African-Americans and Asians, and 11% of non-Hispanic whites (Physicians for a National Health Program, 2001). Moreover, despite the fact that we spend significantly more than any other developed nation, we trail most other nations in the Organization for Economic Co-operation and Development (OECD) on such basic indices as infant mortality and life expectancy. Medicaid, however humane its original vision, is dramatically inadequate in practice, especially with its extreme variations from state to state. Overall, the United States has no bragging rights among developed countries concerning health care delivery or average health care outcomes. According to recent statistics, we spent more than twice as much on health care as the average of other OECD nations, without superior results (Health Care Financing Administration, 2001). Current United States health care delivery, despite the putative efficiencies claimed by the introduction of managed care, remains in disarray, filled with excess in some sectors, while failing to meet the basic medical needs of many indigent as well as the working uninsured.

Thus I begin, impressionistically, by stating the obvious. First, all is not well; indeed, things are far from well with current health care delivery in the United States. Second, only in light of such troubling background features of health care delivery can the urgency of a number of recent proposals for reforming health care be appreciated. Third, the ongoing debate about the legitimacy of health care resource allocation has been quickened by several concerns: the desire to contain costs and provide cost-effective care, the desire to improve the general quality of care delivered, and the wish to expand access to basic care for all who are excluded or marginalized from the current system.

II. Matters of Definition

An initial word is in order about the terms "allocation" and "rationing". "Allocation" has a long pedigree in the literature of public policy. It refers to decisions which determine the amount of resources available for particular kinds of health care services. Examples include how an institution or a nation budgets funds, decisions at the national or regional level with regard to fund tradeoffs between primary and preventive versus curative versus non-medical forms of health care intervention (e.g., environmental spending), and funding choices between medical and other non health-related basic goods. The definition of "rationing" is less clearly defined. For some, rationing means that a person is barred from treatment only by an explicit policy or decision. Others interpret the unavailability of care as rationing, whether or not explicit policies or decisions are involved. A minority of the latter commentators argue that we have sufficient resources to avoid stringent forms of rationing. Most commentators, however, deem rationing as unavoidable. However, rather than maintaining current forms of implicit rationing (most notably, by vagaries of insurance coverage and ability to pay), these commentators favor the development of explicit ethical criteria for a fairer rationing process (Kilner, 1995, pp. 1068-1069).

Recent discussion of health care rationing has identified two issues which are central to the broader discussion of allocation more generally. First, rationing is not equivalent merely to cutting waste or trimming fat in the health care budget. Rather, rationing denotes that we choose not to provide services which are of actual benefit on the grounds that the opportunity costs of such expenditures are excessive when compared with other more effective forms of intervention in pursuit of the designated good or compared with unacceptable funding tradeoffs with other basic social goods and needs. Rationing assumes conditions of finitude – limits upon resources, including the resources of beneficence – and asks us to make coherent societal choices within that context. Assuming limited resources, we will want to get the most for our money, which seems to be a good utilitarian instinct on our part. Yet, such judgments are problematic: we need to know what we mean by and how to measure the *most*. Are we talking about the number of years of life saved, the quality of life after medical interventions, or the sorts of interventions that best contribute to improving overall health outcomes among the general population? It seems a truism among critics, for example, that our present spending priorities are seriously askew. We spend the bulk of our health care dollars on critical interventions rather than on preventive and maintenance care. Big-ticket technologies drive our system to misallocate funds. We devote a great deal to cancer care but far less on environmental medicine. We lavish large amounts on coronary bypasses but paltry sums on screening for hypertension. We spend more than 1% of our gross domestic product on intensive care units, often inappropriately, but have yet to fund effectively long-term and nursing care. We spend disproportionately for neonatal intensive care, but relatively modest sums on prenatal care for indigent mothers. To say, then, that rationing health care resources involves getting the most for our money is hardly a simple calculation. It involves questions of what we mean by quality of care, at what price, and for whom. It is, to be sure, a matter of hard-headed judgment, but only partially. Indeed, what makes rationing troubling within reform proposals is the uncertainty about the values we should invoke to set our health care priorities. Quality of care, cost constraints, and issues of access are three core aspects of allocation debates, and all of them have normative as well as technical dimensions.

III. The Normative Bases of Health Care Delivery

When we consider the moral justification for health care allocation, perhaps the most fundamental matter to address is our society's understanding of what is at stake in restricting access to health care. Some, though clearly now a minority, still consider access to health care to be a matter of privilege. For them, the specter of uninsured Americans going without medical care may be an unfortunate fact of life, like many other unfortunate facts, but not on the face of it unfair. Charity, rather than justice, emerges as the issue here. We may come to the aid of the medically indigent out of our individual or institutional largesse, but that emerges as a response of compassion, not a requirement of justice.

In the good old days, to be sure, the tradition of charity care was a strong one. As the maxim prescribed, charity began at home, and charity underlay a good deal of hospital care when people were too sick to stay at home tended by family but too poor to pay for hospital services. In addition, in an age when medicine was far less sophisticated and, therefore, less able to address many health care needs which today are easily solved, charity care was also a great deal less expensive.

Those good old days (if they ever were that) are gone. With the passage of Medicare and Medicaid, and with the current reality of third-party payers, yesterday's rhetoric of charity moves closer to a claim of justice. More precisely stated, we occupy that overlapping theoretical terrain between the claims of charity and justice. The idea of charity sufficing to meet the health care needs of the indigent and working uninsured is both dubious and anachronistic. It harks back to a simpler time when medicine was far less expensive and far less effective. Moreover, nowadays we have a much more sophisticated profile of who the medically indigent are. In the face of their identified needs – for example prenatal coverage, regular preventive services, and critical care – the discretion we tend to associate with acts of charity seems less appropriate. We move closer to a judgment that certain health care needs must be met, that the actions of individual physicians, however nobly inspired, cannot address the magnitude of the problem, and that a good, or even minimally decent society, should systematically address the most urgent health care needs of its citizens, to the degree that its resources allow, and in keeping with meeting a range of basic needs, among which health care has a central, but not sole, place.

Given this widely shared intuition that something closer to justice than to charity is at stake in health care delivery, many have concluded that individual rights are involved – that everyone has a right to medical care, and that, in failing to have their needs met, persons' moral claims against society are infringed or denied. As has been widely observed, we are very fond of rights language in our current culture. In our litigious society, to label something "a right" is to establish its importance as a matter of definition. Nonetheless, in a media age, when people are prone to proclaim rights to virtually anything under the sun, the vocabulary of rights in relation to health care should be viewed with some skepticism. Claims, after all, are easy to make; determining their legitimacy and scope is far more difficult. Even if a right is at stake in health care delivery, it is a positive right, a claim to assistance from other individuals or institutions. Positive rights are always context-dependent. I cannot demand anything and everything from others. Obviously, my demand will be relative to my needs. Even in a wealthy society, we cannot meet the full health care needs of everyone. Whether we say, therefore, that all citizens have a right to health care (Childress, 1984) or, alternatively, that society has an obligation to provide health care (President's Commission, 1983), the hard questions still remain. What sort of health care is claimed as a right or owed by society at large? Essential health care? A decent minimum of health care? Such terms are difficult to define. They involve macro-allocation choices: how much we will spend to provide medical care vis-à-vis provision for other basic needs. They also involve micro-allocation choices: within medical care, what funds are marked for preventive versus critical care or, within critical care, for particular services and technologies?

And then, perhaps the hardest issue of all, how will we choose among patients when resources are scarce and not all can be helped?

We seek, then, to specify the nature and to limit the scope of the notion of health care as an individual right or a societal obligation. We must, first, place the claim in context, to make sense of that as it has been discussed in the academic and policy literature and, second, understand what is at stake when we speak about allocating health care resources. If medical care is a right, how is it to be allocated and does the idea of allocating rights make sense? On the other hand, if health care is something less than a right, why do we find the discussion of allocation and rationing so difficult and painful?

IV. Five Characteristic Approaches to Justice and Health Care

In the ethics and policy literature of recent years, five different interpretations of what justice requires concerning medical care have been offered, each with a label of its own: an entitlements perspective, a utilitarian calculus, a maximin theory, an egalitarian perspective, and what has been labeled a "decent minimum" approach. In fairly brief compass, I will review representative statements of these positions, list substantive criticisms directed at each, and suggest a synthetic position that may help to clarify what is at stake in the allocation debate.

A. Entitlements

The word, "entitlement", is associated in recent justice theory with the work of Robert Nozick. According to Nozick, most allocation schemes actually redistribute assets which individuals already own without taking account of the way in which such assets have been acquired and transferred – that is, most tax redistributions, to fund health care or any other need, fail to take seriously the idea that individuals are entitled to their personal holdings, when these have been justly acquired and transferred (Nozick, 1974, pp. 225-226).

Nozick's entitlement theory has specific implications for health care provision. Essentially, he argues for a market model of health care delivery. Physicians should be free, he argues, to contract with individual patients for their services and medical consumers should be free to purchase health care directly or by insurance. For Nozick, distribution based on any other principles, including notions of individual rights or social duties, inevitably violates the prior rights of medical providers and consumers. In considering the physician, then, Nozick poses the following question: "Just because he has this skill, why should *he* bear the costs of the desired allocation, why is he lessened title to pursue his goals, within the special circumstances of medicine, than everyone else?" (Nozick, 1974, p. 234, emphasis in the original).

The central criticism of Nozick's perspective is that, with very little by way of argument, he proposes the market as an adequate model for health care delivery. Medical needs, however, are noticeably different from other needs met through market mechanisms. Neither in theory nor in practice is there a free flow of information between medical providers and medical consumers. There are also significant restrictions on the distribution of health care resources, such as entry barriers to the health care professions, licensing requirements, and so forth. Finally, Nozick's contention that doctors and consumers are independent contractors for health care services totally overlooks the significant social resources expended on the training of physicians.

B. Utilitarian Calculus

A utilitarian approach tries to apply the maxim "do the greatest good for the greatest number" to health care delivery with a hard-headedness which seems appropriate in an era characterized by renewed medical inflation. For example, Tom Beauchamp and Ruth Faden recommend that we determine the scope of the right to health care through "cost benefit analysis constrained by a decent minimum criterion" (Beauchamp & Faden, 1979, pp. 127-128). As a society, we should therefore assess the opportunity costs of various types of health care and particular services within discrete categories. Beauchamp and Faden express confidence that such comprehensive and ongoing assessment is a realizable policy goal.

Their utilitarianism has much to recommend it. If we commit ourselves to providing a decent minimum of health care for individuals, we must be willing to operationalize the meaning of that decent minimum at the policy level. If we are to allocate health care resources in a fair and equitable manner, we must adopt the sort of structured overview that cost-benefit and cost-effectiveness analyses entail. Yet, cautions are also in order here. Utilitarianism has a nuts-and-bolts character that is often very appealing to decision makers, but it fails to provide a firm foundation for the notion of an individual entitlement to medical care. Judgments about social utility and justifications of individual rights are, after all, quite separate matters. There is no obvious way that increasing utility generates a right. Although Beauchamp and Faden speak of cost-benefit analysis "constrained by" a decent minimum criterion, it is unclear that appealing to social utility can, of itself, safeguard a decent minimum of medical care as an individual entitlement.

C. Maximin Theory

A third perspective draws on the spirit, if not the letter, of John Rawls's theory of justice. Norman Daniels offers a recent example of the attempt to apply Rawls's framework to health care (Daniels, 1985, 1988, 1994). Daniels's central question is this: How should we pattern just distributions of health care resources among individuals of different ages? In response, he develops what he calls the "prudential life-span account." This model asks us to consider how we would allocate social goods, if we considered age groups not as classes of distinct individual but rather as stages of our own lives, i.e., a self-interested procedure for identifying our duties to others.

If successful, Daniels's prudential life-span account goes a long theoretical way toward resolving issues of apparent conflict between generations – the young and the middle aged verses the elderly. Rather than viewing age-based entitlement programs as transferring benefits from younger to older persons, Daniels suggests that such programs should be reconceptualized as "savings" schemes which allow prudent allocation of resources for different stages of the representative individual's life. On his account, rationing can be viewed as a form of prudence rather than as a choice between persons – assuming that one can generalize about the way in which health care funds are likely to be spent over the course of a "typical" individual's lifetime.

Nonetheless, Daniels's approach can be criticized on two grounds. First, he fails to deal with issues of equity which arise between and among individuals within the same age group. One may be unable to generalize easily about the "average" of care needs and allotments due individuals because of the different health needs of persons within particular birth cohorts. Moreover, as Daniels admits, his is an ideal theory: the range of justifiable compromise with real world variations remains unclear. Yet, in the give-and-take of debates about allocation, access, and rationing, the non-ideal nature of real world circumstances may render Daniels's framework unworkable.

D. Egalitarianism

Other commentators have offered egalitarian arguments for a right to health care (Outka, 1974; Veatch, 1981). Gene Outka views health care needs as discontinuous from other basic needs (Outka, 1974). Medical needs are randomly distributed, to a large degree "unmerited," often catastrophic, and to a great extent unpredictable. Outka, therefore, views critical health care emergencies as having an immediacy and urgency different from other sorts of deprivation. However, in situations where allocation is required, Outka allows exclusions by disease category. The exclusion comports with his egalitarian perspective: he would exclude all members of a given disease category, rather than allowing ability to pay to determine who receives treatment. In effect, Outka would "out-ration" the rationers, because medical need would be the sole criterion for receiving treatment. In certain hard cases, all stricken individuals, rich and poor alike, would therefore be denied treatment.

Stalwart libertarians, of course, object that any curtailing of an individual's options to purchased desired treatment, regardless of the excluded poor, is a violation of liberty. Moreover, an egalitarian approach fails to consider the possible desirability of certain competitive inequalities among provider arrangements which may actually contribute to better overall health care delivery. Moreover, economies of scale may, over time, improve the general quality of health care by extending benefits initially too costly to be available to all.

E. "Decent Minimum"

Finally, Charles Fried argues for what he terms a "decent minimum" approach to health care delivery (Fried, 1975, 1976). Fried's perspective combines Nozick's entitlements emphasis upon personal liberty with Outka's stress on equality. According to Fried, all persons, regardless of their ability to pay, have a right of access to a decent minimum of health care. But, as with other basic goods, persons with greater resources should be free, as they are now, to purchase additional coverage for medical care. Fried's approach differs from egalitarianism. A guarantee of equal access for all to all available services, after all, does not of itself entitle the individual to a decent minimum. Equal access to inadequate services might only guarantee that misery loves company by providing an indecent minimum for all. By contrast, Charles Fried's emphasis on decent minimum assumes that a substantive baseline of medical care can be determined by public discussion and political decision-making.

Although the language of a "right" to health care poses difficulties unless carefully circumscribed, that notion captures, I believe, the emerging sense in our society that some *decent* minimum of medical care is indeed an entitlement of citizens, i.e., that Fried's claim is correct. But a decent *minimum* also expresses necessary limits upon that entitlement and, within such constraints, implies that allocation and, indeed, rationing may be ethically acceptable. Much will depend, of course, on the values that inform the setting of priorities between and among medical services which are the focus of allocation.

A fair allocation process must assume, within the context of limited medical resources, that individuals are entitled to equal consideration. This requires that allocation embodies fairness: treating persons as equals while knowing full well that, in the context of choices to be made at the macro- and micro- levels, equal respect need not imply equal treatment. Treatment as moral equals entails procedural equality, but it need not generate equal substantive results. By definition, allocating resources means that some persons with high-priority medical needs will be covered for treatment, while others with lower priority needs may not be.

In his arguments for the decent minimum approach, Fried underscores what emerges as the central point if allocation decisions are to approximate an ideal of fairness – namely, that the process of defining the decent minimum or, in the context of limited resources, the process of "rational rationing" – is an inherently political one. Thus, to ration rationally – to treat persons fairly – requires that we attend to the procedural values which make democratic policy-making possible and meaningful. Only through a fair political process will we ensure that the unequal substantive results of allocation do not express indifference to or disdain for persons who may be excluded from coverage.

V. The Legitimacy of Two (or more) Tiers of Health Care Delivery: "Rational Rationing": The Oregon Medicaid Example

In 1989, the Oregon State legislature passed the Oregon Basic Health Services Act. The Act established a Health Services Commission, which was charged to develop a priority list of health services, ranging from the most important to the least important for the entire Medicaid population. The purpose of the act was to permit expansion of Medicaid coverage to all Oregonians up to 100% of the federal poverty level, and to do so by covering only those services judged to be of sufficient importance or priority. In effect, rather than providing more extensive medical coverage for only some Medicaid recipients, Oregon chose to provide rationed medical services to *every* qualified Medicaid recipient, as measured by the federal poverty standard.

Recent versions of the Oregon list ranks about 700 medical procedures according to their effectiveness. Depending on how many procedures can be financed from the Medicaid budget annually, the state will draw a line – paying for every procedure above the line but none below it. Initially, Oregon agreed to underwrite the first 568 procedures, thereby excluding, for example, treatment of common colds and infectious mononucleosis.

A number of important features to the Oregon proposal require attention. First, the Oregon Basic Health Services Act of 1989 was proposed not as a rationing effort targeted solely at Medicaid recipients, but as the beginning of a process that would, if successful, establish a unified system of setting health care priorities that would eventually cover the vast majority of Oregon's citizens. The Act also was meant to establish statewide managed care through prepaid plans and other mechanisms designed to contain costs while ensuring access to and coordination of care. A second Senate bill, the State Health Risk Pool Act, was to be aimed at establishing a Medicaid insurance pool program for "medical uninsurables," that is, persons who do not qualify for Medicaid or who do not now qualify for coverage because of preexisting conditions. The Act set out the ways that state and private insurers were to subsidize the pool. To date, however, this second bill has never passed the Oregon legislature. Finally, the proposed Health Insurance Partnership Act mandated that four years after the implementation of the Basic Health Services Act, employers were to provide health benefits to be purchased through the state insurance pool. The package offered by employers was to provide coverage equal to or greater than that provided in the Medicaid benefits package. Any employer who failed to provide insurance to all permanent employees and their dependents by a specified date was to be taxed at a rate which would approximate what would otherwise be the employer's contribution toward health insurance. To date, however, this third bill has also failed to be passed by the Oregon legislature.

Some may believe that limiting medical services for the Medicaid population, while allowing those with adequate insurance or private wealth to receive medical treatment denied the indigent, is socially and morally unacceptable. To understand, however, why it may not be unfair to deny hip replacements or infertility treatments to the poor while allowing them to the rich, one need only take seriously the distinction between private and public dollars, and to appreciate that communal resources, unlike private funds, remain properly at the disposal of the community. Given a utopia of unlimited resources, of course, no hard decisions or tragic choices need ever be made. But short of utopia, the United States seems currently disposed to maintain a two- (or more) tiered system of health care delivery. However much some may argue for a single-tiered system, there apparently are factors unique to the United States experience and national psyche which make a single-tiered system of coverage for all highly unlikely. At the same time, the Oregon example also exemplifies certain problems which may face us as we try to allocate health care resources in a fair and principled fashion. In a pluralistic society, we cannot determine or defend a univocal ranking of social goods, therefore, we are inevitably left to define justice in procedural terms. Politics is not only the art of the possible; it is also, if properly pursued, the collective version of *phronesis*, or practical wisdom. The politics of allocation must emphasize a fair and open process if we are to brace the conclusions or deliberations as ethically and socially acceptable.

Given the desideratum of procedural fairness, there is some evidence that Oregon's legislative decision-making has been flawed from the first. To be sure, Oregon's legislative efforts, beginning in 1987, followed several years of the Oregon Health Decisions Project, a grassroots effort of town hall meetings and reports concerning the future of Oregon's health care. These meetings, involving more than 5,000 participants, may have served well, in many respects, as a model for other states concerned with the same issues. Some commentators, however, have criticized the limited presence and role of actual representatives of the Medicaid community in Oregon's efforts to set priorities (Children's Defense Fund, 1990). If this criticism is even partially borne out, there is an obvious lesson to learn from Oregon's pilot project: we must make greater efforts to include the actual voices of the poor in our common deliberations, rather than assuming that bureaucrats or others, no matter how well intentioned, speak accurately for their interests.

Moreover, there are substantive criticisms of the Oregon experience which call into question the idea of targeting particular groups such as the Medicaid population. Oregon's plan was touted as the first step toward more systematic reform of health care delivery, in that it would concretely specify for the Medicaid population the basket of medical services which comprise adequate basic care. Rather than rhetoric, the scope of the entitlement was specified. Every poor person, and ultimately those who, while not poor, are uninsured or underinsured, would be able to claim a meaningful entitlement. However, as noted above, to date Oregon's allocation efforts have been limited to the Medicaid population. Thus, Oregon rationing remains targeted at the Medicaid population, with little in the way of extending the same basic benefits to the non-Medicaid medically indigent and without the "better off," especially the business community, assuming their share of the burdens and extending coverage to employees. Had the Basic Health Benefits Act actually led to passage of the other two bills, the extension of priority setting beyond the Medicaid population would have done much, as a comprehensive strategy, to improve the lot of all who would gain access, finally, to a meaningful entitlement to basic care. But the record of the past fourteen years suggests otherwise. Hence the debate continues as to whether limiting hard allocation to particular target populations, such as the Medicaid population in Oregon, meets the requirements of providing a fair distribution of burdens that is just to all citizens.

Still, if allocation or rationing is to be done fairly, Oregon's fledgling efforts, however limited, may yet indicate the appropriate directions for ongoing societal discussion, because Oregon's efforts are concentrated on the three fundamental goals of allocation listed above: the development of effective strategies for cost containment, careful attention to quality of care issues, and increased access to basic health care for those persons currently underserved or excluded. In the context of limited resources, considerations of equity will support extending basic medical care to greater numbers of people, even if some smaller number may be denied coverage, so long as such judgments can be applied fairly to all members of a given medical cohort. An effective system of rationing will make tradeoffs based upon an accurate measurement of the cost-effectiveness of comparable forms of therapy. In turn, judgments of cost-effectiveness will be based on careful measurements of the quality of particular modalities of care. If rationing is to be the core feature of future policy decisions, we will need an ongoing and broad-based public discussion of the technical and the normative aspects of health care delivery, to assure that difficult, perhaps even tragic, choices can be made in a fair way.

VI. The Clinton Plan and Its Demise: Implications for Reform

In 1993, the Clinton administration proposed a major restructuring of health care delivery in the United States. In a process which occurred rapidly and with little public accountability or input, the administration developed a lengthy legislative proposal and presented it to the 103rd Congress as the "Health Security Act" in November of that year. The act, which was subjected to major criticisms from both Congressional opponents and lobbies for the health insurance industry, was never passed.

In light of the plan's subsequent defeat, it is useful to rehearse the reasons, both theoretical and practical, for its demise. In both its broad outlines and its intricate details, the Health Security Act provoked significant debate, one which casts into stark relief the deeply entrenched conflicting views about both the nature of the problems facing us in health care delivery and the values to be accorded priority in developing consensus policy solutions.

The problems the Health Security Act sought to address were the spiraling costs of health care services (primarily medical services) and the lack of access for many persons, including both those who have no health insurance and those who are underinsured for the sorts of medical care they require. While the Clinton proposal focused on both values, the primary reality it engaged was health care inflation. Central to the Clinton Task Force's judgment was the recognition of "market failures" in the context of health care delivery. According to one analyst, six such failures were deemed especially problematic (Rainbolt, 1995, pp. 91-96). First, the way in which health insurance is currently configured: after deductibles, such insurance is insufficiently sensitive to the costs of particular options. Second, in the then extant fee-for-service models of delivery, increased provider revenues were tied to maximizing available services and procedures. Third, there are "asymmetries of knowledge" between health care provider and consumer, whereby the obvious differential in knowledge between physician and patient can generate physician-induced demand. Fourth, there are tax subsidies for health insurance, whereby companies that offer health insurance are allowed deductions, while the value of the insurance to employees is not treated as taxable income. Fifth, the high costs of health care administration. (For example, private insurers in the United States spend nearly 12% of their costs on administration, while public insurers such as Medicare and Medicaid spend only 3.2% on administrative overhead.) Sixth, the presence of what has been called "the physician cartel." That phrase suggests that physicians, as a professional group, control the supply of doctors and often work politically to restrict the availability of alternative practitioners that have been shown to restrain the rising costs of care. Until quite recently with the dramatic extension of managed care mechanisms, physicians had "an economic incentive to preserve the [status quo] because another name for 'cutting costs' is cutting 'provider income'" (Rainbolt, 1995, p. 95).

Reactions to the Health Security Act were often the results of ideological posturing rather than careful analysis. Even those disposed to be skeptical of the top-down restructuring of health care through purchasing cooperatives with national standards imposed did acknowledge certain desirable features of the reform proposal. First, they noted its commitment to the idea of universal coverage. Indeed, fully seven years after the defeat of the Clinton proposal, the continuing lack of health care insurance for nearly 43 million Americans remains a very troubling and unresolved feature of health care delivery in the United States. Other reforms proposed in the Health Security Act were also generally seen as desirable by most commentators, regardless of their support of or opposition to full implementation of the Health Security Act. Such favorably judged reforms include the elimination of preexisting condition clauses in insurance coverage, recommendations for reducing administrative overhead and unnecessary duplication of paperwork and billing across different plans, greater transparency of information regarding the quality of services by different providers, especially with regard to outcome data, and some efforts toward tort reform (Zelman, 1994).

At the same time, significant criticisms have been lodged against the Health Security Act. In a perceptive analysis, Gail Wilensky probes five general areas of concern raised by the *range* of recommended benefits called for in the plan and the financing mechanisms recommended for achieving universal coverage. First, Wilensky notes that the Health Security Act, while promising to move toward universal coverage by increasing the overall efficiency of the system, at the same time was recommending major new benefits – especially to early retirees and the underinsured – which were unlikely to be funded merely by economies of scale introduced by purchasing cooperatives or by reductions in inefficiencies across plans. As a result, such increased benefits were likely to lead to significant tax increases in an era when general public confidence in broad governmental solutions remains mixed. Second, Wilensky concluded that the Health Security Act's support of market-based strategies was largely rhetorical, since a central feature of the plan is its reliance on centralized regulatory mechanisms for controlling spending, especially the use of global budgets and price controls. Like many fiscal conservatives, Wilensky adduces evidence that such a "mixed market" model would be both less efficient in the short term and unlikely to increase coverage without major reductions in the quality of overall services in the longer term. The third concern, which Wilensky finds the "most serious issue," is that of employer mandates. The Health Security Act called on employers to finance "80 percent of the average price of the health care plan in their region" and for employees "to purchase a plan and pay the difference" (Wilensky, 1994, p. 182). Wilensky challenges the idea that purchasing cooperatives (not yet formed) would adequately replace the increasing activity of employers in market-based negotiations of coverage and prices; this criticism is a practical expression of her second concern about centralized interference in the activities of the market. The Clinton plan, in order to limit the impact of mandated insurance on smaller businesses, recommended that subsidies be extended to low-wage small businesses in order to limit projected job loss from the injunction of required coverage. Wilensky and others conclude that such subsidies would have further distorted market forces in two ways which undercut the Clinton plan's rhetorical allegiance to market mechanisms: first, because such requirements will lead to job losses and, second, that mid-size companies will seek to downsize in order to take maximum advantage of the progressively higher subsidies available to smaller employers (Wilensky, 1994, p. 182).

Beyond the complexity and centralization of the proposal in its particulars, there were more fundamental problems with the process of deliberation that resulted in the plan. Daniel Yankelovich notes the lack of realism which characterized the attitudes of the general public, especially in its misunderstanding of the core factors responsible for health care inflation and in its unwillingness to address the necessity of hard choices and tradeoffs. Given those attitudes, Yankelovich criticizes the Clinton process of deliberation as a failure of leadership: "The Clinton administration, for its part, failed to disabuse the public of the notion that the no-free-lunch law of economics had not miraculously been suspended for health reform" (Yankelovich, 1995, p. 16). The core features of that failure of public education concerned three fundamental issues. First, how shall we reform the health care system in ways that retain (and even improve) health care benefits for those who are currently covered, which extends access to health care to those who currently lack access to basic care and simultaneously controls costs? Second, how do we control costs without rationing high-technology medicine, which remains the largest factor in driving health care inflation? Third, how do we, as a society, confront the tradeoffs to be made between reducing costs and "doing everything possible to save lives" (Yankelovich, 1995, p. 19)?

More broadly, the lack of sustained public deliberation about the Clinton plan reflects the fundamental tension between the different normative priorities at work in discussions of health care reform. As George Khushf notes, the language of liberty – as reflected in the emphasis by opponents of the Clinton plan about retaining choice of doctors – works against the claims for equality of access (Khushf, 1994). While a close reading of the Clinton plan suggests that both values might have been accommodated through political compromise, the political will to identify commonalities was lacking.

VII. Conclusion: Lessons Learned for the Future

It is difficult to predict the future of theoretical and policy discussions of health care reform in general and allocation issues in particular. In the wake of the failure of the Clinton proposal, however, a number of general lessons, tentatively offered, may suggest the likelihood of certain "trends" to that ongoing debate and discussion.

A. The Need for Sustained and Broad-Ranging Debate

There is obvious need for sustained public debate about health care reform, including the need for explicit tradeoffs and the rationing of resources. Polling data clearly show that debates about health care reform suffer from a pervasive lack of realism (Yankelovich, 1995, p. 14). Health care consumers fail to appreciate the three core factors that drive medical inflation: shifting demographics to an older population, high technology medical advances, and a "payment system that systematically hides the costs of health care from consumers" (Yankelovich, 1995, p. 16). Their lack of realism, in turn, leads the general public to blame the health care system itself, attributing medical inflation to "waste, fraud, greed, and inefficiency" (Yankelovich, 1995, p. 16). This widespread belief puts the general public at odds with the majority of expert opinion.

In addition, there are quite different general social and economic judgments at work among various groups of U.S. citizens. A recent unpublished survey reveals the characteristic values among different socio-economic groups in the United States with reference to health care reform. Three groups were surveyed: the well-educated affluent, those with high school educations, and the poor and less well-educated. The well-educated affluent express verbal support for universal health care coverage but reject increased taxes to pay for it. Those with high school educations express concern about the costs of health care, but judge the current health system to be "controlled by elitists" and resent the poor who receive Medicaid coverage. The less well-educated poor place high value on universal health care coverage (O'Connell, 1994, p. 421). The differences among the groups are unlikely to be bridged without careful attention to the pervasive underlying attitudes, some of which may be ideologically based, which are brought to assessments of health care reform.

B. An Incremental Approach

Incrementalism appears as the strategy likely to be adopted in future efforts to honor the three core values at stake in health care reform and rationing: maintaining or enhancing the quality of medical care, increasing access to basic care for the uninsured and underinsured, and controlling spiraling health care costs. Polling data suggest that the general public, in contrast to attitudes expressed in 1992-1993, no longer support comprehensive approaches to health care reform but do support more modest plans which do not increase governmental control of the health care system. For example, the Health Insurance Portability and Accountability Act, passed in 1996, protects health insurance coverage for workers and their families when they change or lose their jobs. In addition, recent efforts to extend health care coverage for children are widely supported.

C. The Need for Rational Rationing

Virtually all serious commentators – ranging from those who espouse universal coverage according to single-payer mechanisms to those who prefer enhancing current market-based mechanisms – acknowledge the need to face hard choices, including forms of explicit rationing, as core features of health care reform. Moreover, most commentators identify prevalent U.S. attitudes about health care reform as based on a false ideology – that all citizens can receive the best of care, while retaining their choice of health care provider, and without runaway costs. For most critics, the Clinton plan was dishonest in failing to acknowledge explicitly the costs, tradeoffs, and alternatives to be considered. In fact, core features of the Clinton plan, such as global budgets and "certification of need" strategies, did entail implicit rationing. For reasons of political expediency, however, the Clinton administration failed to acknowledge those features as crucial to the plan's implementation. In the future, most commentators emphasize the importance of open deliberation about such tradeoffs. As Leonard Fleck observes, "A just and caring society must make rationing decisions publicly, painful as that may be, in order to protect the fairness of those decisions" (Fleck, 1994, p. 442).

D. Determining the Appropriate Mix of Public and Private

The Public Agenda and Kettering Foundations have identified three major dilemmas of health care reform: (1) How shall we retain (and improve) the health care benefits of those who now have them, extend some of these benefits to those who now lack them, and at the same time keep public costs under control? (2) How shall we curb the growth of health care costs and at the same time continue to enjoy the benefits of state-of-the-art, high-technology medicine? (3) How do we address the conflict between reducing costs and doing everything possible to save lives? (Cited in Yankelovich, 1995, p. 19).

In each instance, the practical focus of the debate reflects differences in the way in which health care is understood (as a public or a private good), differences in expectations about the appropriate role of the public and private sectors, and differences in the normative emphases upon liberty and equality as first principles. Recently, we have seen a dramatic increase in the mechanisms of managed care, which have engaged issues of cost control, though with mixed results. Supporters of managed care insist that, in the context of incrementalism, market solutions may be appropriate in health care as with other basic goods (Patricelli, 1994; Glaudemans, 1994; Greaves, 1994; Lane, 1994; Roper, 1994).[2] At the same time, the American public overwhelmingly perceives lack of access to medical care to be an unfair denial of a "basic right" of citizens (Yankelovich, 1995, p. 12). How to bridge these differences in public perception – differences that are both philosophical and practical – remains the core challenge in future deliberations about health care reform and rationing. After all, controlling costs should, in principle, help to fund increased access to services. And extending access should, in principle, be discussed in the context of explicit allocation criteria, in order to extend benefits responsibly. To date, however, neither private nor public insurers have sufficiently engaged the hard choices which will be required to extend access in cost-conscious fashion.

Notes

1. The first three sections of this chapter rely heavily on my earlier discussion of the same issues (Lustig, 1994).
2. According to one commentator, "a free market is valuable because it allows people to make their own choices regarding how cost-beneficial certain goods are; it registers true costs, and thus avoids hiding or shifting the burden of decisions; it enables society to calculate the actual costs of providing health insurance to the poor and allows for a fair distribution of that care, rather than cost shifting to those privately insured individuals who are ill; it works in a decentralized way and thus does not require the massive collection and dissemination of information needed in a command and control approach; and it rewards individuals for their contribution by direct financial remuneration. In sum, a free market advances truth and justice" (Khushf, 1994, p. 402), summarizing the argument of Robert Moffit (1994).

Bibliography

Beauchamp, T. & Faden, R. 1979. The right to health and the right to health care. *The Journal of Medicine and Philosophy* 4(2): 118-131.

Callahan, D. 1973. The WHO definition of health. *The Hastings Center Studies* 1: 77-88.

Children's Defense Fund. 1990. *An analysis of the impact of the Oregon Medicaid reduction waiver proposal on women and children*. Washington D.C.: Children's Defense Fund.

Childress, J. 1984. Rights to health care in a democratic society. In: J. Humber & R. Almeder (eds), *Biomedical ethics reviews 1984* (pp. 47-70). Clifton, NJ: Humana Press.

Daniels, N. 1985. *Just health care*. New York: Cambridge University Press.

Daniels, N. 1988. *Am I my parents' keeper?* New York: Oxford University Press.

Daniels, N. 1994. The articulation of values and principles involved in health care reform. *The Journal of Medicine and Philosophy* 19(5): 425-433.

Engelhardt, H.T. 1981. Health care allocations: responses to the unjust, the unfortunate, and the undesirable. In: E. Shelp (ed.), *Justice and health care* (pp. 121-137). Boston: D. Reidel Publishing Company.

Engelhardt, H.T. 1994. Health care reform: a study in moral malfeasance. *The Journal of Medicine and Philosophy* 19(5): 501-516.

Fleck, L. 1994. Just caring: health reform and health care rationing. *The Journal of Medicine and Philosophy* 19(5): 435-443.

Fried, C. 1975. Rights and health care – beyond equity and efficiency. *New England Journal of Medicine* 293(5): 241-245.

Fried, C. 1976. Equality and rights in medical care. *Hastings Center Report* 6: 29-34.

Glaudemans, J. 1994. The case for local budgeting. *Health Affairs* 13(1): 243-246.

Greaves, R. 1994. Concerns of an HMO executive. *Health Affairs* 13(1): 247-248.

Health Care Financing Administration. 2001. Health care statistics. Washington, D.C. Available online: <www.hcfa.gov/stats>.

Health Security Act: 1993, 103 Congress, 1st Session. Washington, D.C.: U.S. Government Printing Office.

Kass, L. 1985. *Toward a more natural science: biology and human affairs*. New York: The Free Press.

Khushf, G. 1994. Ethics, politics, and health care reform. *The Journal of Medicine and Philosophy* 19(5): 397-405.

Kilner, J. 1995. Health-care resources, allocation of. In: W. Reich (ed.), *Encyclopedia of Bioethics* (revised ed.), *volume two* (pp. 1967-1084). New York: Simon and Schuster Macmillan.

Lane, J. 1994. A workable framework for health reform. *Health Affairs* 13(1): 248-250.

Lewis, C., Fein, R. & Mechanic, D. 1976. *The right to health*. New York: John Wiley & Sons.

Lustig, B.A. 1994. Needy persons and rationed resources. In: C.S. Campbell and B.A. Lustig (eds), *Duties to others* (pp. 217-233). Dordrecht: Kluwer Academic Publishers.

Moffit, R. 1994. Personal freedom and responsibility: the ethical foundations of a market-based health care reform. *The Journal of Medicine and Philosophy* 19(5): 471-481.

Nozick, R. 1974. *Anarchy, state, and utopia*. New York: Basic Books.

O'Connell, L. 1994. Ethicists and health care reform: an indecent proposal? *The Journal of Medicine and Philosophy* 19(5): 419-424.

Outka, G. 1974. Social justice and equal access to health care. *The Journal of Religious Ethics* 2: 11-32.

Patricelli, R. 1994. Why do we need health alliances? *Health Affairs* 13(1): 241-242.

Physicians for a National Health Program. 2001. Proposal of the physicians working group for single-payer national health insurance. Chicago. Available online: <www:pnhp.org>.

President's Commission for the Study of Ethical Problems in Medicine and Biomedical and Behavioral Research. 1983. *Securing access to health care*. Washington D.C.: U.S. Government Printing Office

Rainbolt, G. 1995. An evaluation of Clinton's health care proposal. In: J. Humber & R. Almeder (eds), *Allocating Health Care Resources* (pp. 85-120). Totowa, NJ: Humana Press.

Roper, W. 1994. Quality measurement and improvement. *Health Affairs* 13(1): 250-251.

Veatch, R. 1981. *A theory of medical ethics*. New York: Basic Books.

Wilensky, G. 1994. Health reform: what will it take to pass? *Health Affairs* 13(1): 179-191.

Yankelovich, D. 1995. The debate that wasn't: the public and the Clinton plan, *Health Affairs* 14(1): 7-23.

Zelman, W. 1994. The rationale behind the Clinton plan. *Health Affairs* 13(1): 9-29.

4 Ethics Committees and Consultation in the United States

Brendan P. Minogue

The Joint Commission on Accreditation of Health Care Organizations is the national agency that grants accreditation for hospitals and other health care institutions in the United States. Since January of 1992, this accrediting agency has required that hospitals and other health care organizations establish institutional ethics committees, which address questions concerning patients' rights and organizational ethics. This requirement reflects in a formal way what has been taking place within hospitals throughout the United States for the past forty years, since the dawn of the modern bioethics movement. Hospital ethics committees have already become commonplace within the United States and are playing a vital role in addressing bioethical questions within the hospital setting. These ethics committees not only educate institutions and health care professionals regarding major bioethical issues but they also offer consultation services to patients and health care professionals who are grappling with difficult cases.

I. Historical Origins of the Health Care Ethics Committee

Emerging medical technology, which posed new ethical problems during the 1960s, was the chief causal factor that explains the development of the modern ethics committee in the United States. Kidney (renal) failure and heart/lung (cardio-pulmonary) failure nearly always caused death prior to the emergence of renal dialysis technology and cardio-pulmonary resuscitation technology during this period. When these technologies emerged, death could be postponed or avoided, sometimes for a very long time. These seemingly miraculous benefits, however, precipitated new philosophical and ethical problems. For example: Under what conditions is it inappropriate to use these technologies? Sometimes using these technologies prolonged death in addition to prolonging life and for many the harm of prolonged death outweighed the value of prolonged life. As soon as these technologies emerged, problems became evident within hospitals where the technology developed and ethics committee developed as a means of responding to such problems.

These committees were developed as a "first attempt" at addressing the difficult problems that arise when one must evaluate whether to use a given life-sustaining technology in a given case. It soon became evident, however, that the philosophical, religious, social and legal challenges that were spawned by such technology were incapable of being managed by hospital-based, local committees. The great bioethical conversation of the second half of the twentieth century had begun and it continues without interruption.

II. Description of the Hospital Committee

What then is a hospital ethics committee or, more broadly, what is an institutional ethics committee? In general terms, it is a group of professionals and lay persons associated with a hospital which meets regularly to address and advise members of the hospital staff, patients, and the wider community regarding ethical problems that emerge within the health care institution. These committee members come not only from professional medicine but also include philosophers or other humanities scholars, lawyers, and clergy representing a variety of religious traditions. These professionals provide the contrasting perspectives of their disciplines and thereby enrich the ethical perspectives of these committees. Throughout the United States, bioethics has become not only a theoretical inquiry but also a practical activity that committees practice within health care institutions. The hospital ethics committee is the setting in which modern bioethics is practiced as a profession.

What is crucial to note is that these committees approach bioethics as a multi-disciplinary exercise. The discipline of philosophical ethics is central to bioethical inquiry but, *by itself, philosophical ethics is not sufficient*. Practical bioethical decisions require communication among individuals who have expertise in different areas – disciplines such as clinical medicine, nursing, law, and social work, in addition to the traditional areas of philosophy, religion, and literature. Furthermore, lay persons are also represented on the committee. The voice of the lay person is *vital* because, for the most part, the patients are lay persons. In short, modern, technological medicine must hear the opinions, values and feelings of those it serves. The committee provides the setting in which dialogue concerning the management of ethical dilemmas which arise in the institution takes place.

III. The Functions of the Hospital Ethics Committee

Perhaps what is most important to recognize about ethics committees is their significant variation. Not only do they vary in composition and size but they also vary with respect to the procedures they follow. Some, for example, do not act until they achieve complete consensus or agreement, while others will act on the basis of less than complete agreement. However, despite these variations, ethics committees can be functionally defined as having the following purposes.

First, all such committees take some responsibility for staying informed on the major issues involved in medical ethics. Committees have an informational function or responsibility. For example, committees will often organize educational programs aimed at both the institution's staff and the wider community. The purpose and style of these educational programs vary but they have a common goal, namely, to inform those who participate in ethical decision-making about the central scientific and ethical factors that influence choices.

Second, such committees function to develop, review and apply the ethics policies or guidelines of the institution. In hospitals, the most common form of ethics policy is the DNR or "Do Not Resuscitate" policy. This policy sets out the institution's guidelines for withholding or withdrawing life-sustaining treatment. However, many institutions have also developed policies on euthanasia, informed consent, and "comfort measures only" orders, the treatment of severely handicapped newborns, and the rationing of scarce medical resources. These are the "well traveled roads" of hospital ethics committees and they are widely discussed throughout the country. It is essential to point out that there is a great deal of diversity with respect to how these matters are resolved and on some questions there is far less consensus and more uncertainty. For example, there is great debate regarding the management of scarce life-sustaining resources. Some hospitals have clear and precise policies, while others leave the questions open to answers that differ on a case by case basis. Furthermore, there are also a newly emerging set of questions that ethics committees are being asked to address. While the above issues may be referred to as "patient-based" ethical issues, these new questions center around institutional ethical questions, which are known as organizational ethics. In this last domain the questions may be characterized broadly as the organization's values with respect to business ethics.

Most hospitals see that these first two purposes must be connected. Such committees aim to educate the staff on the policies that are in place within the institution. For it makes little sense for hospitals to develop sophisticated ethics policies and then fail to educate their staff on issues falling within such policies. Without education, ethics policies have little hope of improving the quality of patient care. Furthermore, policies that are not taught are frequently not used or acted on in real life settings and if these policies are not acted on, they cannot be "tested." Without such "clinical" testing, ethics policies can never be evaluated and redesigned in the light of experience.

Third, such committees are responsible for case consultation. The kind of review that occurs varies. Frequently, the committee is *directly involved in prospective case review*. In prospective review, the committee identifies a member or group of members who function as case consultants. They assist in the ongoing management or care of specific patients who offer ethical challenges to the caregivers. For example, Mr. John Doe, may be a patient on the third floor of the hospital. He may have a treatable disease that is terminal, if left untreated. Furthermore, Mr. Doe is refusing treatment. The committee may be asked to offer specific recommendations concerning this ongoing case. In such a context, the committee is functioning as a "quasi-medical consultant."

Committees, however, may also function to offer *retrospective case review*. These are cases that are no longer within the institution. The goal of the retrospective review is to "look back" and examine whether a case might have been better managed. I will have more to say on the role of the consultant following the general review of ethics committees and their roles within the hospital setting.

Finally perhaps the newest challenge faced by ethics committees within the health care setting is the problem of organizational ethics. Generally speaking, organizational ethics concerns itself not with patient care issues directly but with other matters that indirectly effect the overall care of patients. Health care institutions are businesses and the ethical difficulties that face all businesses also affect health care institutions. I will discuss this new area under the category of special problems faced by ethics committees.

IV. Theory and Practice in Ethics Committees

It is natural to ask what philosophy, what theology, or what ethical theory operates within the setting of an ethics committee. Religious perspectives often control decision-making within religious institutions but in public hospitals the approach is usually more diverse. It is not typical of ethics committees within public hospitals to begin their meetings with a discussion of formal ethical or religious value theory. In this axiomatic approach medicine is treated as an applied discipline in which these axiomatic philosophical or religious theories are taken as given and then applied to concrete cases. In this style, ethical theory comes first and then the problems are "solved" by applying the theories.

The difficulty with this axiomatic approach in the public health care setting is that there is great difficulty identifying universal ethical axioms within public settings. This approach may work well within scientific or mathematical contexts where there is strong agreement as to what are the "best" or "right" theories. But this approach is not common within the clinical ethics setting. Thus, the public ethics committee approach is quite different. Practice takes priority over theory because there is substantive disagreement as to the nature of "good" and "evil" or "right" and "wrong". Public hospitals have relied more on the autonomous decisions of the patients and physicians and administrators, who are in a constant dialogue with one another. In the public setting, ethical conflict is perceived as a conversation among the relevant parties and it is this conversation that represents the best means of managing conflict. Such dialogue permits reference to the principles, theories, values, virtues and traditions, both old and new, of philosophers and theologians, but it also allows the traditions of medical and nursing practice to enter into the resolution of ethical conflicts within the medical setting. Thus, there is a feedback between theory and practice, which fertilizes bioethical discussion within the ethics committee. Just as scientific theory and scientific practice interact, and thereby alter one another, so too ethical theory and human practices interact with each other. This interaction produces theoretical and practical change. In summary, while our ethics may alter our practices, it is also true that our practices may also alter our values (for a more extended discussion of ethics committee practice, see Minogue, 1996).

V. The Problems of Ethics Committees

Let us now turn to the problems that have nourished the modern health care ethics committee. The problems faced by ethics committees are as varied as the diseases faced by clinicians. Renal failure and dialysis and cardio-pulmonary resuscitation (CPR) are very different clinical problems and, therefore, they raise different questions for ethics committees. Exploring the following two heuristic examples can greatly clarify the workings of the modern ethics committee.

A. Renal Dialysis
Renal dialysis (a technology that replaces part of the kidney's function) provides an excellent illustration of the way in which technology spawned the modern hospital ethics committee. During the 1960s, when hemodialysis technology emerged, serious shortages developed because the technology was in short supply and was, as a result, very expensive. Few hospitals were able to purchase sufficient equipment and train the staff to provide dialysis services to all those who needed it. Shortages were acute throughout the nation. The administrators and physicians at the Northwest Kidney Center in Seattle, Washington, were the first really to face the problem. In order to address the scarcity problem, the Center created an ethics committee. This committee's function was to decide who would have access

to dialysis and who would not. In other words, they decided who would live and who would die. Almost immediately the committee became known in the hospital as "The God Committee". A firestorm of conflict emerged, for it seemed to many that a hospital ethics committee was not empowered by anyone to decide who shall live when not all can live.

Northwest Kidney Center was not alone. Throughout the nation, hospitals faced the dilemma of allocating dialysis technology. To meet this challenge, hospitals imitated the Northwest Kidney Center and instituted ethics committees charged with solving two problems. First, what criteria should be used to select patients? Second, how should such criteria be applied? The nation quickly discovered that these questions were easier to ask than to answer. This is because dialysis is much like a lifeboat: lives can be saved using this technology and nearly all who are threatened by kidney failure prefer this technology over death. But when the need for a life-saving service is greater than the ability to provide the service, choices must be made as to who should be allowed to stay in the lifeboat and who ought to be left out. But if men and women are in some sense "fundamentally equal," as the Constitution seems to affirm, how can we make choices among equals? The problem, then, at the first stage is how do we square our sense of human equality, the sense that we all deserve access to renal dialysis, with the need to allocate a scarce resource?

The problems faced by hospitals were common enough to philosophers who had been discussing the philosophical problem of dividing up scarce resources for centuries. But Americans were not accustomed to practically facing the problem of scarce medical resources. Consequently, when committees began distributing the dialysis resources, out-cries of discontent erupted: What right do these committees have to make these decisions? Ethics committee members are not gods who can determine who shall live.

Society responded to these outcries legislatively. In the early 1970s, the United States handled the problem of scarce hemodialysis services by making hemodialysis a right. The government simply sidestepped all the difficulties with respect to rationing by covering all renal dialysis costs under the provisions of social security. End Stage Renal Disease Amendments were added to the Social Security Act of 1973 and these amendments cre-ated a new health care entitlement. The costs of dialysis and transplantation would be paid for by the United States government.

The transformation that took place was almost as fast as a bolt of lightning. Because government financing constituted a nearly limitless supply of funds, medical technology companies responded, and dialysis scarcity ended in a very short period of time. With government providing the funds, the medical marketplace immediately responded and hospital-based renal dialysis centers sprang up throughout the nation. The most signifi-cant relief for hospitals was that now they could disband their "god committees" and pro-vide renal dialysis without appealing to any ethics committees to ration the service. All could live since the government would pay.

From one point of view this was the best of all possible solutions. First, it relieved the early ethics committees from the difficult task of deciding these contentious issues. Second, it put an end to the claims of discrimination by minorities, women, the poor, the aged and anyone else who was denied access to renal service. If no one was denied then no one had a claim of unfair treatment. Poor nations, perhaps even middle income nations, might have an allocation problem, but not the United States. In addition to dissolving a vast amount of conflict among groups within society, this solution allowed for a significant renal technology market to develop across the nation. Corporations began improving the technology and did so because they were confident that the government would buy their expensive technology. On the surface, government involvement not only solved the ethical and social problem of distributing a scarce resource, but also initiated a confident marketplace.

However, this solution has also created new difficulties. Dialysis started out in 1973 covering approximately 11,000 people at a cost of about $280 million. Today over 60,000 patients are receiving hemodialysis at a cost of nearly three billion dollars. What started out as an affordable small cost is now a major expense. This increases medical inflation. Since health care expenditures have historically risen at a rate greater than the rate of inflation throughout the economy these new medical entitlements burden the budget. The United States has begun to recognize this economic fact and this recognition is present in the fact that hemodialysis was the last catastrophic treatment that the government has covered. Hundreds of other diseases have not been covered and the problem of scarce medical resources is again appearing as a major problem faced by hospital ethics committees. This is especially true in areas such as transplantation and treatment for AIDS. Why should we cover dialysis and not these other treatments?[1] Ethics committees continue to grapple with these allocation problems.

B. Cardio-Pulmonary Disease

Dialysis technology was not, however, the only technology that was creating ethical problems for health care institutions. A second set of problems involved cardio-pulmonary resuscitation technology. This technology was more resistant to resolution than renal failure problems, because shortage of money was not the problem. Even if we chose to put vast amounts of money into treatment, the problems persisted. Ethics committees and the consultants associated with these committees continue to play a vital role within the management of these "end of life" problems. Indeed, it is safe to say that *end of life challenges* remain the most common problems faced by ethics committees.

Death traditionally followed cardiac and/or lung failure. Cardio-pulmonary resuscitative (CPR) technology rescues the patient by temporarily replacing or supplementing heart/lung function. While expensive, every hospital could afford the technology associated with CPR. Cost, though significant, was not the key to the problem. The problem involved a set of cultural conflicts surrounding ethical values in end of life care, for sometimes CPR prolongs death as well as life. These challenges mandated that professionals and patients come together to discuss them. Multi-disciplinary committees within health care institutions brought experts in philosophy, ethics, medicine nursing, and the law to struggle with a number of vitally important cultural values challenged by this new technology. These problems are faced by nearly every patient who dies in the United States, because cardio-pulmonary death is the most common *immediate* cause of death. In short, these problems are relevant to everyone who is nearing death.

VI. Ethics Committees and End of Life Resuscitation

The issues surrounding CPR are varied and complex. Rather than try to capture all of them in this limited space, I will focus on four.

A. *Clinical Indications of CPR: The Role of Advance Directives*

First, when is CPR clinically indicated? At first glance this seems like an easy question to answer. One might answer that we should always initiate CPR in order to save the life of a dying person. The difficulty is that while this answer is tempting it often violates some important principles that have influenced the practice of medicine. For example, suppose a patient or a patient's guardian has refused CPR. Giving the patient CPR would seem to violate our duty to respect the wishes of patients and the patients' right to determine the course of their own lives. This is often referred to as the *principle of patient autonomy*. In short, CPR was a challenging technology because it demonstrated that patients' wishes can often conflict with what a physician may believe is in their best interests. This last principle is often referred to as the principle of *patient best interest*. This principle of patient autonomy and the principle of patient best interest often conflict and one of the main tasks of the ethics committee is to *balance* these conflicting principles in a way that benefits the patient and satisfies the values of the society as a whole.

Given the importance of patient self-determination, our first question regarding when we should use CPR must be approached in a more subtle manner. CPR should be employed unless the patient has refused it. In short, American hospital ethics committees have adopted the general rule that CPR should be a standing order within the hospital. The rule of using CPR applies to all patients who go into cardio-pulmonary arrest except those who have refused such treatment. We may refer to this rule as "the standing order". We may further characterize the standing order as an *opt out* rule rather than an *opt in* rule. We appeal to patient autonomy to opt out of CPR rather than using it as the basis for opting into it. We will explore the significance of this later in the essay.

Ethics committee consultants spend vast amounts of time educating staff and patients regarding "end of life" rights as well as consulting on cases involving the advance directives of patients. The advance directive is a legal document used by patients to retain their self-determination even when they are dying. The most common forms of written advance directives are the living will or the durable power of attorney for health care. These advance directives do one of two things. In the case of the durable power of attorney for health care, they stipulate that a given individual has the power to make all health care decisions in the event that a person is terminally ill and becomes incompetent. In the case of the living will, the patient need not name a surrogate decision-maker but specifically states what he wishes to be done in the event that he becomes incompetent and terminally and irreversibly ill. Living will documents usually contain statements asserting that the individual does not wish to be artificially resuscitated in order to extend his or her life. Durable powers of attorney name a specific person to make all health care decisions should the patient fall into an incompetent state at the end of life.

B. *Competence and Foregoing Treatment: Guardianship*

The second problem that dominates ethics committee discussion is the issue of competence. The choice to refuse CPR must be made prior to going into cardiac or pulmonary arrest or CPR will be provided. If the patient is incompetent then he cannot articulate this choice, and therefore he must rely on someone else to speak for him. The concept of competence is central to the ethical use of CPR technology and is therefore of special importance to the hospital ethics committees and their consultants. This concept plays an essential role within hospital ethics policy, because it is generally considered to be unethical to provide medically beneficial treatment to a competent patient who refuses it. However, it is not generally considered to be unethical to provide such treatment to the incompetent patient who has expressed no advanced preferences on the matter.

It is therefore vital that ethics committees have a solid grasp on the difficulties associated with patient competence and there are two reasons why competence is one of the most difficult areas of medical ethics. First, the definition of competence is subject to significant debate. Second, even if competence could be precisely defined, many people are neither competent nor incompetent. Many patients have "diminished levels of competence" but do not satisfy any specific rigid criteria of incompetence and, therefore, it is often difficult to manage such patients. Within these difficult areas hospital ethics committees are often called upon to offer advice. Ethics committees and their consultants often approach competence questions with the following broad definition:

(1) The competent person has the ability to reason in a fairly coherent manner and is able to communicate their preferences by some means.
(2) The competent person can appreciate the consequences of his or her actions or inactions.
(3) The competent person can make decisions on the basis of relatively stable values.

For example, if a competent person is refusing resuscitation efforts, then we should be able to communicate with that person about the issues involved. Furthermore, we should be relatively confident that the individual has deliberated about the consequences of rejecting resuscitation, i.e., that he may well die, if CPR is not provided. We should also be relatively confident that the decision was reached in a manner which is not distorted by mental or physical pathology. These issues remain perplexing problems within the ethics committee setting and committee consultants are called upon to manage these challenges with equal amounts of communicative art, ethical sensitivity and clinical science.

Another problem associated with the issue of competence involves patients who are neither competent nor incompetent. These patients have diminished competency in the sense that they have some cognitive capacity but this capacity may be insufficient to manage the difficult ethical questions involving CPR. Such cases must be treated on a case-by-case basis and special weight should be attached to the professional opinions of psychologists and psychiatrists, who have specific training in competency judgments. However, most ethics committees hold that physicians should typically assume that their patients *are competent*, and if health care professionals decide otherwise, then they bear the burden of proof to establish incompetence. Strong evidence is required before overriding the wishes of the patient.

Hospital ethics committees often grapple with the problem of guardians because the majority of patients do not have advance directives and, therefore, the committees must turn to their guardians or surrogates in order to determine their wishes with respect to CPR. The guardian or surrogate is crucial to many problems in bioethics. The primary function of surrogates is to express the wishes of adults who have fallen into incompetence. Guardians speak for individuals who cannot speak for themselves. In the case of babies, parents are considered the guardians or surrogates of their children and in this context the guardian also helps to determine their best interests. When adults who are terminally and irreversibly ill are incompetent but have not issued a living will or a durable power of attorney, their guardians must cooperate with the physician to determine both the wishes of the patient and what is best for the patient. In most instances the hospital looks to the next of kin, such as a spouse, an adult child, or other relative. Many of the most pressing issues of medical ethics focus around the guardian who must speak in the absence of an advance directive. While it is impossible to address all the relevant issues surrounding guardianship, it is vital to identify the functions of guardianship so that we can evaluate guardians in terms of what purpose they serve.

To summarize, the function of the guardian is twofold. First, the guardian must express the wishes of the patient insofar as they are known by the guardian. Second, the guardian must decide what actions or inactions would maximize the welfare of the patient. Both of these functions are, however, riddled with complexity. For example, many individuals never express their wishes concerning "end of life treatments" such as resuscitation. Frequently, even their next of kin do not know their wishes. Or individuals may express their wishes but express them to people other than their next of kin. The classic problem that then emerges for the ethics committee consultant is: "To whom should I listen when there is conflict among the family or other potential surrogates?" Managing such conflict is one of the single most difficult challenges of the ethics committee consultant.

Another crucial problem within the concept of guardianship is the difficulty of evaluating whether the wishes of the patient are necessary for purposes of withdrawing life-sustaining treatment. In cases involving infants, it is obviously unnecessary, since infants do not have wishes on these matters. The "best interests" are often the sole criterion. In cases of adults, there is more heated debate. Many individuals (as well as courts) have argued that guardians do not have the right to withdraw treatment based completely on the "best interests" of the patient. In the absence of explicitly expressed wishes, withdrawal is problematic. The Nancy Cruzan case illustrates this issue.

In this case, a young woman was injured in an auto accident that left her in a persistent vegetative state (PVS). Her family had convinced a lower Missouri court to permit withdrawal of treatment including nutrition and hydration. However, the case was appealed to the Missouri State Supreme Court and the lower court's ruling was overturned. The State Supreme Court ruled that it was not permissible to withdraw hydration and nutrition from Miss Cruzan even though she was in a persistent vegetative state, because the family had not provided "clear and convincing evidence" that it was Nancy's wish to do so. Nancy's guardians (her parents) thought that it was not in her best interests to be kept biologically alive in the absence of any chance of regaining her cognitive life, but the guardians were unable to convince the Missouri Supreme Court that it was Nancy's specific wish to have nutrition and hydration removed in these circumstances.

Here the question is whether guardians have the right to make welfare or best interest judgments in the absence of a proven expression of wishes. The Missouri high court was reluctant to permit withdrawal because it found "no principled legal basis" for permitting the withdrawal. It decided that there was a compelling state interest to protect individuals who were suffering from PVS from possible harms and ruled that Nancy's parents could not remove the nutrition and hydration if they had not offered "clear and convincing evidence" that this was Nancy's wish. The family could not act on what they considered Nancy's "best interests" because such action might, the court ruled, undermine the state's interest in preserving life.

The *Cruzan* case was then brought before the U.S. Supreme Court and the court ruled that Missouri had the constitutional right to require a very high standard of evidence (clear and convincing) to establish that it was Nancy's wish to refuse treatment. Other states may employ weaker standards but Missouri did have the right to adopt a standard that required a high degree of evidence. However, while the Supreme Court rejected the Cruzan's request, the decision did recognize that there was a constitutional basis for the right to die. The court rested this claim on the Fourteenth Amendment's liberty interest and not on the question of the right to privacy, which was the basis of the *Roe v. Wade* decision regarding abortion. What is crucial about this decision for ethics committees was that it was the first time that the Supreme Court formally recognized the right to die.[2]

C. *Futility*

The third problem associated with CPR technology is called *the problem of futility*. This is a common problem faced by hospital ethics committees and their consultants because guardians often choose to have futile treatment continued in the face of solid evidence that such treatment cannot benefit the patient. We usually take patient or guardian consent as necessary for foregoing treatment, but this, in conjunction with the standing order of the hospital, makes it impossible for the hospital to ever refuse to provide life-sustaining services. Hospitals' ethics committees have noticed this difficulty, for it obligates them to provide even futile treatment. Committees have been influenced by the President's Commission Report on foregoing life sustaining treatment, which asserts that "a decision ... not to try predictably futile endeavors is ethically and legally justified" (1983).

What then is futile treatment? Hospital ethics committees must make their definition explicit. In the case of CPR it involves the inability of the procedure to achieve its physiological objectives of contributing to the interests and recovery of the patient. One could also define a futile treatment as a treatment whose goals cannot be achieved no matter how many times the treatment is repeated.

Such definitions have both virtues and vices. They have the virtue of being patient-centered, in the sense that futility is viewed as something that is defined in terms of a patient's best interests. This "best interests" approach excludes any attempt to offer a complete catalogue of futile treatments. The policy adopts the idea that futility should be judged on a case-by-case basis. On the other hand, these definitions have the weakness of being somewhat inexact and imprecise. Such definitions leave ethics committees with some difficult clinical and ethical judgments to make, including many borderline cases to manage. Indeed, some critics of the futility criterion have argued that because of the haziness of the concept of medical futility, we must never make withdrawal and withholding judgments based on futility alone. Such critics argue that we must always supplement futility judgments with the consent of the patient or a surrogate.

Despite these problems associated with the definition of futility, Hospital Ethics Committees often reject the notion that hospitals have a duty to provide what they consider to be futile treatment, especially in cases that involve maintaining only biological existence and nothing else. Patients who are in a persistent vegetative state meet this criterion, and so many hospital ethics committees do not accept any obligation to maintain merely biological existence.

This position on futility represents a major ethical decision for the hospital, because our society's medical, legal, and ethical traditions lean heavily toward the view that consent is necessary in order to forego treatment; and in the absence of patient or surrogate consent, foregoing futile treatment is unethical.

Four arguments can be offered against these traditions, especially as they relate to persistent vegetative state (PVS). For this class of patients, ventilation, nutrition, and hydration are non-beneficial treatments. The concrete case that forms the backdrop for this discussion is the *Wanglie* case, in which the husband of an 80 year-old PVS victim demanded life-sustaining treatment from health care professionals who thought that such treatment was futile.

The first argument involves counter-examples. When medical resources are scarce, foregoing treatment is permissible, even if consent is absent. If Mrs. Wanglie, for example, were in an intensive care unit and if others needed her bed, it seems clear to many that we would have the ethical right, and perhaps the duty, to withdraw life sustaining services from her. The justification for this decision is based on the desire to save the lives of acutely ill patients who have a chance to recover. PVS patients have no reasonable hope of recovery, therefore, to favor PVS patients over recoverable patients is unjust.

A second argument appeals to the everyday practice of nurses and physicians who serve on resuscitation teams. Such teams often forego resuscitative efforts, even when surrogates dissent and there is no scarcity. Consider the patient with advanced metastatic lung cancer who wants "everything done" and the resuscitation team who has provided five resuscitative efforts on the patient in the last twenty hours. Are they moral monsters for giving up after five resuscitative efforts? Or ten or twenty? To suggest that one can never give up if consent is missing contradicts common medical practice. Such multiple resuscitative efforts are often incoherent because they are futile and few of us would call nurses or physicians moral monsters for giving up. Quitting is justified when professionals cannot *in good conscience* continue to "batter their dying patients" with futile treatments.

The issue of professional conscience takes us to the third argument. Making guardian consent unconditionally necessary transforms the health care professional into a slave of the potentially irrational patient or surrogate. The provider of treatment is not obligated to give a futile treatment merely because a patient or surrogate wants it. Patients often request non-beneficial treatments such as antibiotics for their viral infections. The mere request does not obligate the provider to obey. Patient autonomy is not patient dictatorship. In the *Wanglie* case, Mr. Wanglie demanded treatment for his wife that health care professionals deemed to be futile. They interpreted nutrition, hydration and ventilation as useless for recovery. From their viewpoint, these treatments served merely to prolong her biological existence. As such, nutrition, etc., did not secure the interests of the patient. To coerce these professionals into providing treatment violates the professional's right to conscience. Furthermore, this requirement involves transforming Mr. Wanglie's right to be free from interference into a right to receive from the hospital any treatment he wants and these two rights are substantially different.

The fourth argument has to do with standards of care for PVS patients. In layman's language, this argument concerns determining what is good for the PVS patient. It has been the standard of care to provide ventilation, nutrition and hydration to PVS patients. Should it remain so? For some philosophers and physicians, the answer is "yes," because air, food and water are ordinary necessities of life. They are not medications and therefore we cannot withdraw them. The Society for Critical Care Medicine, in its report on foregoing life sustaining medicine, refers to nutrition, hydration, and ventilation as "treatments that offer no benefit and serve only to prolong dying should not be employed." Food and water are provided by gastric tubes, and IVs are common. Ventilation is often secured by complex machinery that forces air into the lungs. These ordinary necessities become highly technological services within the context of PVS patients. This society of critical care professionals has argued that "in the light of a hopeless prognosis, the indefinite maintenance of patients diagnosed as being in a PVS state raises serious ethical concerns both for the dignity of the patient and for the diversion of limited medical resources." The report is clear that critical care physicians are under no obligation to provide futile therapy.

There is, however, an important criticism of the futility rule, which is especially relevant to hospital ethics committees. Allowing futility judgments seems to transform physicians into gods who have ethical as well as medical expertise. Surely doctors are not omniscient and therefore we should not give them this authority to say that a patient will die without the consent of the patient or his surrogate. This is a powerful argument, but its force can be reduced in three ways. First, we may admit that futility judgments are value judgments but this does not by itself mean that the value decision can *only* be made by the surrogate. Society may authorize physicians to refuse futile treatment if they judge that there is a compelling state interest (such as avoiding the waste of resources) to allow refusal. Second, the physician approaches godhead status when he or she acts in isolation. But if futility decisions require significant consultation with other professionals, the hospital's ethics committee and the administration of the hospital, then the potential for unethical decisions is reduced. In short, a futility decision should be a conscious institutional decision as well as a conscious professional decision. Finally, granting the institution the right to say NO! does not require that surrogates stand by and do nothing. Those who desire the futile treatment remain free to petition the court for an injunction against the hospital or the professional and they are free to seek a transfer to another institution.

D. DNR Orders

The fourth problem associated with CPR is the problem associated with "do not resuscitate orders" (DNR). It is one thing for a patient to fill out an advance directive. It is another to execute that wish by writing a medical order that accomplishes that desire. Some physicians continue to be reluctant to fill out these orders, and one particular study[3] documents that this is a persistent problem within the hospital setting. The possible reasons for this reluctance are many. Some doctors feel as if terminal illness is difficult to define and that hope for recovery should always override the desire to avoid a prolonged death. Some feel that they are at increased malpractice risk if they sign these orders. Choosing life is always the safest course to take. There are many possible reasons for explaining the resistance to filling out DNR orders and for that reason ethics committees are recently spending more time on educating health care professionals on the ethical and legal aspects of DNR.

VII. Organizational Ethics

Recently a new area of concern has been emerging within modern health care ethics committees. It involves what we may refer to as organizational ethics. The business of medicine has radically changed over the past ten years in the United States, due to the nation's desire to control the spiraling increases in the costs of providing medical care. Managed care[4] has emerged as a system of health care delivery that imposes significant market constraints on the practice of medicine. Managed care organizations which control vast sums of medical funds often impose significant demands on hospitals. This causes a great deal of ethical tension in the hospital setting and conflict between medical benefit and the demands for economic efficiency emerges. For example, managed care has created a new form of medical practitioner which we may call the case manager. The case manager reviews the decisions of doctors and hospitals and determines whether the managed care organization will pay for the recommended procedures and medications. In addition, hospitals may be pressured by managed care organizations to develop new "practice guidelines" which may challenge the hospital's commitment to the best interests of the patient. This same pressure may influence the contracts into which hospitals enter with managed care organizations. Such contracts may contain "gag clauses", which impose requirements on doctors to withhold information regarding alternative treatments, procedures, and medications that are not covered by the managed care organization. These "gag clauses" conflict with the principle of informed consent and therefore ethics committees are challenged to manage the conflict that these business practices produce.

VII. Conclusion

The skills of ethics committee are constantly being called upon to manage these patient based and organizational dilemmas within the hospital setting. There is little reason to think that we can even imagine what a modern hospital would look like without the presence of an active and involved ethics committee.

Notes

1. For a more thorough discussion of problems concerning the allocation of scarce resources, see: President's Commission for the Study of Ethics Problems in Medicine and Biomedical and Behavioral Research, 1983a; 1983b; Rawls, 1971; Rescher, 1966; Sandel, 1982.
2. For a more complete discussion of issues surrounding end of life decision making see: Blackhall, 1987; Capron, 1991; Childress, 1983a; 1983b; Council on Ethical and Judicial Affairs, American Medical Association, 1991; Dworkin, 1976; The Hastings Center, 1987; Miles, 1991; President's Commission for the Study of Ethical Problems in Medicine and Biomedical and Behavioral Research, 1983c; Schneiderman, Jecker, and Jonsen, 1990.
3. For an insightful discussion of the problems faced by hospital ethics committees with respect to DNR, see: Lynn, 1995.
4. For a good discussion of the ethical issues associated with managed care see: Council on Ethical and Judicial Affairs, American Medcial Association (1995, p. 330).

Bibliography

Blackhall, L.J. 1987. Must we always use CPR? *New England Journal of Medicine* 317: 1281-1285.
Capron, A.M. 1991. In re Helga Wanglie. *Hastings Center Report* 21(5): 26-28.

Childress, J.F. 1983a. *Who should decide?* New York: Oxford University Press.

Childress, J.L. 1983b. Must patients always be given food and water? *Hastings Center Report* 13: 17-21.

Council on Ethical and Judicial Affairs, American Medical Association. 1991. Guidelines for the appropriate use of do-not-resuscitate orders, *Journal of the American Medical Association* 265: 1868-1871.

Council on Ethical and Judicial Affairs, American Medical Association. 1995. Ethical Issues in Managed Care, *Journal of the American Medical Association* 273: 330.

Cruzan v. Director, DMH 497 US 261 (1990).

Dworkin, G. 1976. Autonomy and behavior control. *Hastings Center Report* 6: 23.

Hastings Center. 1987. *Guidelines on the termination of life-sustaining treatment and the care of the dying.* Bloomington: Indiana University Press.

Miles, S.H. 1991. Informed demand for "non-beneficial" medical treatment. *New England Journal of Medicine* 325: 512-515.

Minogue, Brendan. 1996. *Bioethics: a committee approach.* Boston: Jones and Bartlett.

Lynn, J., et al. 1995. A controlled trial to improve care of the seriously ill hospitalized patient. *Journal of the American Medical Association* 274: 1591-1598.

President's Commission for the Study of Ethical Problems in Medicine and Biomedical and Behavioral Research. 1983. *Securing access to health care: the ethical implications of differences in the availability of health services, Vol. 1: report.* Washington D.C.: U.S. Government Printing Office.

President's Commission for the Study of Ethical Problems in Medicine and Biomedical and Behavioral Research. 1983. *Securing access to health care: the ethical implications of differences in the availability of health services, Vol. 2: appendices, sociocultural and philosophical studies.* Washington D.C.: U.S. Government Printing Office.

President's Commission for the Study of Ethical Problems in Medicine and Biomedical and Behavioral Research. 1983. *Deciding to forego life-sustaining treatment.* Washington, D.C.: U.S. Government Printing Office.

Rawls, J. 1971. *A theory of justice.* Cambridge: Harvard University Press.

Rescher, N. 1966. *Distributive justice.* Indianapolis: Bobbs-Merrill.

Sandel, M. 1982. *Liberalism and the limits of justice.* Cambridge: Cambridge University Press.

Schneiderman, L.J., Jecker, N.S. & Jonsen, A.R. 1990. Medical futility: its meaning and ethical implications. *Annals of Internal Medicine* 112: 949-954.

U.S. Supreme Court. 1990. *Cruzan v. Director, Missouri Dept. of Health.* U.S. 580 SLW 4916, June 25.

Part II: South America

5 Bioethics in Argentina

José Alberto Mainetti, José M. Tau,
Guillermo C. Morello, Héctor H. Pinedo and
Mirta Matínez

I. Introduction

As in other Latin American countries, bioethics flourished in Argentina during the 1980s when the academic discipline and public discourse were institutionalized throughout the region. With the generalization of new medical technology (e.g., critical care, organ transplantation, assisted reproduction) and the restoration of democracy, public and academic interest in bioethical issues expanded in the 1980s. On the one hand, increasing litigation in medical cases, malpractice claims, and an emphasis on patients' rights imitates American bioethics. On the other hand, there has been an academic rehabilitation of practical moral and political philosophy applied to medicine, following the model of moral pluralism and consensus formation, which has been key to the multi-disciplinary exploration of bioethics in the United States (Mainetti, 1995).

After reception and assimilation, re-creation is the stage of bioethics that has identified our own intellectual and moral traditions since 1990. In most countries of South America, the bioethics movement is organized into three areas: academic (scientific research and higher education), care (clinical and public health consultation, such as hospital ethics committees), and policy (advisory services and recommendations to public authorities on normative and regulative issues). Concurrently with each nationwide network, an international bridge of regional associations propelled the Latin American bioethical movement. Thenceforth, the increasing political will of its ethical identity developed into the Latin American bioethical model (Mainetti, 2004).

Within this context, the region requires a host of legislative and policy responses to the complex realm of today's biomedicine. This report compasses major legislation, court rulings, regulatory changes, and policy announcements issued by the government and professional associations on bioethical topics in Argentina. It is based on research undertaken at our Institute of Bioethics and Medical Humanities. Earlier versions of this report appeared in *The Bioethics Yearbook*, volumes 2 and 4 (Mainetti, et al., 1992; Tealdi, et al., 1995).

II. Professional-Patient Relationships and Health Care Ethics

As with other issues in bioethics, Latin America reveals characteristic tendencies in its approaches to issues of confidentiality, consent to treatment and experimentation, health care financing, and concepts of a right to health care. Although new regulations are appearing through both public policy and professional guidelines, it is also the case that there is a wide gap between theory and practice in bioethics.

The field of bioethics, born in the United States, has tended to give priority to the principle of autonomy rather than to the principle of beneficence. Thus, respect for confidentiality and the requirements of informed consent reflect the priority of autonomy. In contrast, research and practice in Latin American health care has tended to emphasize the principle of beneficence.

As a result, the relationship between medical professionals and their patients, as well as health care policy more generally, still exhibits a strongly paternalistic character, despite the ever-growing record of new legislation. If in North America there remains an opposition between theoretical autonomy and practical beneficence, in Latin America there emerges a tension between the priority of practical beneficence and a theoretical principle of justice, which endorses an equal right to health care. Many Latin American societies, because of inadequate social and economic development, are not able to guarantee a right to basic health care.

There is no doubt, however, that recent legislative initiatives, health policy decisions, and updated professional codes are efforts to reduce the distance between beneficience and justice in practice. The paradigm of this transformation has been AIDS, both in its impact on the professional-patient relationship and on health care policy.

Having made these preliminary comments, we will now analyze recent rules concerning the ethical aspects of confidentiality, consent, equal access to health care, and control of health expenditures in Argentina.

A. Confidentiality

In May 1991, the authorities of La Plata Military District disclosed the blood-test results of 5,407 teenagers who were about to join the Army. One in every 160 persons tested positive for HIV infection. Disclosure of these results prompted significant public debate. National Act Number 23.798 on AIDS, which had been passed in 1990, states in Article 2 that the law's provisions are in no case meant to:

> (a) affect personal dignity; (b) cause discrimination, stigmatization, degradation or humiliation; (c) exceed the background of legal exceptions limiting medical secrets ...; (d) trespass the privacy of any inhabitant of the Argentine Nation; or e) individualize people through cards, records or databases which, for this purpose, [would] be codified (Argentina, 1990).

When the above case occurred, this statute was not yet fully in force. Today, however, Article 2 is viewed as fundamentally safeguarding confidentiality, despite its numerous critics.

Of special regional significance is the creation of the National Genetic Databank in Argentina, formed after the disappearance of many people during the military governments of the late 1970s and early 1980s. The purpose of the Databank is to store genetic information belonging to presumptive relatives in order to identify children through genetic techniques. Despite the crucial importance of confidentiality in these cases, the law which created the Data Bank addresses the issue only briefly in the eighth of ten articles: "The records and files of the National Genetic Databank shall be kept inviolable and unalterable" (Argentina, 1987). The Genetic Databank has so far proved essential in identifying a great number of missing children. Yet, given the harmful consequences that could follow if such genetic information were used for other questionable purposes, there exists a significant need to guarantee confidentiality (Drane et al., 1991; Tealdi, 1991, 1990).

Decree 1244/91 promulgates regulations for the implementation of the 1990 Law 23.798 on AIDS (Decree No. 1244/91), with special attention to the problem of confidentiality. Physicians and other health professionals are required to refrain from disclosing any information about HIV-positive or AIDS patients except to the following persons or institutions: the infected person or his proxy, another physician, the National Blood System, the director of the hospital or of the hemotherapy department, judges, and any person under the physician's responsibility who requires such information to avoid serious harm. In such cases, only the patient's initials and date of birth are used as identifiers.

B. Consent to Treatment and Experimentation

1. *Involuntary Treatment.* On his journey to Colombia, Bolivia, Chile, Argentina and Brazil in 1990 to inform the Pan American Health Organization on the state of bioethics in Latin America, North American bioethicist James Drane concluded that review committees for scientific research did not function effectively in any country, nor was informed consent generally obtained from patient or research subjects, despite some existing regulations (Drane, et al., 1991). Drane thus noted the gap between theory and practice to which we have already referred. This situation has not yet been remedied, although nongovernmental organizations are making important efforts.[1]

In Argentina, the National Supreme Court had the opportunity to rule with regard to an already famous case, which has important implications for determining the scope and limits of compulsory treatment when the patient refuses consent on the basis of personal beliefs (*Corte Suprema de Justicia*, 1993). In 1989, Marcelo Bahamondez, a Jehovah's Witness, was admitted to the Regional Hospital of Ushuaia with a gastric hemorrhage. Because of his religious beliefs, he refused to consent to a blood transfusion prescribed by physicians. The hospital appealed to the court and obtained authorization for transfusion despite the patient's refusal. The Federal Appellate Court subsequently confirmed the lower court's ruling on the grounds that the defendant's refusal constituted a gradual and non-violent form of suicide, though not by his own hand. Bahamondez appealed to the Supreme Court, claiming that his decision was not an attempt at gradual suicide but a refusal of treatment based on his personal religious convictions; he argued, that such refusal should be protected under Articles 14 and 19 of the Constitution which guarantee freedom of worship. Meanwhile, the clinical situation changed for the better and Bahamondez was discharged on June 19, 1989.

The defendant applied for a revocation of the lower court judgments before the Supreme Court. In April 1993, the Supreme Court ruled that a judgment would be improper since the cause for the lawsuit – i.e., the clinical circumstances which led to confinement and treatment – had disappeared. Nonetheless, six members of the Court raised a number of important considerations relevant to the basic question at issue.

Despite agreeing that the Court's intervention was inappropriate, Judges Barra and Fayt reasserted the right of a fully competent adult patient to have his refusal of treatment honored, based on the fundamental constitutional principle of the inviolability of the human person. Judges Boggiano and Cavagna Martínez analyzed the case from the perspective of the guarantee to freedom of worship and thought enunciated in Article 14 of the Constitution. They based the right to exercise conscientious objection on that freedom. Although suicide is deemed illicit, because no one may legally consent to serious injury or harm, conscientious objection to treatment is respected, since an individual's liberty and dignity prevail over concerns about bodily injury. Whereas physician collaboration in suicide is illicit, it is quite appropriate in cases involving conscientious refusal of treatment. Thus, Judges Barra and Fayt accepted the plaintiff's appeal and voted to revoke the lower courts' judgments. Judges Belluscio and Petracchi also ruled in favor of the plaintiff. They rejected the foundation of the Appellate Court's judgment by denying that the plaintiff's action was an instance of suicide or euthanasia. Invoking Articles 14 and 19 of the Constitution, they reasserted the principle of individual autonomy and concluded that the right to accept or refuse all bodily interventions is an essential requirement of autonomy. They also advocated the right of a competent adult person to be left alone, a right that may not be curtailed on grounds that a person's decision appears to be unreasonable according to prevailing opinion. They held that a medical intervention is not justified without the consent of a competent patient, especially when the rights of third parties are not affected. For these reasons, they found no grounds for restricting the plaintiff's freedom.

Further jurisprudence has endorsed the trend to respect the legally competent adult patient's decision to reject specific treatments. A paradigmatic example is the "Parodi" case (*Juzgado de Primera Instancia en lo Criminal y Correccional No. 3 de Mar del Plata*, 1995). Here, the judicial authority decided that doctors had to honor the patient's decision and refrain from amputating his gangrened left leg. The court took into account subsequent concerns regarding treatment rejection as well as the "right to die with dignity" in part because this patient had undergone the amputation of his right leg a month earlier.

The "Law of the Patient's Rights" is, without doubt, the most highly evolved enactment of bioethical legislation. Enacted on April 11, 1997, in the Province of Río Negro, Law 3076 is the first normative legislation within the Argentinean juridical order, which establishes in its 2nd article and eighteen sections, a complete catalog of patients' rights; and in the 3rd article decrees the healthcare professional's and institutional responsibility to fulfill them (Province of Río Negro, 1997a).

2. *Consent to Experimentation.* Law number 11.044, "The Protection of Persons Involved in Scientific Research", is the first Argentinean law to deal broadly with consent (Argentina, 1990d). As a provincial statute, it has already encouraged legislative initiatives based on its text, one at a national level and another in the province of Tucumán. According to Article 3, "All research involving study of human beings shall conform to the criteria of respect for their dignity and protection of their rights and welfare." And subsection (e) of Article 40 states that research involving human subjects requires "the consent of subjects under research or their respective agents through public documents which specify the risks they face."

The requirement of consent is also emphasized in other articles of the law. Research subjects are entitled to halt their participation in the research at any time (Article 70). The consent document must explain "the nature of the procedures the participant will be subject to, eventual risks rising from them, the participant's free choice, and the exclusion of all forms of coercion towards him" (Article 90). In cases involving incompetent persons, consent will be given "by the agent under authorization of a qualified judge in expeditious lawsuits [*juicio sumarísimo*]" (Article 110). Ethics and research committees are entitled to adjourn any research that may affect the psychophysical or psychosocial well-being of incompetent participants (Article 120). Consent requirements are also specified for pregnant and puerperal women, newborns, fetuses and embryos (Article 140), special populations (Article 220), research where new methods of prevention, diagnosis, treatment, and rehabilitation are studied (Article 240), and pharmacological research (Article 32). The statute created ethics committees to supervise consent procedures (Article 360).

A bill on the protection of human subjects in biomedical research has been submitted to the House of Representatives by legislators Estévez Boero, Zamora, and Neri, (Estévez Boero, et al.).

C. Equitable Access to Health Care

The right to equitable access to health care has been proclaimed a human right in Article 25 of the "Universal Declaration of Human Rights," adopted by the United Nations General Assembly on December 10, 1948. In the same year, the Organization of American States (OAS) adopted the "American Declaration of the Rights and Duties of Man," proclaiming (although vaguely) the right to health in Article XI. "The Americas Convention on Human Rights" (1978), signed by most Latin American countries, promises gradually to achieve full implementation of economic, social, and cultural rights, including a right to health. Such a right was first proclaimed in the Protocol of Buenos Aires (OAS, 1967). In this general sense, the right of equal access to health care as a "human right" has been elaborated as a matter of international law for more than four decades.

In Latin America, however, the present debate on equitable access to health care exemplifies, once again, the gap between theory and practice. Although different constitutions and statutes in Latin American countries affirm the concept, the economic conditions necessary to guarantee that such a right can be exercised are not always present. Thus, the idea of the "progressive fulfillment" of the right to health care relative to the material conditions of each country has developed. In practice, of course, this idea may sometimes be used as an excuse not to fulfill a basic moral obligation. Nonetheless, the statement of norms in the delivery of health care remains fundamental because norms help to guide the possibility of effective social transformation.

The first right which the current Argentinean Constitution (ratified in 1853 and amended in 1994) recognizes and guarantees is the right to life. The Constitution has no express reference to the right to health care, probably because it is so implicitly understood. The Agreement of San José de Costa Rica ("the Americas Convention on Human Rights") was endorsed by Argentina's Law 23.054, which recognizes, with an emphasis on autonomy, the right to life. This is set in Article 4, first section, which rigorously points out that every person has the right to life. This right will be safeguarded by the law and, in general, from the very moment of conception. Nobody can arbitrarily be deprived of this right. Article 5 states the right to personal integrity, and it reads: "Every person has the right to his/her personal physical, psychical and moral integrity."

It is also worthwhile to mention the provincial constitutions' amendments (particularly those of Salta and Córdoba sanctioned in 1986 and 1987, respectively). The former encloses under Title II "About social security and health". Article 40 titled "Right to health" prescribes: "Health is an inherent right to life and its preservation is a personal obligation. But as a social good, the state is responsible for the physical, mental and social health care of the people as well as for securing equal access to health care before equal needs" for everybody. The latter centers the analysis on Article 4 which edicts the "inviolability of the person": from conception, the physical integrity and the moral integrity of a person are inviolable.

The 1994 amendment of Buenos Aires Province's Constitution decrees in Article 36 that the province will promote the overcoming of economical, social or any other kind of obstacles which might affect or hamper the exercise of the constitutional rights and guarantees. Health being one of these rights, the province warrants all its inhabitants the access to health care, prevention, treatment, medicines, and professional support. As regards this constitutional article, the province's legislature is about to sanction a law which would further develop the provincial system for organ and tissue procurement for therapeutic purposes. For the first time this article would provide the normative framework and subsequent legality to the activities performed by the Sanitary Administration since the practice of organ transplantation began.

In Argentinean law, the notion of police power presumes that the state has the authority to limit personal rights to protect the public health. Policies of various governments, therefore, define the meaning of equal access accordingly. Two national statutes, passed in 1989, set forth a new system of social and national health security (Argentina, 1989a; Argentina, 1989b).

Law 23.660 regulates social security as an important sector of the Argentinean health system. The social security organizations are funded through employer and employee contributions: employers contribute six percent of employee income and employees contribute 3 percent (Article 16). The purpose is to devote those resources to health services, although other social benefits should be provided for as well (Article 3). Public and private sector workers, retired workers (Article 8), families and dependents, are included as beneficiaries (Article 9). Social security organizations are required to devote at least 80 percent of their resources to health care. Those with centralized collection are to distribute funds according to a principle of solidarity, to assure equitable access to health care (Article 5). The organizations are only allowed to devote up to 8% of their resources to administrative overhead. Social security organizations, as part of the National System of Social Security, are subject to regulative norms (Article 3).

Decree 358/90 (Argentina, 1990a), which regulates Law 23.660, defines "other social benefits" as those not encompassed by the medical coverage regulated by articles 25, 26, 27, and 28, and those concordant of Law 23.661, which we will discuss below. According to Article 3 of Law 23.660, social security organizations must guarantee the provision of health services according to norms set by the Health Authority and the Social Security National Administration.

It is clear that Law 23.660 and its accompanying Decree are fundamental to the legal framework that assures equal access to health care in Argentina. Nonetheless, the major instrument for this purpose remains the National System of Social Security.

Law 23.661 created the National System of Social Security "with the purpose of assuring the full exercise of health to all inhabitants without social, economic, cultural or geographic discrimination" (Article 10). Its "fundamental aim is to provide for equitable, comprehensive and humanized health provisions, directed to the promotion, protection, recovery and rehabilitation of health, which shall respond at the highest quality available, and which shall assure the beneficiaries [a uniform] level of services, based on a criterion of distributive justice, without any form of discrimination" (Article 20). These social organizations are agents of health security (Article 20). They must conform to Health Ministry policies aimed at coordinating social security, public health services, and private suppliers (Article 3). Security services are supplied according to national health policies based on a strategy of primary health care, decentralized operation, and freedom of choice of suppliers by beneficiaries (Article 25).

Decree 359/90 (Argentina, 1990b), which regulates Law 23.661, broadens the concept of equal access. Article 50 states that the population will be classified into categories according to their income levels to assure equity. In Argentina, Laws 23.660 and 23.661 provide the main legal framework for egalitarian access to health care. Among their goals, these laws were to modify substantially the existing legal framework by allowing free choice in social security insurance, independent of the worker's occupation. Law 24.445 specified that some social security insurance must be compulsory so as to finance the health services system and welfare practices which Laws 23.660 and 23.661 create. Covered services include medical and pharmacological treatments for HIV and the use of stupefacient. Law 24.754 went even further and established a uniform minimum threshold of practices, including private medical insurance.

In 2000, appealing to reasons of "necessity and urgency," the National Executive Power's Decrees 446/00 and 1440/00 started an ambitious deregulating project of social security services. These decrees aimed at giving beneficiaries free choice among the social security services of the system as well as among the adhering private medical insurance. With the present contribution (8 percent of income), services ought to ensure a minimum obligatory coverage similar to the current "obligatory medical program" (OMP). Adding a uniform minimum contribution per beneficiary, the National Treasury should guarantee the availability of resources through the current Solidarity Fund of the Health Services Superintendence. Though the new system should have been implemented gradually, beginning January 1, 2001, the socioeconomic context, the eventual workers' unions opposition, and the lack of private adhesion, due to the reduced minimum amount guaranteed per beneficiary, it is fair to doubt that the project will go forward as it was originally designed.

This issue has had considerable political impact with regard to organ transplantation. To serve disadvantaged patients without Social Security, Article 49 of Law 24.193 created a Transplantation Solidarity Fund from the following sources: a contribution from the State, fines from the imposition of administrative and criminal penalties, and money collected from public or private donations and taxes used to underwrite transplantation. The latter would amount to one peso (1 U.S. dollar) for each national or international purchase by credit card. Although the Congress passed this law in March 1993, Decree 773, signed in April by the President and his Minister of the Economy, vetoed part of Law 24193. The Decree states that national tax policy has been directed towards the elimination of direct tax revenue. Although the Transplantation Solidarity Fund is important, there are other social needs of equal or greater priority. Thus, if the number of such funds were to multiply, the impact on the allocation of social resources would be severe. The Administration of National Health Insurance warrants Law 23.660 beneficiaries that the practices will be covered through specific assignments allotted to each social security insurance, in order to overcome questions regarding access to transplantation derived from the Executive Power veto of several articles of the law.

In the province of Buenos Aires, however, Decree 3309/92 requires the provision of economic aid to every inhabitant who lacks access to organ transplantation because of limited resources (Provincia de Buenos Aires, 1992). The Decree creates the Agency for Funding Organ Transplantation, to be directed by representatives of the Executive Power, the Ministry of Health and Social Welfare, the Ministry of Economy, and the Coordination Center of Ablation and Implantation (*Centro Único Coordinador de Ablación e Implante*, or CUCAIBA). The Organ Transplantation Financing Fund has been created from the following resources: sums assigned in the provincial budget, the sum assigned by the Ministry of Health and Social Welfare, the resources allotted by the Agency for Funding Social Programs (a public agency with specific funds), percentages from gambling receipts, donations and bequests, publication sales, and other incomes. The decree establishes as a goal equitable access to transplantation for all inhabitants of that state.

D. Ethical Concerns Raised by Cost Containment Measures

In Argentina, the debate on cost-containment measures may be regarded as a choice between high-technology interventions and primary health care. The cholera epidemic in Latin America has provided evidence of the need to place greater emphasis on primary and preventive health care strategies. Several legislators submitted an important draft of a law on the regulation of high-technology medicine and the creation of a national record of high-technology medical resources in October 1991 (Honorable Cámara de Diputados de la Nación, 1991). The bill aims at limiting the use of high-technology in favor of primary health care.

III. The Beginning of Life

A. New Reproductive Technologies

Although ethical principles have generally been observed in the practice of new reproductive technologies (NRTs), there is no official legislation on the subject. In Argentina, however, the national government shows increasing interest in responding to the ethical issues raised by NRTs. In 1989, the National Senate created an interdisciplinary commission to study NRTs to produce appropriate legislation. As a result, artificial insemination and *in vitro* fertilization (IVF) have recently been regulated (Argentina, *Código Civil*, Arts. 243 and 234 bis.). The Penal Code added an article that set penalties for married women who are artificially inseminated without the consent of their husbands. In the Province of Buenos Aires, Law 11.044 guides "medical practices such as assisted fertilization of proven efficacy in human beings" (Argentina, 1990d). Article 5 explicitly refers to informed consent and it reads: "Patients will give their written consent on a pre-printed form where the methods and possible risks the proposed treatment may offer [will be listed]." This same law requires the formation of a provincial ethics committee whose function is to advise the Application Authority on the medical practices it oversees.

Since mid-1991, there have been at least nine bills that, while not yet enacted, are designed to regulate the techniques and practices of assisted human reproduction. Thus far, because the bills have been subject to extensive congressional discussion, Argentina still lacks any statue on the matter. However, the Argentine Society of Sterility and Fertility, in a recent serious discussion of assisted reproduction, has expressed its support of one of the bills.

We will briefly analyze the bills of legislators Gómez Miranda (1991); Storani and Lafferrière (1991), Natale and Antelo (1991), Orquín (1992), Cafiero (1993), Ruckauf (1993), and Britos (1993). In drawing comparisons, we will discuss the position taken in each proposal, regarding the most important aspects of assisted reproduction and related practices.

1. *Access to Assisted Reproduction.* Each bill allows assisted reproductive techniques only as a means of relieving human infertility or sterility. The bills vary in their conclusions about who should have access to such techniques. Ruckauf, Orquín, and Gómez Miranda allow the use of these techniques only by married couples. Britos extends access to all couples, not only those who are legally married. Storani and Cafiero grant access to any adult or emancipated minor.

2. *Assisted Fertilization with Spouse's Sperm or with Donor Sperm.* All the bills permit assisted fertilization using the husband's sperm, but they differ in their recommendations on heterologous assisted fertilization. Cafiero, Natale and Antelo, Orquín, and Storani accept sperm donation from a third party; Britos, Gómez, Miranda, and Ruckauf reject it. In all cases where third-party donation is allowed, the anonymity of the donor is required. All the bills forbid the marketing of gametes and embryos.

3. *Consent from Recipients and Donors.* All the bills discuss the requirements of informed consent by couple. The conditions for repealing consent are specified for some cases of heterologous donation; the donor's informed consent is always required and is revocable at any time. Storani and Laffrerrière's bill introduces the notion of conscientious objection by physicians working in public institutions.

4. *Cryopreservation of Sperm, Eggs, and Embryos.* Ruckauf's bill allows gamete cryopreservation only when one or both spouses have undergone sterilizing procedures or treatments; otherwise fresh gametes must be used. In general, the period allowed for cryopreservation is from two to five years for sperm and from two to three years for ova; however, Gómez Miranda rejects cryopreservation of ova because he deems it unsafe. Opinions about cryopreservation of embryos and pre-embryos differ. While Britos and Orquín forbid the procedure, Gómez Miranda and Lafferrière accept it.

5. *Confidentiality of and Access to Records.* Gómez Miranda's bill sets forth the requirements for confidentiality of clinical data for those involved in assisted reproduction. The bill by Natale and Antelo does the same, although when donation is heterologous, access to data is allowed for medical reasons in some cases. By contrast, Cafiero's bill establishes only "relative" anonymity for a third-party donor. Storani and Lafferrière allow only the offspring or offspring's proxy access to records. However, their bill establishes a centralized record of complete data on recipients, donors, and offspring. Orquín's bill also specifies that records should be sent to a National Center of Genetic Data, even as it defends strict preservation of the donor's anonymity. Ruckauf's draft also proposes to send records to a centralized data bank.

6. *Status of the Human Embryo.* The bills of Britos, Orquín, and Ruckauf declare that human life begins at the moment of conception, regardless of whether it takes place within or outside the womb. These bills do not recognize the category of "pre-embryo".

Lafferrière also considers conception within the womb or implantation of the embryo to constitute the beginning of human life. The drafts of Cafiero, and Storani/Lafferrière do recognize "pre-embryo" as a category.

7. *Fertilization of Eggs and the Transfer of Embryos.* The bills of Ruckauf, Britos and Orquín allow a maximum of six eggs to be fertilized *in vitro*. Embryo selection is not allowed; thus, all fertilized eggs must be transferred to the womb at one time. According to the Cafiero and Gómez Miranda drafts, decisions about the number of embryos to be transferred should be made by the medical team. With regard to the number of pregnancies to be allowed using sperm from the same donor, Cafiero leaves that determination to an oversight agency. Storani and Lafferrière set four pregnancies as a maximum.

8. *Disposition of Gametes and Embryos.* In general, the various bills, except those by Storani and Lafferrière, call for the destruction of gametes when the consent is repealed or when the storage time has elapsed because consent has not been renewed or because of the death of one or both spouses.

9. *Surrogate Motherhood.* All the bills reject the practice of surrogate motherhood and declare surrogate contracts void. In disputed cases, all the bills favor the gestational mother by declaring that motherhood is determined by childbirth.

B. Abortion

Abortion remains punishable by law in the countries of the region with two exceptions: (1) so-called "therapeutic" abortion, when the mother's life is in danger and she consents to the abortion, and (2) if pregnancy is the result of rape. In the latter cases, legal actions – by the victim or her legal representative – should be undertaken prior to the abortion. In the last several years, Argentinean legislation has revealed a variety of attitudes with regard to the range of allowable exceptions (García Marañón et al., 1990).

The situation with regard to abortion has not undergone basic changes in Argentina, perhaps because true public debate on the issue has not yet occurred. Various opinions expressed during the last decade about which abortions may be justified tend to reflect the ideological views of legislators rather than the general trends in public opinion.

Nevertheless, during the last two years, a number of court decisions have raised interesting considerations about confidentiality in abortion cases. A judgment issued by an Appellate Court in November 1991 states the following:

> No legal action can be taken against a woman who has caused her own abortion or consented to another person causing it based on a report made by a physician who knew that fact through medical practice, but proceedings are allowed when the report involves co-authors, instigators, or accomplices (*Capital Federal*, 1991).

This legal immunity, based on the confidentiality of the physician-patient relationship, has been even more strongly supported when the woman's life is in danger. A recent judgment asserts that a woman cannot be asked:

> ... to risk her own life for lack of medical cares in exchange for silencing the fact [of abortion]. Otherwise, she would be required to choose between her

life and a lawsuit ... which the legislature has not required an ordinary person to do without infringing Article 18 of the National Constitution (*Provincia de Buenos Aires*, 1990a).

From these judgments, we can infer that in Argentinean jurisprudence, the privacy of persons is deemed a good that must be strongly protected. However, the general trend among legal experts is to continue to regard life as a supreme good. Thus, in cases of abortion, discussion of exceptions is limited to situations where the mother's life is in danger or when the pregnancy is the result of rape, provided that the woman is disabled.

C. Maternal-Fetal Conflicts

In Latin American countries, there are no records of specific legislation concerning maternal-fetal conflicts. However, some recent general legislation contains normative principles that, in addition to safeguarding the rights of patients, also state that patients have an obligation to take preventive measures necessary to preserve their health. The latter, undoubtedly applicable to pregnant women, suggests that in the future cases are likely to arise which will pose conflicts between maternal and "fetal" rights.

In Argentina, on January 11, 2001, the Supreme Court had the opportunity to rule on a resounding case given by a 26-week pregnant woman who, when she was informed she was carrying an anencephalic fetus, went to the judicial authority to get the court's consent to allow the public hospital doctors to stimulate birth labor or to perform a cesarean section. The Superior Tribunal of the Autonomous City of Buenos Aires issued a temporary restraining order in favor of the plaintiff. In its turn, the National Court would have to decide about an extraordinary emergency protective order forwarded by the General Adviser of the Disabled. The verdict disregarded the extraordinary protective order in favor of the plaintiff, thus ratifying the permission to practice abortion by the vote of five of the eight Ministers (one Minister absent abroad). Though providing different reasons, dissenting Ministers Julio S. Nazzareno, President of the Tribunal, and Antonio Boggiano voted against the plaintiff and in favor of the anencephalic fetus' status of person. Nazareno argued that the pathological alteration appeared after the conception, which is the moment the Argentinean law recognizes the character of person, so he decided to respect the fetus' right to life in the mother's womb during all pregnancy until natural delivery. Boggiano believed that the justification of early parturition, which holds that an anencephalic has little to no possibilities of life after birth, neglects the immeasurable value of the person to be born, because it supposes that the infant's life has less value than the lives of others with better chances. Moreover, it holds that the value of the infant's life is even inferior to the mother's or family's suffering. Enrique Santiago Petracchi considered the plaintiff's temporary order inadmissible because the appealed verdict was grounded on constitutional national common legislation.

In item 13 of the sentence, the Tribunal made it clear that it was not a case of abortion, eugenic abortion, or euthanasia, nor was it a case of freedom for procreation, nor did they consider the fetus other than a person. However, they considered the mother's demands legally reasonable and the juridical authorization to stimulate birth legitimate; it thereby became a novel and emblematic verdict in maternal-fetal conflicts.

D. Care of Severely Disabled Newborns

Latin American countries have not yet passed any specific legislation on severely disabled newborns. Nevertheless, other legal norms, especially those concerning minors and disabled persons, offer a context for interpreting the issues raised by treatment decisions involving disabled newborns, even in the absence of specific legislation.

Law 10.592 establishes the basic legal rights for disabled persons in the province of Buenos Aires. It guarantees health care, education, and social security services for disabled persons who cannot afford them (Provincia de Buenos Aires, 1987). This law was subsequently modified by Law 10.836, which makes transportation available to disabled persons (Provincia de Buenos Aires, 1989), by Decree 1149, which regulates several articles of Law 10.592, especially Article 3 about the issuance of certificates of disability (Provincia de Buenos Aires, 1990b), and by Law 11134, which encourages the purchase of goods produced by disabled persons (Provincia de Buenos Aires, 1991). These laws are meant to protect disabled persons from early childhood through old age, as well as to promote their optimal social integration. Tacit commitment to provide disabled newborns with all possible care could be inferred from such protectionism legislation.

IV. Death and Dying

A. Care of the Dying and Euthanasia

Argentina still awaits a frank discussion of euthanasia. Nevertheless, the Penal Code was slightly modified to lessen penalties for those who help others, with their consent, to terminate irreversible physical suffering (Article 73).

Since October 1996, there is a proposed law waiting to be sanctioned by the National Congress. The House of Representatives has already favorably esteemed this bill (Proposed Law, 1996). It supports a rank of rights of the terminally ill, including those who are irreversibly ill, with an illness for which no cure exists, and who are in a terminal phase or have had an accident which puts them in a similar situation. The bill that made the prohibition of euthanasia explicitly clear was not warmly received by the local bioethical doctrine, because the exceedingly complex regulation for decision-making seemed to safeguard the professional's responsibility rather than the patient's right to dignified care and assistance or the assurance of euthanasia if desired.

B. Definition of Death

Since 1977, when the first legislation on transplants was sanctioned, Argentina accepted total and irreversible absence of encephalic activity as death certification, co-existing with the "traditional" verification of cardiorespiratory arrest.

The process of normative adequacy produced the current regulation called "encephalic death." The former phrase "brain death" was removed, but the regulation retained the requirement of at least two physicians (a neurologist or neurosurgeon), who are alien to the transplantation team, to corroborate the absence of encephalic activity during a given period of time and according to specific methods. This reflects the outcome of the bioethical debate that gave rise to this way of diagnosing death within the context of perfuse organ transplantation activities. Also, from the sanction of Law 24.193 onward, the

National Commission for the Revision of Neurologic Death Diagnosis – integrated by members of the national health authority – has the task of updating the clinical and instrumental methods adapted to the diverse clinical situations in which such a diagnosis could be made. Bolivia, Chile, Ecuador, Panamá, and Perú have also adopted these criteria for brain death.

C. Organ Donation and Transplantation

The initial regulation of transplantation practices previously mentioned (Argentina, 1977) approved a first generation of rights, which, because of their relationship with bioethics, were considered to be the expression of a new "biolaw". Such rights focused on the need to protect the patient (i.e., the principles of beneficence and nonmaleficence) and to guarantee the patient's autonomy. Almost completely forgotten were questions related to the principle of justice, which is closely linked to organ and tissue procurement and transplantation.

It was within the framework of transplantation matters that informed consent had a broader and more specific legislative reception. Article 11 of that law compelled (for the first time in Argentinean Positive Law) chairmen and associate professionals of the transplant team to obtain the patient's informed and documented consent. The new law (Ley 24.193) regulated in article 13 that the reach of this obligation now extends to the patients' relatives – according to a rank established in the same law – that the information must be clear, sufficient, and adapted to their cultural level, encompassing not only the ablation and implant risks but the physical and psychological sequelae as well, including certain and possible foreseen evolvement, outcome limitations, and the true possibilities of the recepient's improvement. A document must be drawn up at least forty-eight hours before the procedure.

This last law on organ transplantation involves a provocative provision on "presumed consent" to the procurement of organs, undoubtedly aimed at relieving the chronic scarcity of organs for transplantation. Article 20 states that officials of the Registry of Vital Statistics will be required, whenever adults come to the Registry for any purpose, to record information about their willingness to donate organs; individuals may also refuse to express their preference. Registry officials will then be required to a) record the result of the inquiry on the document which certifies the particulars and b) communicate affirmative responses to the national office which regulates procurement and distribution of organs. In all cases, certified records must be kept of the limitations specified by presumed donors about the disposition of their organs. In addition, Article 29 states that the Executive Power shall engage in a long-term campaign of public information through the mass media to promote public solidarity on the need for donation. However, Article 62 states that, beginning on January 1, 1996, those who have not expressed their unwillingness to donate organs under the provisions of Article 20 will be presumed to have granted their tacit consent to the donation of their useful organs to other persons. In an effort to reach consensus on Article 62, the Executive Power will carry out an intense educational campaign to inform the general populace about the implementation of "presumed consent," and evidence will be required to show that 70 percent of adult citizens have been consulted according to the prescribed procedure.

The low degree of accomplishment of the opinion poll or the "obligatory consultation" for organ donation, which was carried out by the Enrolling Registry Office in February 2001, completely diminished this law's efficacy. This is why explicit consent is routinely sought from the deceased's family or, if absent, the judicial authority, each time the procurement team is called, after the death has been reported.

Another of the novelties of the 1993 law was the commitment of medical doctors who ought to report encephalic death cases. Not fulfilling this requirement in article 32 would end in a severe penalization with both a fine and professional license withdrawal. Nevertheless, in practice, deficient regulation by the Executive Power and the risk that its application would hamper effective implementation has led even the Sanitary Authority to avoid utilizing article 32.

Presently, in Buenos Aires Province, there is legislative debate over the creation of a procurement system that would provide the State with authority to act not only as prosecutor but also as coordinator and regulator of all transplant activity. It would also endorse the juridical and functional individuality of the different agents involved in it, as well as the non-governmental organizations of patients, recognizing their right to participate in its administration.

D. Commercialization of Organs and Tissues

Not all of the countries in the region have adopted regulations prohibiting commerce in organs and tissues, despite the likelihood that such trafficking will disproportionately burden those who live in poverty. Moreover, the failure to distinguish commerce in organs from compensation of donors for related costs has created a significant legislative and regulatory vacuum. The absence of a legal basis for donor compensation discourages potential donors, frustrates efforts to inform and educate the public about organ donation, and leaves the matter of compensation to private agreements between donors and recipients (Mainetti, 1987).

V. Other Issues

A. Ethics Committees and Commissions

A National Commission of Bioethics, chaired by the Ministry of Health and Social Welfare of the Nation, was created in December 1992 (Ministerio de Salud y Acción Social de la Nación). The Commission will consider general aspects of the impact of science and technology on the health care field and the development of bioethics as a discipline. Several public and private institutions were invited to send their representatives as members: the Supreme Court of Justice, the National Congress, the Secretariat of Science and Technology of the Nation, the National Academy of Sciences, and other academic and professional institutions. The goal of the Commission is to advise the Health Secretariat on specific issues in bioethics and medical ethics.

In 1996, Law 24.742 (Argentina, 1996) dictated that in every hospital of the public health system and social security there should exist, as long as its complexity allows it, a hospital ethics committee, which would provide assessment, study, teaching, and supervision functions of the research regarding ethical questions which might emanate from medical practice at the hospital.

The process of bioethics institutionalization has been growing in the different provincial states of the Argentinean Republic through laws that create Provincial Bioethics Commissions. For example, in Río Negro, Law 3099 (Provincia de Río Negro, 1997) created and regulated a Provincial Bioethical Committee, which then made judgments regarding bioethical research, analysis, and information in relation with the people's health "of social and sanitary interest" in that Province's territory.

Law 6507 of the Congress of the Province of Tucumán created hospital ethics committees in the six most important hospitals in the province. It stipulated that half of the membership of such committees should be physicians, with the other half professionals "related to ethics" such as philosophers, clergymen, lawyers, psychologists, and nurses. All should be "related" to the hospital. The committees will perform educative, consultative, and normative functions. They will not act as courts or be able to impose penalties (Provincia de Tucumán, Honorable Legislatura de Tucumán, 1993).

In like manner, Jujuy (Provincia de Jujuy, 1995) and Santa Fe are among the states that have legally permitted the creation of hospital ethics committees.

B. Ecosystem or Environment

The Province of Entre Ríos made a decisive step forward to the defense of the environment and the preservation of the ecosystem through a specific emergency protective judicial order against ... any decision, action, deed or omission of authority – administrative, judicial or legislative – public official or individual who might unlawfully harm, restrain, alter, hinder or impair the inhabitants' collective or diffuse interests with relation to the preservation, protection and conservation of the environment in an ample frame of possibilities for the defense of public health and environmental values recognized by the community (Provincia de Entre Ríos, 1996, article 1).

The action foreseen in the Law called "Of Environmental Protection" has a double end: protection and restoration. It is characterized by the broadness of active legitimization (any citizen) as well as by the expertise (any Judge or Chamber, without distinction of statute with jurisdiction in the place), and its course is short and simple; hence it would be positive that the remaining Argentinean provinces adopt analogous procedural remedies.

C. Argentina's Bioethics Directory

Asociación Argentina de Bioética
Facultad de Derechu, UNMDP
Fax: +54-223-491-1786
25 de Mayo 2855, piso 3
7600 Mar del Plata, Buenos Aires
www.aabioetica.org
hooftpf@infovia.com.ar

Centro Cuyano de Estudios Bioéticos
Ph: +54(361) 4291-1302; 4261 4835
Fax: +54(3 61)4261-532; 452 066; 211
Avellaneda 488
5221 Guaymallén
Mendoza

Centro de Estudios Bioéticos
Ph: +54(11) 4201-3153; 4201-7563

Av. Belgrano 763
1870 Avellaneda
Buenos Aires

Comisión Nacional de Etica Biomédica
Ph: +54(11)4438-16004

Secretaría
Av. 9 de Julio 1925, Piso 2-Of.209
Buenos Aires

Consejo de Médicos de la Prov. de Córdoba
Ph: +54(351) 4226-752/220-718

Comisión de Bioética
Ph: +54(351) 255-923
Obispo Trejo 661
5000 Córdoba

Consejo Latinoamericano de Ciencias
Sociales
Ph: +54(11) 4811-7317/4811-6588
Fax: +54(11) 4812-8459
Callao 875, Piso 3, Depto. E
1023 Buenos Aires

Fundación del Hosp. de Emergencia
Clemente Alvarez
Ph: +54(341) 4820- 016; 4 820-017;

Departamento de Etica y Bioética
Ph: +54(341) 4820-018
Rueda 1100
2000 Rosario

Fundación Dr. José María Mainetti
Ph: +54(221) 471-1160 int. 215

Instituto de Bioética y Humanidades
Médicas
+54(221)471-2222
Calle 508 (entre 116 y 118)
Email: elabe@satlink.com
B 1897 GPB Manuel B. Gonnet
La Plata, Buenos Aires

Cátedra de Etica Bioética de UNESCO
Ph: +54(11) 4322-7010
Florida 537, Piso 18
1005 Buenos Aires

Universidad Nacional de Buenos Aires
Ph: +54(11) 4432-2292

Centro de Investigaciones Eticas
Pueyrredón 480, Piso4
1406 Buenos Aires

Universidad Nacional de Córdoba
Ph: +54(351) 4602-918

Centro de Investigaciones en Humanidades
Médicas
Ph: +54(381) 4211-360

Centro de Bioética de Tucumán y el
Nordeste
Balcarce 680
San Miguel de Tucumán
Tucumán 4000

Colegio de Médico Distrito II
Ph: +54(482) 4201-7563; 201-3153

Fundación Fraternitas
Ph: +54(11) 4801-127/ 28/ 29/ 30
Moreno 1056
Email: frater@citynet-net.ar
2000 Rosario

Hospital Dr. José Penna
Ph: +54(291) 4813-300

Area de Bioética
Necochea y Lainez
Email: cracon@intersat-bb.com.ar
8000 Bahía Blanca
Buenos Aires

Hospital Iturraspe Comité de Bioética
Ph: +54(342)553-634
Av. Pellegrini 3551
3000 Santa Fé

Pontificia Universidad Católica Argentina
Ph: +54(11) 4345-5425 / 349-0334

Instituto de Etica Médica
Ph: +54(11) 4349-349-0284
Av. Adolfo Dávila 1400
Puerto Madero
1107 Buenos Aires

Universidad Austral
Ph: +54(341) 4307-307-4822

Centro Argentino de Bioética
Ph: +54(11)4361-1329
Av. Juan Garay 125
1063 Buenos Aires

Universidad del Salvador
Ph: +54(11) 4824-3681
Cátedra de Etica Bioética
Larrea 1234, Piso 5-A
1117 Buenos Aires

Universidad Nacional de Buenos Aires

Facultad de Ciencias Médicas
Pabellón Perú, Ciudad Universitaria
Estafeta 32
5000 Córdoba

Universidad Nacional del Noroeste
Ph: +54(381) 211-360

Facultad de Humanidades. Cátedra de Etica
Las Heras 727
3500 Resistencia
Chaco

Institutio de Bioética
Pontificia Universidad Cathólica
Argentina
Alberto Bochatey, Director
www.bioetica.com.ar
bioetica@uca.edu.ar
Ph: +54(11) 4349-0284

VI. Conclusion

This report presents a picture of some bioethical, biojuridical and biopolitical developments in Argentina, where, as in other Latin American countries, bioethics has become a field of new challenges. The particular historical setting, cultural *ethos*, and social reality of the Latin American region would infuse new life into the global bioethics community. In this sense, a symptom of the new time is the fact that the second World Congress of the International Association of Bioethics took place in Buenos Aires, Argentina, in 1994, and the sixth Congress will be held in Brasilia, Brazil, in 2002. A "New Brazilian Bioethics" or "Hard Bioethics" began to flourish in recent years, inspired by the country's contradictory social reality, in search of alternative perspectives to traditional bioethical currents (Garrafa, 2000). So, in this context, we can expect an increasing normative production throughout the region in the field.

Note

1. In 1990, The *Escuela Latinoamericana de Bioética – ELABE (Fundación Mainetti*, Argentina) organized its First International Seminar on Ethics Committees. This was the first regional effort to train professionals from Colombia, Uruguay, and Paraguay. The antecedent of this seminar in 1989 was a course on Health Care Ethics Committees, taught by Dr. Stuart Spicker, hosted in Gonnet, Argentina. The *Federación Latinoamericana de Instituciones Bioéticas (FELAIBE)* was created in December 1989. One of Dr. Spicker's aims was to foster the development of ethics committees in the region.

Bibliography

Argentina (1977). Ley 21.541.
Argentina (1987). Banco Nacional de Datos Genéticos, Ley 23.511. *Boletín Oficial de la República Argentina.*

Argentina (1989a). Ley 23.660.

Argentina (1989b). Ley 23.661.

Argentina (1990a). Decreto 358/90. Supplement to *Ley* 23.660.

Argentina (1990b). Decreto 359/90. Supplement to *Ley* 23.661.

Argentina (1990c). Ley SIDA, Ley 23.798.

Argentina (1990d). Ley 11.044/90. *Provincia de Buenos Aires*.

Argentina (1991). Decree No. 1244/91 of July 1, 1991. *Boletín Oficial de la República Argentina* July 8, 2.

Argentina (1993). Ley 24.193, March 24. *Boletín Oficial de la República Argentina*, April 26.

Argentina (1996). Ley 24.742. *Boletín Oficial de la República Argentina*, December 23.

Argentina. *Código Civil*, Articles 243 and 234 bis.

Britos, O. 1993. Proyecto de ley sobre fecundación humana asistida [Proposed law on IVF]. *H.C. Senadores* DAE, 151 (November 11), 1771.

Cafiero, J.P. 1993. Régimen legal para la procreación médicamente asistida [Legal regimen for medically assisted procreation]. *H.C. de Diputados*, 45 (July 1), 2272.

Capital Federal. 1991. *Cámara Nacional de Apelaciones en lo Criminal y Correccional, Sala 4, Fallo Plenario*, 91060552, November 29.

Corte Suprema de Justicia. 1993. *Causa B.605 XXII, Bahamondez, Marcelo s/Medida Cautelar*, April 6.

Drane, J.F., et al. 1991. Medical ethics in Latin America: a new interest and commitment. *Kennedy Institute of Ethics Journal* 1(4): 325-338.

Estévez Boero, G., Zamora, F. & Neri, A. Ley de protección humana en la investigación biomédica [Law for human protection in biomedical research]. *H.C. de Diputados* TP No. 44, 1686.

García Marañón, E., et al. 1990. *Aborto e Infanticidio. Aspectos Jurídicos y Médico – Legales*. Buenos Aires: Editorial Universidad.

Garrafa, V. 2000. A bioethical radiograph of Brazil, *Acta Bioethica* Año VI 1: 177-182.

Gómez, Miranda F. 1991. Régimen de técnicas interdisciplinarias de reproducción humana asistida [Regimen for interdisciplinary technique in assited human reproduction]. *H.C. de Dipuados* TP, 56 (July 23), 1949.

Honorable Cámara de Diputados de la Nación. 1991. Expediente 3369-D/91. *Trámite Parlamentario* 120, 3659.

Juzgado de Primera Instancia en lo Criminal y Correccional No. 3 de Mar del Plata. 1995. Emergency protective order dictated in: *Hospital Interzonal General de Agudos de Mar del Plata s/presentación*.

Mainetti, J.A. 1987. Bioethical problems in the developing world: a view from Latin America. *Unitas* 60, 238-248.

Mainetti, J.A., Pis Diez, G. & Tealdi, J.C. 1992. Bioethics in Latin America: 1989-1991. In: B.A. Lustig (ed.), *Bioethics yearbook: volume 2. Regional developments in bioethics: 1989-1991* (pp. 83-96). Dordrecht: Kluwer Academic Publishers.

Mainetti, J.A. 1995. Medical ethics, history. The Americas, Latin America. In: W. Reich (ed.), *Encyclopedia of bioethics* (pp. 1639-1644). New York: Macmillan.

Mainetti, J.A. 2004. Development of bioethics in Latin America. In: L.B. McCullough and R. Baker (eds), *A history of medical ethics*. Cambridge: Cambridge University Press.

Ministerio de Salud y Acción Social de la Nación, Secretaría de Salud (1992). Resolución No. 450, December 4.

Natale, A. & Antelo, J. 1991. Régimen de regulación de las técnicas de procreación que tengan por finalidad fundamental paliar la esterilidad humana [Regulation of reproductive techniques developed to palliate human sterility]. *H.C. de Diputados* TP, 145 (November 20), 4155.

Orquín, L. 1992. Proyecto de ley para regular la técnicas de reproducción humana [Proposed law to rule human reproductive techniques]. *H.C. Diputados* TP, 108 (September 29), 5784.

Proposed Law. 1996. Régimen de los derechos de los enfermos teminales [Regimen of terminal patients' rights], with favorable ruling by *Comisiones de Acción Social y Salud Pública, Legislación General y Legislación Penal de la Cámara de Diputados*. October 9, sanctioned by a minority *Diputados Dumon, Banzas de Moreau y Carrió*.

Provincia de Buenos Aires (1987). Ley No. 10592, October 22.

Provincia de Buenos Aires (1989). Ley No. 10836, September 28.

Provincia de Buenos Aires (1990a). *Suprema Corte de Justicia*. Fallo No. 90011057, April 3.

Provincia de Buenos Aires (1990b). Decree No. 1149 of April 6. *Boletín Oficial de la Provincia de Buenos Aires*, April 27, 2218-2221.

Provincia de Buenos Aires (1991). Ley 11.134, September 12.

Provincia de Buenos Aires (1992). Decree No. 3309 of November 11, 1992. *Boletín Oficial de la Provincia de Buenos Aires*, December 24, 7065-7066.

Provincia de Entre Ríos (1996). Ley 9032, sanctioned November.

Provincia de Jujuy (1995). Ley 4861, enacted November.

Province of Río Negro (1997a). Ley 3076. *Boletín Oficial de la Provincia de Río Negro*, April 4.

Provincia de Río Negro (1997b). Ley 3099, enacted June.

Provincia de Tucumán, Honorable Legislatura de Tucumán (1993). Ley No. 6507, November 29, 3298.

Ruckauf, C. 1993. Proyecto de ley de regulación de la aplicación de las nuevas técnicas de diagnóstico, terapéuticas, industriales y de investigación en la evolución biológica de la esp ecie humana y de su medio ambiente [Proposed law to rule new diagnostic, therapeutic, industrial and research techniques in biological evolution on humankind and environment]. *H.C. Diputados* TP, 81 (August 23), 3340.

Storani, C. & Laferrière, R.E. 1991. *Proyecto de Ley por el que se establecen normas para el uso de técnicas de reproducción humana asistida* [Proposed bill to establish normative for the use of reproductive assisted techniques]. *H.C. Senadores* DAE, 152 (November 20), 1718.

Tealdi, J.C. 1990. Proyecto Genoma Humano. ¿Quién nos Mide?, Submitted to: *II Jornadas Marplatenses de Bioética*. Mar del Plata, Argentina.

Tealdi, J.C. 1991. Banco Nacional de datos genéticos: El caso Laura/Laura, Presented at: *Ética en el Principio de la Vida, II Curso Internacional de Bioética, Escuela Latinoamericana de Bioética, Fundación Mainetti*. Argentina: Gonnet.

Tealdi, J.C., Pis Diez, G. & Esquisabel, O. 1995. Bioethics in Latin America: 1991-1993. In: B.A. Lustig (ed.), *Bioethics yearbook: volume 4. regional developments in bioethics: 1991-1993* (pp. 113-136). Dordrecht: Kluwer Academic Publishers.

Part III: Europe

6 Bioethics in France

Anne Bernard and Anne Fagot-Largeault

I. Introduction

In France, bioethics has become one of society's major challenges. Hundreds of books and articles on the subject provide ample evidence of this situation, as do the many conferences and debates organized every year.[1] A forthcoming revision of an innovative piece of legislation passed by the French Parliament in 1994, known as the "bioethics laws", is presently at the center of public debate and has intensified discussion. Discussion was already heated because of several events which mobilized public opinion: a nurse was brought to trial for committing euthanasia on some of her elderly patients; the National Consultative Ethics Committee for Health and Life Sciences (CCNE) published a report on euthanasia; the law on elective abortion was revised; and a judgment was pronounced by the *Cour de Cassation* (supreme court in the civil and criminal judicial system), the so-called "Arrêt Perruche" (2000).

The *Cour de Cassation* ruled that reparation should be made for prejudice suffered by a seriously handicapped child following his mother's undetected bout of rubella during pregnancy (2000). The alternative to that judgment, in the event compensation for the prejudice of a severely handicapped life, was the non-birth of the person concerned, since the mother could have considered termination of her pregnancy, if she had known she had rubella. By this action, the *Cour de Cassation* instigated a debate on the recognition of the rights and position of the handicapped in French society through an appeal for solidarity by a demonstration of effective support. However, the judgment prompted highly emotional reactions, since its enforcement raises many dilemmas and paradoxes, which no one had really thought through until then.[2] The handicapped themselves, their families and loved ones, and the associations representing them are all directly concerned and hurt by this injury to their dignity. They point out that the very existence of those born with a disability has been challenged.[3] The rules of conduct and practices of health care workers whose work involves them with parents during pregnancies will be directly confronted with the consequences of the judgment (Bienvault & Gomez, 2001; Dossier, "Arrêt Perruche", 2001). In some quarters it was thought that perhaps there should be legislation to prohibit certain handicapped lives from receiving compensation, so as to avoid discrimination. Others wondered whether the emerging right not to be born handicapped was acceptable, with its attendant risks of excessive elimination of fetuses and possibly of eugenic trends.[4] The Minister for Employment, Solidarity and Health referred the matter to the CCNE.[5]

II. Background

In the last twenty years, whenever the life sciences have advanced, researchers, physicians, and lawyers have been moved to call for the commitment of the political authorities on some of the issues arising. The first step was the creation of a National Consultative Ethics Committee for Health and Life Sciences (CCNE) in 1983 by the President of the French Republic. Later, after numerous preparatory studies starting in 1987-88, three "bioethics" laws were promulgated in 1994. These laws naturally attracted the attention of civil society so that there were calls for new changes in various fields, some of which will be raised in this article.

As regards bioethics, the most important institution is the CCNE, established by a decree signed by the President of the French Republic in 1983 and then enacted by law (Loi no. 94-654, 1994). The Committee's mission is "to give opinions on ethical problems raised by progress in the fields of biology, medicine and health and to publish recommendations on this subject". In March 1999, Didier Sicard was designated as its third president since CCNE's creation. All CCNE's Opinions are translated into English as a contribution to the international debate. The publication of CCNE's opinions and reports give rise to lively debate on the part of public opinion and professional circles. The various themes broached by CCNE will be referred to under each heading.

III. Topics

A. Bioethics in General

In July 1994, France gained bioethical legislation when Parliament approved a set of three laws on bioethics: a law regarding respect for the human body; a law on the donation and use of components and products of the human body, medically assisted reproduction and prenatal diagnosis; and a law on processing nominative data for use in health related research (Loi no. 94-548, 1994; Loi no. 94-653, 1994; Loi no. 94-654, 1994). These laws seem to be among the first items of legislation adopted on these subjects throughout the world.

The aim of French lawmakers was to define a set of principles and circumscribe practices. The guiding principles for the protection of human beings were given constitutional consecration by a decision of the *Conseil Constitutionnel* (in charge of verifying the conformity of laws with the French Constitution). They are now enshrined in the *code civil*, and they deal with the dignity of the person, the status of the human body, and the integrity of the human species.

The first principle underlying the laws on bioethics is safeguarding the dignity of the human person: "The law ensures the primacy of the person, prohibits any assault on a person's dignity, and guarantees respect for the human being from the beginning of his or her life."

The second principle establishes the rule that the human body is inviolable and is not a commodity: "The right to respect for the body is universal. The human body is inviolable. The human body, its components and products are not subject to property rights".

A final principle governs the aims of genetic research: "The integrity of the human species must always be respected. Any eugenic practice aiming at human selection is prohibited. With the exception of research intended to prevent and treat genetic diseases, no change can be made to genetic characteristics with the aim of altering human descent".

Legislators applied these three principles to several domains: the use of organs, tissues, and cells of human origin, research on the embryo, organizing medically assisted reproduction, and genetic studies.

Taking into account the evolutionary nature of science, the bioethics laws include a legal exception requiring that they be reviewed after five years, thus underscoring the difficulty of reconciling the progress of the life sciences and respect for the essential values necessary for the preservation of human dignity. Consequently, the bioethics laws were to be reviewed in 1999. This revision, still pending, was delayed for several reasons, and is eagerly awaited by doctors, researchers, and also society as a whole. There has been much protest over this delay, the consequences of which are tragic for patients awaiting organ transplantation who could be saved by live donors. Furthermore, the delay could be disastrous for French research teams which have been prevented so far from exploring new avenues such as embryonic stem cell research.[6]

The law provides that revision must start by an evaluation of the enforcement of existing laws by a Parliamentary bureau for the evaluation of scientific and technological decisions (OPECST, which is a new kind of structure within Parliament composed of Senators and Members of Parliament in equal numbers). This phase was completed in good time (Office parlementaire d'évaluation des choix scientifiques et technologiques, 1999). The consultative bodies, i.e., the *Conseil d'Etat* (supreme court of the administrative judicial system) (Conseil d'Etat, 2000), CCNE (Comité Consultatif National d'Ethique pour les sciences de la vie et de la santé, 1998), the *Académie de Médecine* (Académie nationale de médecine, 1998), and the Consultative Commission for Human Rights (CNDH) (Commission Nationale Consultative des Droits de l'Homme, 2000), also sent in their contributions. A fact-finding mission, preparatory to drafting the bill for the revision of the bioethics laws, was set up in the *Assemblée Nationale* (French Parliament) in May 2000.

On November 28, 2000, when he spoke at CCNE's annual ethics symposium, Lionel Jospin, the Prime Minister, described the main lines of a preliminary draft bill for reforming the bioethics laws (Jospin, 2000). In this document, reproductive cloning and the creation of embryos for the purpose of research are still prohibited. Research on the embryo is permitted in two cases: first, to improve medically assisted reproduction technology; and second, to seek new treatments using stem cells from spare embryos which are no longer wanted for planned parenthood. It authorizes therapeutic cloning and creates an Agency for Reproduction, Embryology, and Human Genetics. As regards transplantation, it relaxes existing restrictions on the use of live donor organs.

The main body of ethical debate raised by this draft bill is connected to research on human embryos and therapeutic cloning. Analysts have remarked that the government's text is rather pragmatic (and thus closer to British-style practicality), and that it officially opens the route to the reification of the embryo (Nau, 2001a; Nau, 2001b; Verspieren, 2000).

The government submitted the draft bill to CCNE and CNDH. CCNE (Comité consultative national d'éthique pour les sciences de la vie et de la santé, 2001), in a reply focusing on embryo research, repeated categorically and unanimously its previously stated position in favor of explicit prohibition of human reproductive cloning. With a broad consensus, CCNE made three points: the principle of prohibition of creating human embryos for research purposes, the introduction of an exception to that principle within the framework of evaluation of new medically assisted reproduction techniques, and the regulated possibility of using spare embryos for research, in particular as regards research on embryonic stem cells. On the issue of therapeutic cloning where the proposed text transgresses existing legislation (which posits that the creation of human embryos for any other purpose than their own development is prohibited), opinions within CCNE diverged. A majority was in favor of therapeutic cloning, mainly because of therapeutic expectations, a duty of solidarity with the ailing, and the globalization of research (Kahn, 2000; Petitnicolas, 2001). CNDH will accept authorizing supplementary, regulated opportunities for research on spare embryos, when the aim is evaluating new medically assisted reproduction techniques (Commission Nationale Consultative des Droits de l'Homme, 2001). However, in contradiction to CCNE, it is opposed to therapeutic cloning on the grounds that there is a need for caution and because of the pressure that might be exerted on women to supply oocytes.

In a speech delivered on February 8, 2001, however, Jacques Chirac, President of the French Republic, stated that he was hostile to therapeutic cloning, because he feared mercantile developments and the lures of reproductive cloning (Chirac, 2001). In opposition to the government view, this statement moves bioethics onto the political scene (Nau, 2001c, 2001d). After consulting the *Conseil d'Etat*, whose considerations were not made public, the government submitted a modified draft bill (Projet de loi relatif à la bioéthique) to the Ministers on June 20, 2001. The most salient change is the exclusion of therapeutic cloning and a proposal to authorize only research based on frozen spare embryos if they are no longer required for planned parenthood. On July 10, 2001, the group set up by the *Assemblée Nationale* produced a report, which concluded that research on the embryo under the control of an independent authority should be allowed, and that a public debate on therapeutic cloning should be organized (Mission d'information commune préparatoire au projet de loi de revision des "lois bioéthiques", 2001).

Present plans are that the *Assemblée Nationale* should give a first reading to the government's June 20 bill in early 2002.

B. *Professionalism*

The obligation of physicians to inform their patients is not new. It has long been part of the medical code of deontology (Ordre national des Médecins, 1995, 1998). However, there have been major changes in recent years, and doctor–patient relationships have evolved towards a spirit of greater partnership, based on increased respect for the patient as a person, solicitude in securing consent, and the patient's active participation in the selection of therapeutic options. These changes evolved originally because patients wanted them. Nowadays, patients are more knowledgeable about health and are more demanding than they used to be regarding the information provided to them. A general discussion on health in 1999 and a large number of public statements expressed complaints about the shortcomings of information supplied to patients, or of the role reserved for them, and patients claimed various kinds of rights, including access to medical files. This is one of the main demands at the moment (Etats généraux de la santé, 1999; Ligue nationale contre le cancer, 1999). The issue of information to patients is one of the principal themes contained in plans for a draft bill on modernization of the health care system (see below, section E).

Many publications, court decisions, reflections and writings have recently demonstrated the importance, and also the complexity, of this question, which can be considered from several angles and does not always give rise to a consensus.[7]

The medical code of deontology (Ordre national des Médécins, 1998, 1995) outlines the main principles of the obligation to inform. Physicians have a duty to provide faithful, clear, and appropriate information regarding the state of health, the medical investigations, and the treatment they intend to offer to those they examine, treat, or advise. The code states some limitations for certain patients who, in their best interests and for reasons which the physician must evaluate in all conscience, may be left in ignorance of an ominous diagnosis or prognosis.

Recent court decisions, the importance of which cannot be denied in view of the controversy and the changes in practices which ensued, established the obligation on physicians to inform patients even about severe or exceptionally rare risks. By these decisions, courts have reminded doctors and hospitals that they are under an obligation to provide evidence of their competence and that patients, in the name of the principle of autonomy, must be informed and recognized as actual participants in medical decision-making. The *Conseil d'Etat* has modified and refined its position on the obligation to inform patients in the public health care system (Conseil d'Etat, 2000). As regards private practice, which is within the jurisdiction of the *Cour de Cassation* (2000a), several decisions since 1997 have been influenced by evolving jurisprudence, along the same lines as in the *Conseil d'Etat*. Physicians are only relieved of the obligation to inform in cases of emergency and impossibility, or refusal by the patient to be informed. Recent jurisprudence, therefore, demands clear information giving the patient full freedom of choice based on knowledge of both his chances of recovery and any risk of disability or death connected to the treatment offered. In case of litigation, it is up to the physician – not the patient – to provide appropriate proof that he informed the patient of any risk connected to the treatment. The medical profession's problem at this point is pre-establishment of proof.

CCNE's Opinion no. 58 (1998) and the recommendations made by the *Agence Nationale d'Accréditation et d'Evaluation en Santé* (2000) (ANAES, National Agency for Accreditation and Evaluation in Healthcare) are reference documents on these issues. In its Opinion "Informed consent of and information to persons accepting care or research procedures" (Comité Consultatif National d'Ethique pour les sciences de la vie et de la santé, 1998b), CCNE wrote on the duty to inform. It emphasized that several factors at this time converge in the direction of total transparency for medical acts: official documents and evolving jurisprudence, the growing interconnection between research and care, the risk inherent to any medical act, and the demand for information from patients. It proposed a study on the possibility of giving everyone the right to choose for themselves a "representative" or agent whose task would be to speak for them to doctors at any time when they are unable to speak up for themselves and make decisions. CCNE stated that everyone should be presumed capable of being informed and giving free and enlightened consent to whatever the medical profession was proposing, unless it had been duly established that they were not competent to do so. Doctors and, more generally, health care providers must inform sufficiently, clearly, and appropriately for people to be able to exercise their freedom of choice and decision. As regards written proof of information provided, CCNE underlined the danger of excessive bureaucratization of the patient–doctor relationship.

The ANAES published recommendations for physicians concerning information to patients (Agence Nationale d'Accréditation et d'Evaluation en Santé, 2000). The object of these recommendations is to help the medical profession provide pertinent and high quality information. The ANAES sees information as a pivotal component of the physician–patient relationship, enabling the latter to make an active contribution to the care provided. Patients must receive clear, comprehensible, and appropriate information regarding their treatment and their state of health. Consent from patients and/or their loved ones is required for any procedure which concerns them. In an analysis of methods of information, the ANAES prefers oral transmission and sees written information as a possible complement. Information must meet quality criteria, i.e., be based on validated criteria, set out the expected benefits of treatment before possible drawbacks and risks, and include a list of critical risks, however exceptional.

C. Reproduction

1. *Termination of pregnancy.* The French government was concerned about rising figures for terminations and deemed it necessary to update the law on birth control (1967) and the one on elective abortion (called the *loi Veil*, 1975), since they are no longer completely adequate as regards social and medical realities.

In France, more than 200,000 elective abortions are performed every year. Nearly 10,000 adolescent girls are confronted with unwanted pregnancy, and 7000 of them resort to elective abortion. Up to 5000 women go to neighboring countries, because they are determined to terminate their pregnancies but are past the legal time limit which is presently in force as regards that procedure (Bajos, 2000).

After having requested research on the difficulty of access to elective abortion and the deficiencies of contraceptive action (Nizand, 1999; Uzan, 1998), the government produced a draft bill which *inter alia* included deferring the time limit from ten to twelve weeks of gestation and modified rights of access for minors. This initiative led to a flood of reactions from various philosophical, religious, medical, and political sources.[8] The government ascertained from the ANAES that there were no medical or safety objections to the limit being extended to twelve weeks (Agence Nationale d'Accréditation et d'Evaluation en Santé, 2001).

The Presidents of the Chambers of Parliament referred to CCNE very specifically as regards the risk of eugenic abuse as a result of this extension. This is because, for certain opponents to the draft bill, the ethical dimension of the legal extension from ten to twelve weeks resides in the fact that, as of the twelfth week, it becomes possible to use prenatal diagnosis to discover the sex of the child. In its reply (Comité Consultatif National d'Ethique pour les sciences de la vie et de la santé, 2000c), CCNE pointed out that this risk seemed unfounded, since an action which is limited to satisfying individual requests cannot be confused with eugenics. Arguing that knowing the sex of the child or of the existence of a minor anomaly is reason to refuse an extension of the legal limit, in the eyes of CCNE, is an insult to the dignity of women and couples. In response to some proposals preferring to broaden the scope for termination of a pregnancy on medical grounds, rather than to extend the time limit for termination, CCNE objected that this approach would be contrary to the spirit of the 1975 law which gave women the freedom to decide on terminating a pregnancy (Nizand, 2000).

The draft bill provided for a modification of rights of access to the possibility of termination for minors, to overcome difficulties encountered when parental consent is unavailable or for those who prefer to keep their condition secret. In such cases, the under-age girl could choose and designate an adult to accompany her.

When the draft bill was discussed, parliamentarians brought up the issue of sterilization for contraceptive purposes. Two CCNE reports in 1996 (Comité Consultatif National d'Ethique pour les sciences de la vie et de la santé, 1996a, 1996b; Giami & Leridon, 2000) had given spectacular impetus to this debate. The draft bill outlines a framework for masculine and feminine sterilization for contraceptive purposes for the benefit of any adult who so wishes, based on an expression of free, motivated, and deliberate will, on the basis of clear and complete information as to consequences. The procedure would be authorized for mentally retarded incompetent adults, if no other contraceptive method were possible. Sterilization could only be performed once a decision was made by the magistrate in charge of the case and after consulting with various authorities. This suggestion has caused much alarm among non-governmental organizations, who feared that this would be opening the door insidiously to sterilization of the disabled without their consent (Monroe, 2001).

The draft bill was adopted by the *Assemblée Nationale* on November 30, 2000, and was sent to the Senate, who opposed it in March 2001. They suggested that the more pathetic cases could be dealt with by medical termination of pregnancy. However, parliamentarians did not adopt the modifications requested by Senators, and after a second shuttle between *Assemblée Nationale* and *Sénat*, the bill was finally adopted by the lower house on May 31, 2001 (Projet de loi relative à l'interruption volontaire de grossesse et à la contraception, 2001).

Meanwhile, to avoid adolescent termination of pregnancy, a law which was definitively approved on December 13, 2000, permits the prescription and delivery of emergency contraceptives to under-age girls who do not wish to reveal their condition. In high schools, nurses may provide emergency contraception to under-age or adult pupils in compelling or clearly distressing situations (Loi no. 2000-1209, 2000).

"Therapeutic" termination of pregnancy is legal in France since the entry into force of the 1975 law on this subject, which was modified on May 31, 2001 (Loi no. 75-17, 1975; Projet de loi relative à l'interruption volontaire de grossesse et à la contraception, 2001). The law says that termination can be performed at any time providing two physicians testify that the pregnancy is a serious threat to the mother's health, or that there is a strong probability that the child will be born with a particularly severe impairment, known to be incurable at the time of diagnosis. One of the two physicians must be employed by a multi-disciplinary prenatal diagnosis center. The other must be on a list of experts recognized by the *Cour de Cassation* or an appellate court. The word "medical" has now in practice replaced "therapeutic", which puts more emphasis on the medical dimensions of the decision and the fact that no treatment is involved. In fact, the law on termination of pregnancy voted on May 31, 2001, gave the word legal recognition. Medical termination of a pregnancy implies the mother's freedom of decision, once she has been informed clearly, faithfully, and precisely by her doctor of risks involved if gestation continues. In some cases, the decision to terminate does not raise any special ethical issue when the prognosis is obviously lethal or particularly severe. However, when there is uncertainty as to medical diagnosis or prognosis, or in situations that are not purely medical, there are sometimes extreme individual ethical dilemmas, as can be seen from the reports of practitioners and moralists.[9] From a collective viewpoint, the most complex ethical problem that arises in cases of medical termination, because of the development and breakthroughs of prenatal predictive medicine and society's lack of acceptance of many of those who suffer from severe disability, is the connection with eugenics. This debate was given new impetus by the *Cour de Cassation's* recent judgment in the Perruche case (Cour de cassation, 2000b; Dossier "Arrêt Perruche", 2001).

Medical studies and the experience of parents have shown that the bereavement following the death of an unborn child (Authier-Roux, 1999; Delaisi de Parseval, Lett, Carbonne, et al., 1999; Haussaire-Niquet, 1998) is a very distressing consequence of medical termination, and that it requires sympathy and consideration. Reports of first-hand experience have shown the extent to which social and legal denial in this respect cause grief and aggravate the feeling of loss. (According to French law, no birth certificate can be issued for children born dead at less than six months of gestation: they are null and void, they are things that have no owner, their birth cannot be registered, and a funeral is out of the question.) Maternity wards are beginning to deal with the pain that the death of a child causes to the psyche, in particular when death occurs during pregnancy and by medical termination. Groups that include parents and health care professionals are working on how to get society to see things in a different light (Dupont & Fourcade, 2000; Fellous, 2001).

2. *Medically assisted reproduction (MAR)*. This section will only refer to the following subjects: preimplantation diagnosis, post-mortem embryo transfer, and anonymity.

(a) *Preimplantation diagnosis*. The 1994 law on bioethics authorizes the preimplantation diagnosis procedure, but it is very strictly controlled:

> Biological diagnosis based on cells sampled from *in vitro* embryos is only exceptionally authorized, and on the following conditions: a physician practicing in a multi-disciplinary prenatal diagnosis center must testify that the couple, in view of their family background, will very probably give birth to a child suffering from a particularly severe genetic disease, recognized as incurable at the time of diagnosis. Before diagnosis, the anomaly or anomalies causing such a disease must be identified in one of the parents. Diagnosis can only be performed in a facility specially approved for that purpose (Loi no. 94-654, 1994c).

There has been controversy at intervals on the ethical pertinence of this method, which is based on a classification of embryos (Glorion, 2000; Milliez, 1999; Munnich, 1999; Testard, 1999). It has been emphasized that such embryo classification is really eugenics and could be the prelude to more sophisticated procedures for the selection of individuals, but the majority opinion in France which believes that judicious use of this technique, keeping well within the legal framework and in connection with individual decisions, should avert the possibility of eugenic practices. In its Opinion no. 60, CCNE recognized the exceptional nature of this diagnosis. However, it noted the apparent contradiction in the text of the law between reference to the incurable nature of a disorder and the possibility of treating it (Comité Consultatif national d'Ethique pour les sciences de la vie et de la santé, 1998c). As much time passed before enabling documents were forthcoming, pre-implantation diagnosis is only just starting in France, and only three centers are authorized for the purpose. The first birth in France in November 2000 of a healthy baby after using this technique was unanimously applauded.

(b) *Reproduction post-mortem*. The debate on medically assisted reproduction post-mortem, which is a very special and extremely rare case but does give rise to philosophical and legal controversy, has resumed now that the bioethics laws are being revised. In spite of reluctance on the part of professional health care providers (Clément, 2001; Delaisi de Parseval, 1998; Salat-Baroux, 1998), CCNE, the *Conseil d'Etat*, and OPECST (Comité Consultatif National d'Ethique pour les sciences de la vie et de la santé, 1993, 1998c; Conseil d'Etat, 1999) all consider it permissible for a widow to request the transfer of frozen embryos, provided that the couple had already started medically assisted reproduction procedures before the death of spouse or partner. The circumstances surrounding the woman's request must be such that they guarantee a fully independent decision, unimpeded by any psychological or social pressures. CCNE's argument is mainly based on the notion that no person or authority can have equal or stronger rights than the mother over her own embryos. However, in the draft bill for the revision of the bioethics laws, the government does not reverse the decision made by the law in 1994, according to which medically assisted reproduction is reserved for the use of a couple composed of a living man and woman, and adds that if the couple no longer exists, this is sufficient to bar insemination or embryo transfer (Projet de loi relatif à la bioéthique, 2001).

(c) *Anonymity*. The bioethics laws, as regards medically assisted reproduction, stipulate that donors of gametes shall remain anonymous. Discussion is animated on this subject and simultaneously there seems to be a notable erosion of the principle of anonymity in public opinion.[10] Several reasons for this seem to converge. Efforts to keep secret the identity of the donor of gametes or of the couple donating the embryo create secrecy of affiliation for which anonymity is partly responsible. In particular, those who favor a psycho-analytical approach consider that anonymity could be harmful since any human being has a right to know where he or she comes from and what genetic identities made up the pattern to which he or she owes his or her life (Delaisi de Parseval; 1998). The obligation of anonymity would then be the ally of deceit and denial. Nevertheless, CCNE in its Opinion no. 60 (Comité Consultatif national d'Ethique pour les sciences de la vie et de la santé, 1998c) considers that there does not seem to be any new fact which argues in favor of removing the veil of anonymity for the gamete donor, but would like to see societal debate conducted on this point. In the same way, the *Conseil d'Etat* and OPECST does not question the principle of anonymity in medically assisted reproduction and call for public discussion (Conseil d'Etat, 1999; Office parlementaire d'évaluation de choix scientifiques et technologiques, 1999). Mandatory anonymity is not an issue in the draft revision of the bioethics laws (Projet de loi relatif à la bioéthique, 2001).

Anonymity and secrecy are particularly integrated in the procedure called "*accouchement sous X*" (both father and mother remain anonymous), which is a practice allowed by French law with the aim of protecting the life of the child and helping mothers to be delivered in a safe environment, albeit secretly. In the last few years, several associations of children born in these circumstances have emerged and they are active in demanding the right for children to be given information on their biological origins. Their arguments are based on article 7 of the International Convention for the Rights of Children. A commission (Dekeuwer-Defossez, 1999) recommends seeking solutions for reversing the

decision for secrecy. However, they also recommend retaining the possibility of anonymous birth in cases of extreme necessity and providing for mandatory dual permission,
from both mother and child, for the secret of biological origins to be lifted. The government has prepared a draft bill concerning access to personal data which recognizes both
the right to secrecy which may be useful to protect the mother giving birth in difficult circumstances, and the right to know one's origins (Projet de loi relatif à l'accès aux origins
personnelles, 2001a). It is based on the creation of a national council for access to personal data. This bill was adopted by the *Assemblée Nationale* on May 31, 2001.

D. Death and Dying

The extension of the life span, death becoming increasingly institutionalized in a medical
environment, the glaring shortage of palliative care facilities, the sometimes tragic situation
of people who have reached the end of their lives, and cases of clandestine euthanasia which
revealed to the public the distress of some health care providers, have combined to put life's
end very much at the center of public debate in France (Etats généraux de la santé, 1999).

The importance of palliative care was recognized in France in 1986 in a circular on the
organization of care and attention for terminal phase patients. A law in 1991 included
palliative care in the tasks incumbent on public hospitals. The authorities have taken steps
to develop palliative care, the most recent being a three-year project to combat pain in
1998. Despite such efforts, supply has continued to lag far behind demand.

There are no specific items of legislation regarding the end of life. In particular,
the criminal code of law does not cover euthanasia as such since it is simply a form of
crime. Since 1998, several events – death by active euthanasia of several public figures,
agitation arising out of prosecution of a nurse for clandestine euthanasia, reports from the
advocates of active euthanasia and assisted suicide (Malèvre, 1999; Montjardet, 1999;
Piccini, 1999), a manifesto signed by 132 well-known people supporting legalization of
euthanasia – have strongly intensified polemical stances adopted on a national scale by
the partisans of legalizing euthanasia and the upholders of palliative care. These two
groups, principally represented by the *Association pour le Droit de mourir dans la Dignité*
(ADMD) (Association for the Right to Dignified Death), on the one hand, and the *Société
Française d'Accompagnement et de Soins Palliatifs* (SFAP) (French Society for Palliative
Care) and the *Association Jusqu'à La Mort Accompagner La Vie* (JALMALV) (Caring for
Life until Death), on the other, are in violent conflict and irreconcilable opposition on their
respective concepts of the dignity of the sick, patient autonomy, respecting the founding
principles of humanity, the consequences of permissivity in ending life and the risk of
social and personal loss of concern for sickness and suffering.[11]

These events have prompted the authorities to ask the *Conseil Economique et Social*
and Senator Newirth to report on the situation as regards palliative care (Decisier, 1998;
Neuwirth, 1999). At the same time, parliamentarians have suggested that time in the
Assemblée Nationale should be set aside for a debate on the end of life, to denounce the
law of silence surrounding euthanasia, and to consider the drafting of legislation on
the subject. Discussion is ongoing in many other forums (Hollender, Pellerin, et al., 2000;
La Marne, Malaquin-Pavan, Nectoux, et al., 2000; Sicard, Denis, Fiat, et al., 1999).

In April 1999, bills were proposed to both Houses of Parliament, which soon led to the
adoption of a law on June 9, 1999, with a view to assuring access to palliative care (Loi

no. 99-477, 1999). The law states that "any sick person whose condition requires it, has a right to palliative care and attention. Palliative care is defined as active and continuing care dispensed by a multi-disciplinary team at home or in an institution. Its object is to alleviate pain, appease moral suffering, safeguard the dignity of the patient and give moral support to friends and family". Devoting a whole law to palliative care was designed to give it more impact in the eyes of health care providers and the public. It was also interpreted as meaning implicitly that euthanasia would not find a place in French law (Loi no. 99-477, 1999). For the partisans of palliative care, the law gives the stamp of official approval to palliative care facilities and to their triple mission, i.e., provide facilities all over French territory, provide training and information, and engage in specific research. They add that palliative care units in hospitals are also highly valuable symbols conveying the message that death is part of life. They insist on the importance of the presence of volunteers as a sign that civil society has become conscious of the need for care and attention with a social and not exclusively medical dimension.

In March 2000, CCNE published a report on "End of life, ending life, euthanasia" (Comité Consultatif National d'Ethique pour les sciences de la vie et de la santé, 2000a), in which it situated these issues in the context of significant changes in Western societies, as regards their outlook on death and their modes of moral or medical support to be provided to the dying. In this report, CCNE began by strongly encouraging convincing efforts to implement policies for palliative care, assistance to the dying, and rejection of aggressive and futile life-prolonging efforts. It went on to examine the question of active euthanasia, and considered that certain extreme cases and twilight situations would continue to be a problem. Finally, it denounced the hypocrisy and stealth covering certain ongoing practices. Distancing itself from the two partisan positions described above, CCNE broached the problem from another angle and suggested a "joint commitment" based on formal respect of the patient's autonomy as evidenced by an authentic request, consensus between the patient, loved ones, and health care providers, and collegial decision. It stated that ending life should remain a transgression and rejected the idea of legalizing euthanasia. However, the adoption of the joint commitment could be translated into law as a "plea for euthanasia", which would give courts the use of a legal instrument to solve the dilemma created up till now by the breach between law and human reality.

Publication of the CCNE report raised an absolute storm in the media (Bernard & Sicard, 2000), gave renewed vigor to controversy on euthanasia, on the medical environment at the end of life, on respect for life, and the right to die with dignity. There was a flurry of comment and reactions of every kind. At one extreme, SFAP, in particular, protested vehemently, as did practitioners and advocates of palliative care who were alarmed by changes in policy which could lead to making euthanasia an ordinary event. At the other, ADMD, in particular, approved the report. Midway, reservations were expressed with varying degrees of forthrightness or reticence by certain political leaders, representatives of the various faiths, and members of the medical profession – in particular medical resuscitation specialists.[12] The headline of a daily newspaper Le Monde (Nau, 2000), "Plea for euthanasia versus palliative care", is a perfect illustration of the crisis brewing around the antagonistic pair: palliative care and euthanasia. The polemic raged for several months but did have the advantage of provoking an effort to gain better understanding of the subject of euthanasia, in particular on the part of those committed to palliative care (Dossier "Euthanasie", 2001; Hérouville, Schaerer, Hocquard, et al., 2000).

The issue of programmed end of life decisions in neonatal care is viewed as one of the most difficult to contend with in the field of biomedical ethics. Until very recently, the matter was not much discussed in France, but it is of particular importance because of the position adopted by French resuscitation specialists that the fetus and neonate, at any gestational age and regardless of birth weight, are fully entitled human beings. As a result, systematic standby resuscitation is the rule (Cuttini, Nadai, Kaminski, et al., 2000). The advantage of that position is to maximize the chances of survival, but the drawback is that it creates the problem of lives for which at some point it may become necessary to decide whether resuscitation should be discontinued. For a long time, physicians involved in such decisions were hesitant about making them known to the public, so that this was a some-what solitary responsibility. Collective reflection gradually developed within neonatal care and pediatric resuscitation teams, supplemented by multidisciplinary groups and various publications.[13] Pediatricians broadened the debate by referring the matter to CCNE. The Committee, in "Ethical considerations regarding neonatal resuscitation" (CCNE, 2000b), suggested preferring a humane non-dogmatic approach to solve dilemmas on a case-by-case basis, depending on the condition of the child and the wishes of parents. It also spoke in favor of responsible ethics and insisted on an obligation for doctors to prevent and limit the occurrence of the more dramatic situations that lead to medical decisions to end life. The role of parents, which the CCNE report considers at some length, is still a crucial and topical problem (CCNE, 2000b; Dehan, Devictor, Grassin, et al., 2001; Fédération nationale des pédiatres néonatologistes, 2001). In conclusion, CCNE underlined the dearth of social investment in caring for handicapped children and called on society to shoulder responsibility in this respect. The national federation of neonatal pediatricians referred to CCNE's thoughts in recommendations they published on perinatal end of life decisions in December 2000 (Fédération nationale des pédiatres néonatologistes, 2001; Ropert, 2001).

The lack of coherence between prenatal and postnatal epochs as regards the contrasted status of a fetus and a neonate in the eyes of the law complicates the matter further. However advanced the gestation, the law authorizes medical termination of pregnancy. But if a severely damaged child is born, the doctor may no longer legally decide to end life. Certain pediatricians plead in favor of ethical equality for the fetus and the neonate and would like legislation regulating discontinuation of resuscitation on the same lines as the law on medical termination of pregnancy (Grassin, 2001).

E. Access to Health Care

Equitable access to care, respect for individuals, and social solidarity are the major principles underlying the health care system of France. Many health indicators (mortality, life expectancy, regression of major pathologies) show that France enjoys a high quality of health care. The system, however, has its faults and is not of consistent quality. In particular, it does not always take sufficient account of regional and social inequalities.[14] The health of the more deprived is still one of the country's major problems. Healthcare for everyone continues to be the crucial cohesive aim of France's social protection system. To achieve this, in 1998 the government presented a law to combat exclusion (Loi no. 98-657, 1998) which confirms the social mission of hospitals and supports systematic regional planning so that the most deprived can have access to preventive medicine and care. On

July 27, 1999, another law came as a complement to provide medical insurance for all (*couverture maladie universelle* – CMU), which gives everyone protection through a mandatory sickness insurance scheme, and, for the particularly needy, there is the added guarantee of complimentary insurance to cover full costs with no advance payment by the insured person. However, access to medical help for certain sectors of the population, such as handicapped adults, impoverished elderly citizens, and foreigners continues to be very limited.

Increasing health care expenditure has made it clear in recent years that, although care for everyone is a necessity, the national health insurance system cannot pay for every possible kind of treatment. National conferences on the subject (see below) are being organized to help government and Parliament define health priorities, on the basis of regular studies made by the *Haut Comité de la Santé Publique* (High level Committee on Public Health), whose mission it is to provide assistance for decision makers to improve public health by enhanced observation of the general state of health of the population and contributing to a definition of the aims of the health care policy (Haut Comité de la Santé Publique, 2000).

1. *Ethics of collective health decisions.* In 1998, CCNE chose to study the collective health decisions from an ethical angle, in other words, how to make the best and most equitable use of resources available for health care. In its report "Technical progress, health and societal models: the ethical dimension of collective choices" (1998a), CCNE noted to begin with that, since health care policy choices must of necessity integrate financial constraints, the principle of cost containment arouses ethical speculation and apprehension. There are fears that economic considerations will dictate policy, and that individual users will be the losers as regards access to health care. CCNE considered that no *a priori* ethical judgment should be made regarding the increasing cost of health, and that it was reasonable to reflect on the optimal distribution and use of health care resources. That need not and should not challenge accepted concepts such as the right to health care, respect for human dignity, nor accepted values of solidarity, justice, and equity to which French society is attached. The Committee proposed several points for consideration:

(a) Rejecting any notion of developing implicit criteria for selection of those who have a right to health care and those who do not;
(b) Organizing a mediation procedure so that citizens could raise health care problems; steps for the correction of any inequality being a priority;
(c) Giving renewed emphasis to prevention;
(d) Refining the definition of health care needs, both as regards the present and predictable future developments in supply and demand. Society should also attempt to analyze the contents of health aspirations;
(e) Evaluating health care needs, the effectiveness of procedures, and the true dimensions of risks, should lead to giving pride of place to the development of medical evaluation, which is absolutely necessary.

2. *Health and democracy.* Publication of a report called *"La santé en France"* (Health in France) by the *Haut Comité de la santé publique* (High level committee for public health) in 1994 was an essential step on the way to increased democracy as regards health. Using this report as a starting point, the Ministry of Health asked each French region to reflect on health priorities. This led to the creation of regional health care conferences, which became official in April 1996 with the publication of an order that contained a section on the "rights

of patients". This was a novelty. The first *Conférence Nationale de Santé* (CNS, National Health Conference) was held in September 1996. It drew on regional contributions and proposed priorities for public health. An examination of ethical issues led to setting three basic principles when health priorities are determined: respect for human dignity, the need to integrate solidarity into the analysis of health needs, and efficiency.

The health conferences referred to above were mostly designed as a forum for health care providers and regional representatives of associations concerned with health and social services, whereas the general conference is the result of a policy which seeks directly to include French civil society in a debate on the organization of the health system along democratic principles. The General Conference on Health took place in 1998-99 (Etats généraux de la santé, 1999). French public opinion took a keen interest, thus demonstrating a strong desire for public debate on these subjects. Regional and thematic summary reports on discussions and events led to various proposals being adopted as a priority, e.g., give the individual rights of health system users the benefit of legal protection and arrive at truly significant user participation. Public opinion is increasingly concerned with reinforcing the rights of users of the health system (Brocas, Le Coz, Ghadi, et al., 2000; Denis, 2000; Durand-Zaleski & Jolly, 1999). When a survey is made of fundamental rights as set out in numerous official documents (the code of medical practices, the code of civil law, the code of criminal law, the code of public health), these rights are not highly visible. There are several reasons for this: references are widely scattered as well as rather obscure and there are many exceptions. In practice, it is difficult to exercise such rights and user associations have had cause to complain.

In the circumstances, and taking into account the conclusions of the general health conference and of the National health conferences, the government has created a working group on user participation at various levels within the health system (Caniard, 2000) and has announced further legislation. The first two headings of a preliminary draft bill on modernizing the health system were published in July 2000. This document reaffirms patients' rights: respect for human dignity, protection of the integrity of the human body with, as its corollary, the right of consent to any medical procedure, the principle of non-discrimination based on state of health, the existence of a handicap, or according to genetic heritage, as well as respect for privacy and medical confidentiality. Procedures for the information of patients include *inter alia* patient access to personal medical files, which is viewed as particularly characteristic of the spirit of the bill (Denis, 2000). The draft also gives recognition to the role and status of patient and user associations within the health system. Title III, which deals with therapeutic risk and compensation for it, was the subject of fierce inter-ministerial discussion, and finally the Prime Minister approved it in principle in June 2001. This draft bill, which is viewed as essential so that the democratic process can move forward, has in fact been pending for months. However, it was finally sent to the *Conseil d'Etat* in July 2001 and could come before Parliament in the fall of 2001.

3. *Safety and health care.* In just a few years, safety has become an important component of health policies, and the same is true of prevention or the organization of care. Following recent medical and industrial tragedies (e.g., contaminated blood and mad cow disease), safety is viewed as a collective right which authorities are duty bound to ensure by appropriate organization and supervision. This being a state priority and one of its essential missions, a law was voted on July 1, 1998. The law aims to reinforce vigilance and

supervision as regards the sanitary condition of products designed for human consumption (Loi no. 98-535, 1998), and sets up various structures for this purpose. These bodies, which are somewhat of an innovation in the public health system, are not univocal. The organizations now existing (<www.sante.gouv.fr>) are:

- The *Agence Nationale d'Accréditation et d'Evaluation en Santé (ANAES)* (National Agency for Health Accreditation and Evaluation)
- The *Institut de Veille Sanitaire* and specific agencies (Institute of Sanitary Supervision)
- The *Agence Française de Sécurité Sanitaire des Aliments* (French Agency for the Safety of Foodstuffs)
- The *Agence Française de Sécurité Sanitaire des Produits de Santé* (French Agency for the Sanitation and Safety of Health Products)
- The *Etablissement Français des Greffes* (French Transplantation Establishment)
- The *Etablissement Français du Sang* (French Blood Transfusion Establishment)
- The *Office de Protection contre les Rayonnements Ionisants* (Bureau for Protection against Ionizing Radiation)
- The *Agence de Sécurité-Environnement* (Agency for the Safety of the Environment)

A national health safety committee comprises all the competent authorities in this field and is in charge of overall coordination of public action.

F. Ethics Consultation and Committees

1. *In research*. In 1998, the Minister for Education, Research, and Technology asked that thought be given throughout the system and at all levels on the possible ethical consequences of various research efforts and their repercussions on the ecology. The potential for risk and acceptability for society (Allègre, 1998) were to be included in the process. He therefore suggested that each of the organizations concerned should set up an Ethics Committee, whose opinions and reports would be made public, and that they should take whatever steps were necessary to organize public debate or information.

As a result, the *Institut National de Recherche Agronomique* (INRA, National Institute for Agronomic Research), the *Centre National de la Recherche Scientifique* (CNRS, National Center for Scientific Research), the *Institut de Recherche pour le Développement* (IRD, Research Institute for Development), and the *Institut National de la Santé et de la Recherche Médicale* (INSERM, National Institute for Health and Medical Research) have each set up their own ethics committee in the last two years.[15] Some of these committees have published reports on subjects which researchers wanted to explore. Others prefer to work on education, discussion, and training policies, in the hope of provoking greater mindfulness of ethical problems arising out of research. These various committees should be able to network with each other and create links with equivalent European bodies. In the same way, whereas there is no institutional link between CCNE and these committees, they would intend to refer to CCNE, in case of need.

As for CNRS, they had created as early as 1991 an operational committee for ethics in the life sciences called COPE, with the mission of identifying and analyzing the ethical concerns of research workers in those fields and helping them to solve any difficulties which might arise, in particular, because of the implementation of the bioethics laws (<www.cnrs.fr/SDV/cope.html>).

As regards biomedical research on humans, clinical tests are governed by the December 1988 law regarding the protection of people who consent to such research. More than ten years after enactment, its usefulness remains undisputed. As a result of this law, consultation committees for the protection of people engaged in biomedical research were created throughout the country. They play a key role for the enforcement of the law, since they must be consulted whenever clinical trials are organized (Fagot-Largeault, 2000; Huriet, 2001).

2. *In hospitals.* In 1996, the Paris public hospitals (AP-HP) created an Ethics Forum (*Espace Ethique*) which is intended for the discussion of the ethical dimension of medical practices. Since that time, the *Espace Ethique* has considerably amplified its activities as regards reflection, training, and education, and has created a great number of groups for discussion and dialogue. To encourage and coordinate the pooling of experience and research on ethics of health care in public hospitals, the Paris hospitals mentioned above and the *Assistance Publique des Hôpitaux de Marseille* (public hospitals in Marseilles) created a national federation for ethics and hospital care.

There are also so-called regional ethics committees and hospital ethics committees. Some of them were created as early as the 1980s. It is difficult to arrive at a full census since they have no legal status.[16] In the main, they have chosen to focus on assisting medical decision making, as well as reflection and information on health and health care. These committees have now all grouped together to form a more permanent organization which could give them better official visibility.

Finally, Bernard Kouchner, Minister for Health, created a mission for the development of clinical ethics in May 2001. This was to respond to aspirations for an authentic doctor–patient partnership when medical decisions need to be made.

IV. Conclusion

Although many subjects not included in this survey (biomedical research, organ transplantation, AIDS, genetics) are in fact the subject of in-depth consideration, public debate has mainly focused – as we have attempted to relate – on the subjects which are the subject of revision in the bioethics laws.

Furthermore, the medical crises that unsettled French public opinion in recent years have triggered numerous discussions on the principle of precaution, which is mentioned in the 1995 law on the reinforcement of protection of the environment and its consequences on public health. The right to respect of the environment is emerging as a demand on the part of civil society. Protection of the environment and environmental ethics is increasingly a concern of French public opinion (Fagot-Largeault, 2000). "Humanistic ecology" could be a policy for the future, based on the definition of collective ethics so that decisions are mindful of the rights of future generations (Chirac, 2001b).

Notes

1. Baud, 2001; Canto-Sperber, 2001; Dinechin, 1999; Ferry & Vincent, 2000; France-Adot, 1999; Gavarini, 2001; Gouyon, Lecourt, Memmi, et al., 1999; Kahn, 2000a; Mattei, 2000a;

Mehl, 1999; Meyer, 2000; Postel-Vinay & Corvol, 2000; Sicard, 1999; Thiel & Thévenot, 1999; Vacquin, 1999.

2. Aynès, 2001; Dossier: Arrêt Peruche, 2001; Dreifuss-Netter, 2001; Gomez, 2001; Labrusse-Riou & Mathieu, 2000; Pedrot, 2000.

3. Barral, Blanc, Chauvière, et al., 1999; Gomez, 2001; Moyse, 2000b; Pech & Sedar, 2000.

4. Dossier: Arrêt Peruche, 2001; Dreifuss-Netter, 2001; Mattei, 2000b; Moyse, 2000b; Pech, 2001.

5. Opinion no. 68 "Congenital handicaps and prejudice", adopted by the National Consultative Ethics Committee on May 29, 2001, was made public on June 15, and is available in English (www.comite-ethique.fr/english/avis_68.htm).

6. Biétry, 2000; Bourguet, 1999; Clément, 2001; Feuillet-Le-Mintier, 1999; France-Adot, 1999; Gobert, 1999; Hirsch, Espace Ethique, 1999b; Levy, Brunet, Bellivier, et al., 2000; Lignieres-Cassou, 2001; Montagut, 1999; Neirinck, 1998; Ordre national des Médecins, 1998a; Salat-Baroux, 1998; Sève, Taguieff, Thomas, et al., 1999.

7. Dupont & Fourcade, 2000; Durand-Zaleski & Jolly, 1999; Hirsch, Espace Ethique, 1999a; Maziau, 1999; Ponchon, 1999; Sicard, Esper, Sargos, et al., 2000; Verspieren, Sargos, Farbre-Magnan, et al., 2000.

8. Bessis, 2000; Canto-Sperber, 2000; Clermont, 2000; CPCEV, 2000b; Sicard, 2000; Sureau, 2000.

9. Glorion, 2000; Milliez, 1999; Moyse, 2000a; Munnich, 1999; Testard, 1999a.

10. Clément, 2001; Delaisi de Parseval, 1998; Gaumont-Prat, 1999; Gosme-Seguret, Golse, David, et al., 1999; Lesaulnier, 1998.

11. Abvien, Chardot, & Fresco, 2000; Dagognet, 1999; Dinechin, 1999; Kahn, 2000a; Kermarec, Natali, Camberlein, et al., 1999; La Marne, Malaquin-Pavan, Nectoux, et al., 2000; Montjardet, 1999; Moyse, 2000a; Sicard, 1999; Sicard, Denis, Fiat, et al., 1999; Verspieren, Sargos, Farbre-Magnan, et al., 2000.

12. CPCEV, 2000a; Legros, 2001; Ricot, 2000; Sicard, Desfosses, Verspieren, et al., 2000; Verspieren, 2000a.

13. Dehan, Devictor, Grassin, et al., 2001; Germain, 1999; Golse, Gosme-Seguret & Mokhtari, 2001; Grassin, 2001.

14. Cayla & Verkindt, 1999; Joubert, Chauvin, & Facy, 2001; Leclerc, Fassin, Grandjean, et al., 2000; Sailly, 1999.

15. Comité Consultatif de déontologie et d'éthique, 2000; Comité d'éthique et de precaution, 2000; Comité de réflexion et d'animation en éthique de l'Inserm, 2000; Toulouse, 1998.

16. Arnoux, 2001; Feuillet-Le-Mintier, 1999; Michaud, 1999; Mino, 1999.

Bibliography

The bibliography is far from being exhaustive. We tried principally to list official texts and some of the most relevant references. The laws are available on the website: www.legifrance.gouv.fr or at *Journal Officiel de la République française*, 26 rue Desaix, 75015 Paris, France (Telephone: 33 1 40 58 76 00). *La Croix, Le Figaro, Le Monde*, and *Libération* are national daily newspapers.

Abiven, M., Chardot, C. & Fresco, R. 2000. *Euthanasie: alternatives et controverses*. Paris: Presses de la Renaissance.

Académie nationale de médecine. 1998. Propositions pour la révision des lois du 29 juillet 1994. *Bulletin de l'Académie nationale de Médecine* 6: 1273-1290. [On-line] Available: <www.academie-medecine.fr>.

Agence Nationale d'Accréditation et d'Evaluation en Santé. 2000. Information des patients: recommandations destinées aux médecins. [On-line] Available: <www.anaes.fr>.

Agence Nationale d'Accréditation et d'Evaluation en Santé. 2001. Prise en charge de l'interruption volontaire de grossesse jusqu'à 14 semaines. [On-line] Available: <www.anaes.fr>.

Allègre, Cl. juillet 1998. "Pour une rénovation de la politique de recherche".

Arnoux, I. 2001. La fonction éthique dans les comités d'éthique hospitaliers: la situation française. *Revue générale de Droit Médical* 5: 9-34.

Authier-Roux, F. 1999. *Ces bébés passés sous silence: à propos des interruptions médicales de grossesse.* Ramonville-Saint-Agne: Eres.

Aynès, L. 2001. Malheur et préjudice, *Le Monde*, 31 janvier.

Bajos, N. 2000. *Accès à la contraception et à l'IVG en France: premiers résultats de l'enquête GINE.* France: Inserm.

Barral, C., Blanc, A., Chauvière, M., et al. 1999. Quelle place pour les personnes handicapées? *Esprit* 12: 5-106.

Baud, J.-P. 2001. *Le droit de vie et de mort – Archéologie de la bioéthique.* Paris: Alto/Aubier.

Bernard, A. & Sicard, M.-N. 2000. Observations et réflexions sur la couverture presse du rapport no. 63 du CCNE. *Les Cahiers du CCNE* 24: 3-10.

Bessis, R. 2000. N'allongez pas le délai d'IVG – Cesbron P.: Douze semaines … seule la souffrance compte. *Libération*, 3 octobre.

Bienvault, P. & Gomez, M. 2001. L'arrêt Perruche inquiète les échographistes. *La Croix*, 7 mars.

Biétry, M. 2000. La révision des lois de bioéthique se fait attendre. *Le Figaro*, 19 avril.

Bourguet, V. 1999. *L'être en gestation: réflexions éthiques sur l'embryon humain.* Paris: Presses de la Renaissance.

Brocas, A.-M., Le Coz, G., Ghadi, V., et al. 2000. La démocratie sanitaire. *Revue Française des Affaires Sociales* 54: 5-126.

Caniard, E. 2000. *La place des usagers dans le système de santé.* Rapport au secrétariat d'Etat à la santé et à l'action sociale.

Canto-Sperber, M. 2000. L'IVG à douze semaines: loi libérale et exigence morale. *Le Monde*, 19 septembre.

Canto-Sperber, M. 2001. *L'inquiétude morale et la vie humaine.* Paris: Presses Universitaires de France.

Cayla, J.-S. & Verkindt, P.-Y. 1999. Santé et exclusion: l'accès aux soins et la politique de santé publique; la santé des personnes les plus démunies et le rôle des organismes sociaux. *Revue de Droit Sanitaire et Social* 35: 407-428.

Chirac, J. 2001. *Allocution lors de l'ouverture du forum mondial des biotechnologies.* [On-line] Available: <www.elysee.fr>, 8 février.

Chirac, J. 2001. *Discours sur l'environnement.* [On-line] Available: <www.elysee.fr>, 3 mai.

Clément, J.-L. 2001. Les dons d'embryons ne se conçoivent pas. *Libération*, 15 janvier.

Clermont, J.-A. 2000. L'avortement ne doit pas être banalisé. *Le Monde*, 14 octobre.

Comité consultatif de déontologie et d'éthique, Institut de Recherche pour le Développement. 2000. [On-line] Available: <www.ird.fr>.

Comité Consultatif National d'Ethique pour les sciences de la vie et de la santé. 1993. *Opinion on the transfer of embryos after the decease of a husband or partner,* no. 40, [On-line]. Available: <www.comite-ethique.fr/english/avis/a_40.htm>.

Comité Consultatif National d'Ethique pour les sciences de la vie et de la santé. 1996a. *Opinion on the contraception for the mentally handicapped,* no. 49, [On-line]. Available: <www.comite-ethique.fr/english/avis/a_49.htm>.

Comité Consultatif National d'Ethique pour les sciences de la vie et de la santé. 1996b. *Report on sterilisation considered as a means of permanent contraception,* no. 50, [On-line]. Available: <www.comite-ethique.fr/english/avis/a_50.htm>.

Comité Consultatif National d'Ethique pour les sciences de la vie et de la santé. 1998a. *Technical progress, health and societal models: the ethical dimension of collective choices,* no. 57, [On-line]. Available: <www.comite-ethique.fr/english/avis/a_57.htm>.

Comité Consultatif National d'Ethique pour les sciences de la vie et de la santé. 1998b. *Informed consent of and information to persons accepting care or research procedures*, no. 58, [On-line]. Available: <www.comite-ethique.fr/english/avis/a_58.htm>.

Comité Consultatif national d'Ethique pour les sciences de la vie et de la santé. 1998c. *Re-examination of the law on bioethics*, no. 60, [On-line]. Available: <www.comite-ethique.fr/english/avis/a_60.htm>.

Comité Consultatif National d'Ethique pour les sciences de la vie et de la santé. 2000a. *End of life, ending life, euthanasia*, no. 63, [On-line]. Available: <www.comite-ethique.fr/english/english/avis/a_63.htm>.

Comité Consultatif National d'Ethique pour les sciences de la vie et de la santé. 2000b. *Ethical considerations regarding neonatal resuscitation*, no.65. [On-line]. Available: <www.comite-ethique.fr/english/avis/a_65.htm>.

Comité Consultatif National d'Ethique pour les sciences de la vie et de la santé. 2000c. *CCNE's response to the President of the Sénat and to the President of the Assemblée nationale regarding extension of the gestational age limit for elective abortion*, no. 66. [On-line]. Available: <www.comite-ethique.fr/english/avis/a_66t.htm>.

Comité consultatif national d'éthique pour les sciences de la vie et de la santé. 2001. *Opinion on the preliminary draft revision of the laws on bioethics (Referral by the Prime Minister)*, no.67. [On-line]. Available: <www.comite-ethique.fr/english/avis/a_67.htm>.

Comité d'éthique et de précaution. 2000. *Rapport d'activités 1999-2000*. Paris: Institut National de la Recherche Agronomique.

Comité de réflexion et d'animation en éthique de l'Inserm. 2000. *Décision du 13 septembre 2000*, Institut National de la Santé et de la Recherche Biomédicale, [On-line]. Available: <www.inserm.fr>.

Commission Nationale Consultative des Droits de l'Homme. 2000. *Avis portant sur la révision des lois de 1994 sur la bioéthique*.

Commission Nationale Consultative des Droits de l'Homme. 2001. *Avis portant sur l'avant-projet de loi tendant à la révision des lois relatives à l'éthique biomédicale*.

Conseil d'Etat. 1999. *Les lois de bioéthique: cinq ans après*, La Documentation française [On-line]. Available: <www.conseil-etat.fr>.

Conseil d'Etat. Décision no. 198530 2000 [On-line]. Available: <www.conseil-etat.fr>.

Conseil Permanent de la Conférence des Evêques de France. 2000. *Un compromis impossible* [On-line]. Available: <www.cef.fr>.

Conseil Permanent de la Conférence des Evêques de France. 2000. *Respecter la vie humaine en ses commencements* [On-line]. Available: <www.cef.fr>.

Cour de cassation. 2000. Arrêt 1157 FS-P, 20 juin.

Cour de cassation: Arrêt no. 457P sur le pourvoi no. N99-13.701, 17 novembre 2000.

Cuttini, M., Nadai, M., Kaminski, M., et al. 2000. End-of-life decisions in neonatal intensive care: physicians' self-reported practices in seven European countries. *The Lancet* 355: 2112-2118.

Dagognet, F. 1999. *La mort vue autrement*. Paris: Synthelabo Les Empêcheurs de penser en rond.

Decisier, D. 1998. *L'accompagnement des personnes en fin de vie*, Conseil Economique et Social [On-line]. Available: <www.conseil-economique-et-social.fr>.

Dehan, M., Devictor, D., Grassin, M., et al. 2001. Commentaires sur le rapport du CCNE Réflexions éthiques autour de la réanimation néonatale. *Les Cahiers du CCNE* 26: 19-35.

Dekeuwer-Defossez, F. 1999. Rénover le droit de la famille : propositions pour un droit adapté aux réalités et aux aspirations de notre temps. *La Documentation française*.

Delaisi de Parseval, G. 1998. Secret et anonymat dans l'assistance médicale à la procréation avec donneur de gamètes. *Médecine et Droit* 30: 23-30.

Delaisi de Parseval, G., Lett, D., Carbonne, B., et al. 1999. *L'euthanasie fœtale*. Paris: Esprit du Temps.

Denis, J.-J. 2000. *L'accès au dossier médical et les droits de la personne malade*. Colloque du 15 mars, Assemblée nationale.

Dinechin, O. 1999. *L'homme de la bioéthique*. Paris: Desclée de Brouwer.

Dossier "Arrêt Perruche". 2001. *La Lettre de l'Espace Ethique*, printemps.

Dossier "Euthanasie". 2001. *Revue de la Fédération JALMALV*, no. 63 décembre 2000 et no. 64 mars.

Dreifuss-Netter, F. 2001. Observations hétérodoxes sur la question du préjudice de l'enfant victime d'un handicap congénital non décelé pendant la grossesse. *Médecine et Droit* 46: 1-6.

Dupont, M. & Fourcade, A. 2000. *L'information médicale du patient: règles et recommandations*. Paris: Doin/Assistance Publique-Hôpitaux de Paris.

Durand-Zaleski, I. & Jolly D. 1999. *L'information du patient: du consentement éclairé à la décision partagée*. Paris: Flammarion.

Etats généraux de la santé. 1999 [On-line]. Available: <www.sante.gouv.fr/egs>.

Fagot-Largeault, A. 2000. *L'éthique environnementale*, Sens.

Fagot-Largeault, A. 2000. Les pratiques réglementaires de la recherche clinique. Bilan de la loi sur la protection des personnes qui se prêtent à des recherches biomédicales. *Médecine/Sciences* 16: 1198-1202.

Fédération nationale des pédiatres néonatologistes. 2001. Dilemmes éthiques de la période périnatale: recommandations pour les décisions de fin de vie, *Archives de Pédiatrie* 8: 407-419.

Fellous, M. 2001. *A la recherche de nouveaux rites*, L'Harmattan.

Ferry, L. & Vincent, J.-D. 2000. *Qu'est-ce que l'homme?* Odile Jacob.

Feuillet-Le-Mintier, B. 1999. Le devenir des comités régionaux d'éthique, *Journal International de Bioéthique* 10: 53-66.

Feuillet-Le-Mintier, B. 1999. *Les lois bioéthiques à l'épreuve des faits: réalités et perspectives*, Presses universitaires de France.

France-Adot 1999. *Motion pour le réexamen des lois de bioéthique*.

Frydman, R. 1997. *Dieu, la médecine et l'embryon*. Odile Jacob.

Gaumont-Prat, H. 1999. Le droit à la vérité est-il un droit à la connaissance de ses origines? *Juris-Classeur* 10: 6-12.

Gavarini, L. 2001. *La passion de l'enfant*. Denoël.

Germain, J.-F. 1999. *La réanimation néonatale: éthique aux limites de la vie*. Presses Universitaires de France.

Giami, A. & Leridon, H. 2000. *Les enjeux de la stérilisation*. INED/Inserm.

Glorion, C. 2000. *La course folle: les généticiens parlent*. Les Arènes.

Gobert, M. 2000. La Cour de cassation méritait-elle le pilori? *Petites Affiches*, 8 décembre.

Gobert, M. 1999. *Médecine, bioéthique et droit: questions choisies*. Economica.

Golse, B., Gosme-Seguret, S. & Mokhtari, M. 2001. *Bébés en réanimation*. Odile Jacob.

Gomez, M. 2001. Préjudice de naissance ou non? *La Croix*, 30 mars.

Gosme-Seguret, S., Golse, B., David, G., et al. 1999. *Assistance médicale à la procréation et filiation: lorsque l'éthique se vit au quotidien*, Doin/Assistance Publique-Hôpitaux de Paris.

Gouyon, P.-H., Lecourt, D., Memmi, D., et al. 1999. *La bioéthique est-elle de mauvaise foi?* Presses universitaires de France.

Grassin, M. 2001. *Le nouveau-né entre la vie et la mort. Ethique et réanimation*, Desclée de Brouwer.

Haussaire-Niquet, C. 1998. *L'enfant interrompu*, Flammarion.

Haut Comité de la Santé Publique. 2000. *Le panier de biens et services de santé: première approche*, <www.hcsp-ensp.fr>.

Hérouville, D., Schaerer, R., Hocquard, A., et al. 2000. Euthanasie: mieux comprendre pour mieux réagir, *La Lettre de la SFASP* 12.

Hirsch, E., Espace Ethique. 1999. *La relation médecin-malade face aux exigences de l'information*, Doin/Assistance Publique-Hôpitaux de Paris.

Hirsch, E., Espace Ethique. 1999. *Pratiques hospitalières et lois de bioéthique: perspectives de révisions des lois du 29 juillet 1994*, Doin/Assistance publique-Hôpitaux de Paris.

Hollender, L., Pellerin, D., et al. 2000. L'accompagnement de la fin de vie. *Bulletin de l'Académie nationale de Médecine* 8: 1765-1774.

Huriet, Cl. 2001. *La protection des personnes se prêtant à des recherches biomédicales. Le rôle des comités: un bilan et des propositions,* Sénat, Les rapports, 267.

Jospin, L. *Discours prononcé le 28 novembre 2000 lors de l'ouverture des Journées annuelles d'éthique,* <www.premier-ministre.gouv.fr>

Joubert, M., Chauvin, P. & Facy, F. 2001. *Précarisation, risque et santé,* Inserm.

Kahn, A. 2000. *Et l'homme dans tout ça?* NIL.

Kahn, A. 2000. Le clonage thérapeutique est-il légitime? *Libération,* 5 décembre.

Kermarec, J., Natali, F,. Camberlein, Y., et al. 1999. Soins palliatifs et accompagnement. *Actualité et Dossier en Santé Publique*: 15-66.

Labrusse-Riou, C. & Mathieu, B. 2000. La vie humaine comme préjudice? *Le Monde,* 24 novembre.

La Marne, P., Malaquin-Pavan, E., Nectoux, M., et al. 2000. Fin de vie, euthanasie ou soins palliatifs? *Soins,* part 1, 647: 29-54; part 2, 648: 33-56.

Lesaulnier, F. 1998. L'enfant né d'une procréation médicalement assistée et le secret de l'identité de l'auteur du don. *Médecine et Droit* 30: 16-22.

Leclerc, A., Fassin, D., Grandjean, H., et al. 2000. *Les inégalités sociales de santé,* La Découverte/Inserm.

Legros, B. 2000. Commentaire de la loi du 9 juin 1999 visant à garantir le droit à l'accès aux soins palliatifs. *Médecine et Droit* 42: 1-9.

Legros, B. 2001. Sur l'opportunité d'instituer une exception d'euthanasie en droit français. *Médecine et Droit* 46: 7-16.

Levy, C., Brunet, L., Bellivier, F., et al. 2000. La recherche sur l'embryon: qualifications et enjeux. *Revue générale de Droit Médical*: 7-249.

Lignieres-Cassou, M. 2001. *Femmes et bioéthique: l'assistance médicale à la procréation,* Assemblée nationale.

Ligue nationale contre le cancer 1999. *Les malades prennent la parole: le libre blanc des 1er Etats Généraux de la santé,* Ramsay.

Loi no. 75-17 du 17 janvier 1975 relative à l'interruption volontaire de grossesse.

Loi no. 94-548 du 1er juillet 1994 relative au traitement des données nominatives ayant pour fin la recherche dans le domaine de la santé.

Loi no. 94-653 du 29 juillet 1994 relative au respect du corps humain.

Loi no. 94-654 du 29 juillet 1994 relative au don et à l'utilisation des éléments et produits du corps humain, à l'assistance médicale à la procréation et au diagnostic prénatal.

Loi no. 98-535 du 1er juillet 1998 relative au renforcement de la veille sanitaire et du contrôle de la sécurité sanitaire des produits destinés à l'homme.

Loi no. 98-657 du 29 juillet 1998 d'orientation relative à la lutte contre les exclusions.

Loi no. 99-641 du 27 juillet 1999 portant création d'une couverture maladie universelle.

Loi 99-477 du 9 juin 1999 visant à garantir le droit à l'accès aux soins palliatifs.

Loi no. 2000-1209 du 13 décembre 2000 relative à la contraception d'urgence.

Malèvre, Ch. 1999. Mes aveux. *Fixot.*

Mathieu, B. 2000. Les comités d'éthique hospitaliers: étude sur un objet juridiquement non identifié, *Revue de droit Sanitaire et Social* 36: 73-86.

Mattei, J.-F. 2000. *Le passeur d'univers: un engagement pour la vie.* Calmann-Levy.

Mattei, J.-F. 2000. Proposition de loi relative à l'interdiction de poursuivre une action en indemnisation du fait du handicap naturellement transmis. Assemblée nationale, décembre.

Maziau, N. 1999. *Le consentement dans le champ de l'éthique biomédicale française, Revue de Droit Sanitaire et Social* 35: 469-492.

Mehl, D. 1999. *Naître? La controverse bioéthique*, Bayard Editions.

Meyer, Ph. 2000. *Philosophie de la médecine*, Grasset.

Michaud, J. 1999. Un avenir pour les comités, *Médecine et Droit* 38: 15.

Milliez, J. 1999. *L'euthanasie du foetus: médecine ou eugénisme?* Odile Jacob.

Mino, J.-C. 1999. La place et le rôle de structures locales d'éthique à l'hôpital: une enquête à l'Assistance Publique-Hôpitaux de Paris. *Santé Publique* 3: 271-285.

Mission d'information commune préparatoire au projet de loi de révision des "lois bioéthiques" de juillet 1994, 2001, <http://www.assemblee-nationale.fr>.

Monroe, L. 2001. Stérilisations: les associations réclament un débat public. *La Croix*, 27 mars.

Montagut, J. 1999. L'assistance médicale à la procréation à l'heure de son réexamen. *Médecine et Droit* 34: 1-6.

Montjardet, A. 1999. *Euthanasie et pouvoir médical: vivre librement sa mort,* L'Harmattan.

Moyse, D. 2001. *Bien naître, bien être, bien mourir: propos sur l'eugénisme et l'euthanasie*, Eres.

Moyse, D. 2001. Naissances coupables? A propos de l'affaire Perruche et d'autres du même genre. *Esprit* 1: 6-17.

Munnich, A. 1999. *La rage d'espérer: la génétique au quotidien*. Plon.

Nau, J.-Y. 2000. L'exception d'euthanasie contre les soins palliatifs. *Le Monde*, 7 mars.

Nau, J.-Y. 2001. Bioéthique: le nouveau pragmatisme français. *Le Monde*, 4 janvier.

Nau, J.-Y. 2001. L'embryon, de la procréation à l'expérimentation. *Le Monde*, 9 janvier.

Nau, J.-Y. 2001. La prise de position de Jacques Chirac projette le débat sur la bioéthique dans l'arène politique. *Le Monde*, 10 février.

Nau, J.-Y. 2001. Le gouvernement ajourne la réforme des lois de bioéthique. La question du clonage oppose Lionel Jospin à Jacques Chirac. *Le Monde*, 19 avril.

Neirinck, C. 1998. L'embryon humain ou la question en apparence sans réponse de la bioéthique. *Les Petites Affiches*, 29.

Neuwirth, L. 1999. *Rapport sur les soins palliatifs et l'accompagnement*, Sénat.

Nizand, I. 1999. *L'IVG en France: propositions pour diminuer les difficultés que rencontrent les femmes*. Rapport réalisé à la demande du Ministre de l'Emploi et de la Solidarité.

Nizand, I. 2000. L'interruption volontaire de grossesse repoussée à quatorze semaines. *Gynécologie Obstétrique et Fertilité* 28: 609-611.

Office parlementaire d'évaluation des choix scientifiques et technologiques, (1999). *Rapport sur l'application de la loi no. 94-654 du 29 juillet 1994 relative au don et à l'utilisation des éléments du corps humain, à l'assistance médicale à la procréation et au diagnostic prénatal.*

Ordre national des Médecins. 1998. *Révision des lois de bioéthique*, <www.conseil-national.medecin.fr>.

Ordre national des Médecins. 1995. *Code de déontologie médicale*, <www.conseil-national.medecin.fr>.

Ordre national des Médecins. 1998. *Commentaires du code de déontologie médicale*, <www.conseil-national.medecin.fr>.

Pedrot, Ph. 2000. Naître ou ne pas naître. *Libération*, 16 novembre.

Pech, M.-E. & Sedar, A. 2000. Cent familles contre l'arrêt Perruche. *Le Figaro*, 3 décembre.

Pech, M.-E. 2001. Arrêt Perruche: un pas vers l'eugénisme. *Le Figaro*, 30 mars.

Petitnicolas, C. 2001. Le clonage thérapeutique divise les sages. *Le Figaro*, 8 février.

Piccini, B. 1999. *Euthanasie: l'hôpital en question*, Michalon.

Ponchon, F. 1999. *Les droits des patients à l'hôpital*. Presses Universitaires de France.

Postel-Vinay, N. & Corvol, P. 2000. *Le retour du Dr Knock*. Odile Jacob.

Projet de loi relatif à la bioéthique. 2001. [On-line]. Available: <http://www.legifrance.gouv.fr>, 20 juin.

Projet de loi relatif à l'accès aux origines personnelles. 2001. Assemblée nationale, 31 mai.

Projet de loi relative à l'interruption volontaire de grossesse et à la contraception. 2001. Assemblée nationale, 31 mai.

Ricot, J. 2000. Un avis controversé sur l'euthanasie. *Esprit* 11: 98-118.

Ropert, J.-C. 2001. Les décisions de fin de vie en période périnatale: Un débat professionnel, une question de société. *Archives de pédiatrie* 8: 349-351.

Sailly, J.-C. 1999. Nécessité et difficultés de la détermination des priorités en matière de santé publique: l'expérience française. *Journal d'Economie médicale* 17: 405-421.

Salat-Baroux, F. 1998. *Les lois de bioéthique*. Dalloz.

Sève, L., Taguieff P.-A., Thomas, J.-P., et al. 1999. La bioéthique a-t-elle force de loi? *Res Publica* 21: 20-59.

Sicard, D. 1999. *Hippocrate et le scanner – Réflexions sur la médecine contemporaine*, Desclée de Brouwer.

Sicard, D. 2000. Ne pas culpabiliser les femmes. *Le Figaro*, 4 octobre.

Sicard, D., Esper, C., Sargos, P., et al. 2000. Accueillir et informer à l'hôpital: information et consentement. *Gestions hospitalières* 394: 171-243.

Sicard, D., Denis, J.-J., Fiat, E., et al. 1999. Fins de vie et pratiques soignantes. *La Lettre de l'Espace Ethique/AP-HP*: 1-122.

Sicard. D., Desfosses, G., Verspieren, P., et al. 2000. L'euthanasie en question. *La Lettre de l'Espace Ethique/AP-HP*: 21-28.

Sureau, Cl. 2000. A propos du projet de loi sur l'interruption volontaire de grossesse et la contraception. *Bulletin de l'Académie nationale de Médecine* 28: 609-611.

Testard, J. 1999. *Des hommes probables. De la procréation aléatoire à la reproduction normative*, Seuil.

Testard, J. 1999. Le diagnostic préimplantatoire: un enjeu pour le XXè siècle. *Médecine/Sciences* 15: 90-96.

Thiel, M.-J. & Thévenot, X. 1999. *Pratiquer l'analyse éthique*. Cerf.

Toulouse, G. 1998. *Regards sur l'éthique des sciences*. Hachette.

Uzan, M. 1998. *Rapport sur la prévention et la prise en charge des grossesses des adolescentes*. Ministère de l'Emploi et de la Solidarité.

Vacquin, M. 1999. *Main basse sur les vivants*. Fayard.

Verspieren, P. 1999. *Face à celui qui meurt: euthanasie, acharnement thérapeutique, accompagnement*. Desclée de Brouwer.

Verspieren, P., Sargos, P., Fabre-Magnan, M., et al. 2000. Le droit des malades à l'information: une évolution juridique? vers quelles nouvelles pratiques?, *Laënnec* 48: 1-31.

Verspieren, P. 2000. L'exception d'euthanasie, *Etudes* 5: 581-585.

Verspieren, P. 2000. La recherche sur l'embryon est-elle légitime?, *La Croix*, 27 décembre.

7 Crossing the Rubicon? The Medical Ethical Debate in Germany in 2001*

Kurt W. Schmidt

In the year 2001, current medical ethical questions had the German public on tenterhooks in a manner almost unprecedented. The role of politics, and in particular the German Parliament, as an important instrument in the guidance of fundamental medical ethical issues was made very transparent. Whatever one's opinion of the final result, the debate about the permissibility of stem cell research was a successful and encouraging example of the shaping of public opinion, of open discussion and of the path towards democratic policy.

The medical ethical debates of 2001 about the permissibility of stem cell research, preimplantation diagnostics and euthanasia were motivated by events within Germany, as well as developments abroad. Famous figures from the worlds of politics and science, like German President Johannes Rau or Hubert Markl, President of the Max Planck Society, made momentous speeches expressing controversial views on topical biomedical issues. Many new boards and advisory committees were set up to provide policy-makers with comprehensive information in these sometimes very complex ethical fields. People spoke of an "ethics boom". At the beginning of the year, even the German Chancellor set up a National Ethics Council, and in so doing subjected himself to loud accusations of having created this body as a way of "creating acceptance" for his new biomedical policies. He was also accused of "deparliamentarizing" the German Lower House, which had to conduct these debates.

To an extent never before witnessed, the media, especially the print media, addressed these complex medical ethical issues for weeks on end, reporting sometimes even daily on the different positions in the debate about, for example, embryo research.[1] Some publications did society a great service, hammering these difficult topics into the public conscience. For a long time it seemed as if no other theme was important in the Summer of 2001 – until the events of September 11th abruptly stole all the attention. It then took many weeks before the permissibility of stem cell research regained political and public interest. In retrospect, for Germany it was to remain the most significant medical ethical topic of the year. Bearing this in mind, this paper will attempt to illustrate not only the different fundamental positions involved, but also the interesting chronology of the embryonic stem cell research debate. Because of its strict embryo protection laws, Germany's position on this issue is significant in the European context, too.

The second topic sparking the German debate was the debate about euthanasia. A new law passed by the Netherlands enabling doctors to perform euthanasia in accordance with the wishes of an incurable patient – without public prosecution – provoked a similar debate in their neighboring countries. The dispute about the permissibility of preimplantation diagnostics, a measure forbidden in Germany, was also ultimately exacerbated by the fact that it is permitted in some neighboring countries, and by the fear that maintaining the prohibition would lead to patient tourism of the kind already observed in connection with differing abortion laws. These three areas all have one thing in common: whether in conjunction with embryo research, euthanasia or abortion, the real issue at stake is no less than the ethical permissibility of ending human life. In 2001 in Germany, there was no shortage of opportunities to debate, argue about or contemplate this point.

I. The Chronology of the German Debate

A. *When does Human Life Begin?*
Regardless of whether embryonic research or preimplantation diagnostics is the theme, the question of when human life – and the nature of its protection – begins is always hovering in the background. Internationally, this debate had been raging for years – especially in the fields of philosophy and medical ethics – and the various positions were well-known. However, the fact that this debate had primarily remained a *specialist debate* and could not simply be turned over to the public as it stood, the prerequisites and philosophical foundations of the positions being too unfamiliar and partly subject to severe accusations, was an experience which the designated Minister for Culture, Julian Nida-Rümelin, was forced to make at the beginning of the year. Just a few days after the New Year, Nida-Rümelin, himself a professor of philosophy and obviously familiar with the medical ethical debate (Nida-Rümelin, 1996), stated that the *human dignity* criterion could not be expanded upon to include embryos. Since *human dignity* is one of the significant features of the German debate (Article 1 of the German Basic Law unequivocally states that: "The dignity of the human being is inviolable"), many received this statement with outrage. It was a taste of the severity that the dispute in Germany would assume if embryo research or preimplantation diagnostics really should come up for serious debate. Even though certain individuals were in favor of an open debate and willing to grant the future Minister the right to his own point of view in this controversial issue, the cries of resistance, concern and outrage were overwhelming, voicing a fear that the floodgates would be opened as soon as it became an option to view human dignity as no longer apportioned from fertilization to death, but reserved for certain human groups – to the detriment of others.

Nobody could have envisaged at this point that an alteration to the strict German embryo protection law of 1991 could really be up for discussion, especially when the Minister for Health at the time, Andrea Fischer (Green Party), announced a bill for a new reproduction law sharply leaning towards the protection of life, which was to maintain the level of protection assigned to embryos to date and – against the wishes of the German Medical Board – not even permitting in special cases, but continuing to prohibit, preimplantation diagnostics. Everyone waited with bated breath to see how Chancellor Schröder (SPD), who was becoming increasingly interested in biomedical topics and had suddenly started warning against "ideological blinkers" and "fundamental prohibitions" in genetic research, would find a common coalitional denominator with his Health Minister. It looked all set for a conflict, especially as the Chancellor was pointing out the "great economic importance" of this branch of research. What happened next was by German standards sociopolitically remarkable. United by the issue of life protection (somewhat later Erika Buhlman, Minister for Research, would announce a "year of the life sciences", not synchronized to start with the calendar year), previously more or less unthinkable alliances began to form: members of the Green Party moved close to the standpoint of the church, especially the Catholic Church, and even members of the CDU attempted to stake out biomedical boundaries of the kind "up to here and no further". In a widely followed *Frankfurter Rundschau* interview with Andrea Fischer (Green Party) and CDU Chairperson Angela Merkel, it became clear just how close these two persons were in their fight to protect life. The expected conflict between Chancellor Schröder and his Health Minister was never fought out in the end, due to a completely unrelated incident. In mid-January, the Minister for Health became caught up in the BSE affair and the lack of sufficient public information about dangers to the German population. Not only the Minister who was chiefly responsible, Agriculture Minister Funke, resigned, but surprisingly also Andrea Fischer. When her successor, Ulla Schmidt (SPD), announced that she would not be pursuing the restrictive reproduction law planned by her predecessor, and that in the future an open debate about the narrowly restricted application of preimplantation diagnostics would be required, it was clear that the Ministry of Health had changed course, seemingly to fall into line with that of the German Chancellor.

B. The Situation Remains Clouded, but the Fronts become Clear

In the weeks that followed, various voices became loud, illustrating a development which was to become typical of the rest of the debate: Apart from members of the FDP, who were "liberal" enough to deem many things permissible which resulted from the free decisions of individuals or which could help to heal individual patients, from embryonic stem cell research to euthanasia,[2] the political parties were no longer to have unified positions. Within the same party, individual members advocated completely opposing standpoints, and the point was made that in these basic issues of life each Parliamentary member ultimately only had to answer to his own conscience. With regard to party political positions, the situation therefore remained clouded; the fronts became clearer, but they ran right down the middle of all parties. The only entities to remain united in their standpoints on life protection were the Catholic bishops and, for a long while, the representatives of the Protestant church. It came as a surprise to many when, in mid-March 2001, despite the professed promise of previously unknown cures, the German Council for the Disabled[3] rejected research on embryonic stem cells.

C. On the High Seas – The Bioethics Debate Departs from its Protective Haven

The middle of the year saw changes coming thick and fast: The Cabinet barely had time to decree the convening of a "National Ethics Council" on May 2nd, when on May 3rd the *German Research Association (DFG)*[4] surprised many by announcing a recommendation with regard to research on embryonic stem cells which amounted to a radical turnabout:

> Point 6: Since the last DFG report on this topic two years ago (March 1999), considerable progress has been made both in embryonic and in tissue-specific (adult) stem cell research. (…) Human embryonic stem cells can now be converted to particular desired cell types much better than before, even if to date only the production of enriched populations is possible. The DFG is therefore

of the opinion that science has now reached a level where neither potential patients in Germany nor German scientists should be excluded from these developments (DFG, 2001).

Whereas before the DFG's rejection of research on embryonic stem cells was partly on moral grounds (!), now suddenly new scientific progress was being cited as an argument for not excluding patients or scientists from the potential benefits of further know-how. What filled so many with consternation was not so much the fact that scientific progress had come so far that in this new light policy-makers saw themselves forced to rethink their previous decisions; far more problematic was the fact that DFG President, Professor E.-L. Winnacker, had asserted all his personal authority in the media to assure the public that the embryo would remain inviolable in its need for protection. The fact that Winnacker personally announced this change of policy left the public in doubt about the assertions of scientists in general. For many it was just further confirmation of a fatalistic belief that "whatever biomedical researchers are capable of doing, they will eventually do".

This feeling of devastation should not be underestimated when evaluating the German ethical debate. The public could only speculate about the exact reasons behind the DFG's change of course. One of its consequences was that the import of embryonic stem cells from abroad, for which Bonn neuropathologists Oliver Brüstle and Ottmar Wiestler had been crying out for months, was no longer only being discussed "in theory", but was suddenly backed by the greatest research authority in Germany. Politicians had to confront this new development and make some decisions which were to have practical consequences.

And after this recommendation at the beginning of May from the most significant research body in Germany, German President Johannes Rau, the most significant political voice in Germany, decided just two weeks later, right in the middle of the raging debate, to say a few words of his own. In his famous "Berlin Speech" he, figuratively, turned the tide of events and called for human life to be treated by medics and researchers with awe, without a departure from established boundaries:[5] There is "so much scope this side of the Rubicon" (Rau, 2001). By using this metaphor, Rau expressed precisely what many citizens had been feeling, asking themselves how on earth a democratic society was to put an end to this "dispute of moralities". What was remarkable was that President Rau did not propose a compromise; instead, he fell back on basic European values to make a clear stand:

> It really does not take a believing Christian to know and to feel that certain possibilities and plans of biotechnology and genetic engineering run contrary to fundamental values of human life. They have been developed over several millennia and not just here in Europe. They also form the basis of the simple sentence which precedes all others in our Basic Law: Human dignity shall be inviolable (Rau, 2001).

What many had been crying out for, the President had now done: He had staked out a boundary. In his speech, Rau clarified why it was important for this "fence" to preserve our culture as it has emerged, turning around a quotation from Hoelderlin, as philosopher Ernst Bloch had done before him in conjunction with the atomic energy debate: "But where there is a rescuing element, danger grows as well" (Rau, 2001).

A few days after the President's speech, representatives of the German medical profession at their annual convention in Ludwigshafen also rejected embryo research. This rejection – it was important to read their resolution carefully – was only, however, "for the present".[6] The medical profession also desired a "process of social clarification" in this matter. Clear positions naturally had to be found for orientational purposes, and in May 2001 standpoints and "fronts" emerged with increasing transparency *between* the DFG, the Chancellor, the President, the church, the medical profession; and yet, *within* the major political parties a clear position was indetectable (and this was to remain). What was to turn the decision about embryonic stem cell research into a touchstone for sociopolitical policy-making, however, was a newly discovered legal loophole concerning the import of embryonic stem cells from abroad.

D. The Import of Embryonic Stem Cells from Abroad – A Possible "Backroute"
It was originally assumed that Germany's strict embryo protection law (EschG) forbade any kind of work on embryonic stem cells whatsoever. According to the usual interpretation of the law, §2 of the EschG prohibited the import of embryos (and of totipotent cells harvested from embryos). On June 1st, however, researchers in Bonn announced their wish to import embryonic stem cells from Israel and were supported in their intention by Northrhine-Westphalia's Prime Minister, Wolfgang Clement (SPD). Several legal reports had concluded that *pluripotent* embryonic stem cells could be imported from abroad since they were *not* subject to the prohibitions of the EschG. According to §9 Par. 2 EschG of the German Criminal Code, such an import is only a punishable offense if the German researchers involved in the import request foreign colleagues to create the embryonic stem cells specifically for this purpose or positively influence them in any other way (Bülow, 2001, p. 46; Wolfrum, 2001). Since these cells were not harvested in conjunction with a request from German researchers and, on the contrary, had already been removed, the researchers were able to import these cells from abroad without committing a punishable offense.

The situation intensified. Criticism of Clement's advance could be heard from all political camps, and even his supporters admitted that Clement's timing, so close to the forthcoming Parliamentary debate, was unfortunate. Researchers were pressuring the DFG, the DFG was pressuring politicians, politicians were imploring researchers to wait for the political result. New policies were heralded in quick succession, only to be postponed at the last minute. In the meantime, news was trickling in from other universities in Germany that they were also interested in researching on embryonic stem cells, that some had already ordered the stem cells, that some cells had even already arrived in Germany and were being stored on ice. They all maintained that they had not embarked on any research as yet.

Following an appeal to the DFG by the Lower House, members of the Government and the National Ethics Council, the DFG postponed its decision – originally expected July 3rd – about Brüstle and Wiestler's Bonn research project involving the import of embryonic stem cells. They were conscious of "their responsibility towards both science and society" and did not wish "to influence the intensive public debate, which they themselves had called for, with a decision to promote a concrete research project". In postponing their decision until December, the DFG appealed to the policy-makers to create the conditions necessary before such a decision can be reached. The DFG expected their action to intensify the public debate, which was already well underway, and at the same time to rob it of some of its ferocity so that from now on it could be pursued with a style of dialog appropriate to the issue in question (DFG, 2001b).

E. Worth, Dignity, Economy – The Parliamentary Debate on 31st May 2001

The German Parliamentary debate on the "Law and Ethics of Modern Medicine and Biotechnology" was keenly awaited as *the* debate of the Parliamentary term. It emerged that the speakers would be giving their personal opinions (especially as the parties themselves could not agree on a common direction) when Gerhard Schröder spoke not as the Chancellor, but simply as an SPD member of Parliament. New coalitions were also formed, however. A "human dignity alliance", for example, was formed across all (!) parties (except the FDP). In the light of the new challenges to medicine and science, their common goal was to safeguard human dignity as guaranteed in the German Basic Law and to organize a petition protesting against the lowering of ethical standards. Amongst other things, this petition would censure preimplantation diagnostics as a new selective practice which, like consumptive embryo research, is incompatible with human dignity (Bündnis, 2001). The five-hour debate revealed deep cracks within the two major parties: SPD and CDU. Everyone agreed that there had to be a boundary, but nobody could agree where.

F. Liberty, Responsibility, Human Dignity: President Markl Fights Back

Three weeks after the Parliamentary debate had been unable to produce any clarity about further policy, Hubert Markl, President of the famous Max Planck Society for the Advancement of Science, entered the debate within a regular general meeting on 22nd June with a speech addressing the principle of research freedom: "The President of the Max Planck Society cannot and must not turn away from the debate, the extent of which reaches far beyond the rather limitedly significant topics of stem cell research and preimplantation genetic diagnosis, because it is also about fundamental questions concerning the inseparable connection between the freedom of science and its mission. Speaking for myself, I quite personally have no desire to back out of it, for I, as a biologist, am the last one who would want to evade the problems associated with that connection."

In a speech full of barbs, Markl attacked the positions held by the churches and President Rau, heftily criticizing the "moral high-mindedness" which – in his opinion – many were all to keen to display:

> I almost feel like a pike in the jam-packed fish pond of moral high-mindedness. Then I thought about what Harry Truman (following an old bit of Talmudian wisdom) is reported to have said: "Who, if not you? When, if not now? Tomorrow you will be gone!" We are fortunate to be living in a country where a modest Max Planck President is allowed publicly to contradict the highly esteemed President of the entire nation, from citizen Markl to citizen Rau, as it were. For, in matters of conscience, morals, freedom, responsibility, and human dignity, every citizen has to be his or her own expert and make use of the freedom of speech themselves to the best of their knowledge and conscience (Markl, 2001).

Throughout his speech, Merckl stayed true to his own style, addressing what so many had accused the DFG of avoiding in its recommendation, namely debating the beginnings of human life:

> After all, it always boils down to one question: *What is a human being?* Although this question has been following humanity since man became conscious of his existence, the heated debate on this question has already progressed so far that some life scientists will soon not dare enter the laboratory unless accompanied by a constitutional expert and a moral theologian. And if that doesn't go for working in the lab, then it at least applies to appearing in public.
>
> Every human being that is born is something new and unique that developed from a fertilized human egg cell. However, the fertilized egg is by far not yet a human being, at least not as an established fact of natural science. It is, at best, only if we assign – completely at will – the concept of "human being" a meaning totally new and different from that which it has had up until now. This has to do with what we mean sensibly, i.e., true to reality, when we refer to an organism as "human". This is not some label attached by nature, but a human expression of self-reference, the meaning of which is not stipulated by nature but by humans themselves (Markl, 2001).

Markl stood up for the freedom of parents, especially mothers, "to decide whether or not to carry a baby to full term after consulting their physician when preimplantation genetic diagnosis or prenatal diagnostic techniques have revealed the possibility of severe developmental disorders in the embryo". And:

> nothing less holds true for the decision made with one's own free will to receive desired assisted suicide. Only those who do not view themselves as free citizens with the right to make their own decisions, but instead as government property with the obligation to live and pay tribute to the bitter end can accept a majority taking it upon themselves to make this most personal of all decisions concerning one's life dependent on government approval. I, for one, openly declare my respect for the Dutch Parliament, which, in spite of all the hostility, had the guts to recognize the high value of a human being's freedom to decide for itself, in other words, his or her human dignity (Markl, 2001).

Markl emphasizes at this point that:

> you will surely have realized that I may be speaking to you as the President of the Max Planck Society, but by no means officially for the Max Planck Society, that is to say about positions voted on in the Society's bodies. Above all, this is a call for freedom, and not necessarily for the freedom of research, though that also plays a role, but it plays the smallest. Instead, this is primarily a call for the freedom of every citizen in a democratic society. For this freedom is under threat from the zealous moral coercion of a moral majority just as much as from the lack of restraint of unscrupulous individuals. If my

conviction is accurate, that politically, more weight must be given in bioethical matters, such as these, concerning the beginning and ending of human life to the carefully thought-out decisions made in line with one's own conscience, since it just isn't possible to take a vote on questions of conscience, then neither can there be an official opinion of the Max Planck Society or of the majority of its members. This is where I, as an individual with all my fallible conviction, have to take the responsibility. I wish to underline that in particular whenever I, as a biologist, state my opinion on the question of the beginning of life, because there are sure to be many Max Planck scientists whose opinions I highly respect even though they may see things differently (Markl, 2001).

The President of the Max Planck Society was expressing here what is true for the leaders of all political parties and the Protestant church: With regard to issues as fundamental as these, all positions voiced have to be *personal* ones – nevertheless expressed with strength and vehemence. The core of Markl's speech was undoubtedly the *freedom of individuals to decide for themselves.*

G. *September 11th*

In the Summer of 2001, it seemed inconceivable in Germany that one single event could overshadow the embryo research debate for any length of time. And yet the events of September 11th put the debate firmly in the shade. Embryo research only reappeared on the agenda when researchers insisted that the DFG finally make a decision. Nevertheless, the original schedule for the debates could no longer be adhered to, and the DFG once again postponed its decision, this time until January 23, 2002. Our Dutch neighbours still managed to reach a political decision, though, and in October *the Netherlands* passed a law permitting research on surplus embryos. The German Parliamentary decision was still to come. As a gauge of the general mood in the interim, the public eagerly awaited decisions from the members of the various advisory boards.

H. *From the Enquete Commission to the National Ethics Council: Fall Moods*

On November 12th the members of the *Enquete Commission*, which had been advising the German Parliament about the legal and ethical aspects of modern medicine for years, voted with a clear majority *against* the import of stem cells (proportion of votes 17:9); two weeks later, on November 29th, the majority of the members in the *National Ethics Council* convened by Chancellor Schröder voted *for* an import with temporal limitations.[7] This ballot, however, as Chairman Spiros Simitis stressed, was to be taken neither as a "decision", nor as a "recommendation", but as a formal representation of current opinion and as information about the various options and arguments involved. The Chairman of the Enquete Commission, Margot von Renesse, had previously also announced that the members of the Enquete Commission had agreed not to establish a joint position, but formally to express the various personal opinions held.

The Central Ethics Commission of the German Medical Board was likewise unable to agree, but voted with a large majority (1 vote against) *for* research on embryonic stem cells harvested from embryos which evolved for the purposes of IVF, but which were never implanted (Zentrale, 2001).

Thus there were no uniform votes. In a manner almost unprecedented, the members of the German Lower House were asked to express their personal opinions and consult their personal consciences. And when the crucial debate and ballot finally did take place in the German Parliament at the end of January 2002 (after being postponed yet again!) Germany's Protestant church spent the two days before it in debate with theologians and politicians in Berlin, an invitation which seemed more than anything to underline the differing opinions held by Protestant theologians (Gemeinschaftswerk, 2002).

Without going into all the details of the German debate here, its core issues and ethical arguments will be summarized.

II. Human Embryonic Stem Cell Research: The Pros and Cons in the German Debate

A. Plurality of Opinions

The embryo research debate illustrates a characteristic of many debates about fundamental ethical values: The arguments put forward cannot be analyzed as "right" or "wrong", and the adversaries cannot be accused of having logical breaks in their chains of thought. In this debate, for example, many of the opinions regarding the start of human life and its need for protection were certainly "coherent", and yet, there were no "better" arguments able to win opponents over. Only when it became clear that the different positions stemmed from completely different *views of humanity*, and that some of the demands being made were incompatible with these views, did it become possible to approach an understanding for why these different standpoints would never win arguments. What can always be achieved, however, is an understanding for why person A with a view of humanity B will assume position C. The political task is then to bring about a consensus within a democratic pluralistic society which will enable these people with differing views to live alongside each other in harmony.

B. The Basic Conflict

Scientists see human stem cell research as a previously unknown opportunity for basic research, promising knowledge about human embryonic development as well as the various tissues and organs. In the long term, such knowledge could help to provide new therapeutic approaches for patients with severe and sometimes even as yet incurable diseases.

This cautious formulation illustrates a problem pervading the entire debate: stem cell research *could* facilitate new therapies, but many scientists have been quick to point out that it is not yet possible to say which therapies these will be or when they might become available. It must be said that in the German debate many are keen to expose the fact that whilst many new therapies are being promised as a result of stem cell research, it is still completely unclear when or even whether these promises will ever be fulfilled. And yet it must also be said that throughout the entire – often very emotional – debate these aspects were not paid much attention, perhaps intentionally so. This often made the adversaries problematic, especially in some of the staged television debates: Anybody in favor of banning embryo research could quickly be presented as opposing new chances to heal and cure. It was especially easy on TV to present this "protector of life" as a "monster", by seating him opposite a patient (often also a spokesperson for a rights group) whose ailment could not be cured using the means currently available and who was now placing all hope in the new stem cell research. By wishing to continue the ban on this form of research, the "embryo protector" was taking away all hope from such a (nice) patient, leaving viewers in doubt about his abilities to feel any kind of empathy at all.

But controversy also remained on the part of the researchers as to whether embryos may be taken and used – and if so which ones, for they can be acquired in all manner of ways – to achieve the different goals of this research. A clear stance on whether the ethically less problematic adult stem cells could be used for research with the same success as embryonic stem cells was not adopted in the course of the debate (or to date).

Different ethical approaches emphasizing various values, anchoring obligations and weighing up consequences, came to bear. Whilst Germany's President Johannes Rau, in his well-received Berlin speech of May 18, 2001, pleaded for not crossing the Rubicon[8] and for first exploiting the (research) options already available, others deemed it irresponsible to withhold from (future) patients possible revolutionary breakthroughs in our understanding of disease development and potential new therapeutic options. Some researchers proposed beginning by researching on *all* types of stem cells, since the various potentials of the different stem cell types are still a complete mystery. A new decision could then be made once these potentials have been sufficiently researched and greater clarity has been achieved as to which stem cell types should be used for further research into which therapeutic applications. Many scientists gave their consensus to this approach on the condition that the research be strictly regulated and controlled.

This "wide" gate to research, as well as some other more narrow approaches, contrasted starkly with positions based on the idea that all embryos merit protection. Here life itself is deemed to be in great danger of being abused and there is considerable doubt as to whether the means required to achieve the desired ends might not be a price too high. Even though the following account may not amount to a comprehensive ethical reflection in all its intricacies, it is nevertheless an attempt to analyze the overall German debate from an angle which exposes the main bone of contention. We shall examine the consequences which individual *views of humanity* and comprehensions of *the protection of life* have for the way in which the permissibility of research on human stem cells is evaluated.

C. *Ethical Evaluation Based on Where the Cells originated*

The stem cell seems to be currently in high demand as an object of research because it is a kind of "original cell", possessing the ability to reproduce almost limitlessly and become many different types of cell. Stem cells are to be found in the human organism at all stages of its development, and yet opinions are divided about their various suitability for research purposes. Even though it was rarely said in as many words, the German debate really revolved around the ethical permissibility of such research with regard to *where the stem cells originated*. Six different harvesting methods are known, and research on each is different from an ethical point of view. They are:

(1) Research on stem cells from umbilical cord blood.
(2) Research on adult stem cells.

(3) Research on stem cells from aborted embryos.
(4) Research on embryonic stem cells from surplus embryos after in-vitro fertilization (IVF) treatments.
(5) Research on embryonic stem cells from embryos created especially for this purpose using IVF (consumptive embryo research).
(6) Research on stem cell lines imported from abroad through possibilities 1-5.

Looking back at this debate, the representatives of the different *protection of life* positions can be divided up into three groups: Group 1 advocates *protection of life from the start*, i.e., from conception. The moment sperm and egg unite, the fertilized egg cell is a life worthy of protection, far removed from any "debates about values" and not to be weighed up against other "goods" (research results, potential new therapies). Group 2, by contrast, advocates a *stepwise increase* in the protection of life. I shall not go into detail here about the wide spectrum of positions within Group 2, wishing instead to focus attention on the tense attempt of individual politicians to reach a compromise in this situation of discord. Politicians from across all parties, particularly women, for example, the former Health Minister (Green Party) Andrea Fischer, developed an additional and – for many of them personally – new group (Group 3). Whilst fundamentally in favor of protecting life from the start, they introduced the idea that research on embryonic stem cells needs to be permitted within a numerical – and possibly temporal – limitation. This would mean weighing up the value of life against the value of other goods, and yet society would still have to acknowledge the peculiarity of this measure and treat life with respect, without any dams breaking or general disparagement ensuing.

Of course it was important for the debate to analyze which consequences the three positions would have for research in Germany.

D. Position (1): Protection of Life from the Start

Human life is comprehended as inviolable from the start; i.e., from the moment of fusion between sperm and egg cell. It cannot become part of a calculation involving other values, goods or goals. Although this stance is a very old one, throughout the course of history the exact moment when human life is thought to start has increasingly been brought forward. One of the greatest influences in the Middle Ages in this respect was Thomas Aquinas, who propounded the Aristotelian notion that a human being only started to exist when God breathed a soul into it. The male embryo was said to receive its soul on the 40th post-fertilization day, the female embryo on the 80th. It was impossible for a human being to evolve purely "biologically", i.e., without God's help. Later, medical research and especially the discovery of the female egg cell led to a rethinking regarding the moment when human life is said to begin, for modern embryology had revealed that nearly all the biological necessities for human development already exist at the point of conception. The Catholic Church duly took up this discovery, and in 1869 Pope Pius IX decreed a "simultaneous giving of souls" to replace the prior "consecutive giving of souls": The soul is given to the embryo not a few weeks into its development but parallel to conception; from this point on the embryo is a developing human being deserving full protection.

This background – which is on no account purely theological in nature, being instrumental to the current legislation in both Ireland and Germany, to name but two examples – gives rise to the following options when evaluating research on stem cells harvested in the different ways:

1. *Option one: Research on stem cells from umbilical cord blood.* Following the birth of a child, stem cells can be harvested from blood in the umbilical cord. Even though the know-how to be gained from research on these cells is limited, there was still a Parliamentary ruling: This research does not infringe upon the protection or moral status of the embryo and there can, therefore, be no objections to it.

2. *Option two: Research on adult stem cells.* Again, this form of research does not represent any fundamental problems for the advocates of protecting life from the start, especially when the donor is an adult capable of making his own decisions. Just as with other medical interventions for research purposes, here too the donor would have to give his informed consent before stem cells could be removed. Since it does not endanger life itself in any way, this type of research can also be permitted.

3. *Option three: Research on stem cells from aborted embryos.* Aborted embryos from the 5th-9th week are a source of so-called *primordial germ cells.* These cells correspond to pluripotent embryonic stem cells, but not to the totipotent stem cells harvested from blastocytes from which complete human life can develop.

Advocates of *life protection from the start* should not have any problems with the pluripotent stem cells themselves, but the abortion *prior to the harvesting* is another matter. Those *categorically* opposed to abortion for moral reasons have to remain consistent and also oppose research on aborted embryos, since no "moral good" can come of an action which is "morally bad". The goals of such research, however desirable they may be, will never change the minds of those with this ethical approach.

Even though some people like to view the whole embryo research debate as a new and previously unknown threat to human dignity, by now it must surely be clear that the issues involved are not at all new. Instead, it is a reminder of how many compromises our society has already entered into: For quite some time now, differentiated cell lines harvested from the tissue of aborted embryos have been used for research purposes and in the manufacture of pharmaceutical drugs. There is no room here to examine why this has never been debated with the same intensity and controversy as stem cell research. Far more important in this context was the fact that it could not be used for the sake of a sound argument. On the contrary, this situation was being exploited by the advocates of stem cell research: If the use of aborted fetuses for these purposes is already permitted and tolerated, then research on pluripotent cells and the creation of embryonic pluripotent stem cell lines should also be possible.

4. *Option four: Research on embryonic stem cells from surplus embryos after IVF treatment.* Stem cells can be harvested from fertilized egg cells which are the product of IVF but which are surplus to requirements and are never implanted in the female patient. Normally they would now be discarded. Advocates of protecting life from the start cannot agree to research on these embryos since this would instrumentalize them; i.e., turn them into objects. The fact that the surplus embryos are being put to "good use" does nothing to alleviate this problematic situation. Since the embryo has not yet entered the protected maternal sphere (where all interventions require the consent of the mother), the State in particular is called upon to offer protection. The alternative proposed would be to put the embryos up for adoption, thus preserving life.

5. *Option five: Research on embryonic stem cells from embryos created especially for this purpose using IVF (consumptive embryo research).* If the embryo is viewed as a

human being, then creating an embryo purely for research purposes means putting the dignity and protection of human life at stake. The prospect of cures being found through stem cell research is a good cause which nevertheless appears in a very unfavorable light when life is created purposely just to be killed again later on. The end does not justify the means.

Research with the positive goal of *healing suffering* undermines human dignity, human life and all things living when the embryo is not comprehended as a person, but as a thing. It is not only the embryo which is instrumentalized, however, but also the woman and the man, reduced to human life "suppliers".

6. *Option six: Research on stem cell lines imported from abroad.* Considering the options above, the decision as to whether the import of stem cell lines should be allowed should depend on how these stem cell lines were harvested (see 1-5). Even if stem cell lines do not require protection to the same extent as embryos, a researcher working with stem cell lines bears at least some of the responsibility for their harvesting.

E. Position (2): Increasing Levels of Protection

Whereas the advocates of Position 1 consider a fertilized egg cell worthy of full protection, from the moment of conception perceiving *a human being which merely has to mature* (ein *Mensch im Werden*; a human being in the making), the advocates of Position 2 assume that the fertilized egg cell first *has to develop into a human being* (*werdender Mensch*; a developing human being) and that the level of protection due to it gradually increases as it does so.

The ethical debate has seen different stages of embryonic development being put forward as meriting an increased level of embryo protection, i.e., the point where responsible research has to stop. Some see *nidation,* i.e., the implanting of the fertilized egg cell in the womb, as the point after which interventions for research purposes can no longer be justified if ultimately leading to the death of the embryo. These people argue that *nidation* marks the start of the bond to the mother which is the prerequisite for development into a human being capable of survival. This position is not only held by some philosophers and biologists, but is also found in some religions, for example, Islam.[9]

Others argued for the point of increased protection being set when twins are no longer a possibility and individuation has thus definitely begun. For still others, the deciding criterion was the formation of neuronal structures and thus the presumed emergence of sensibility. Each of these cut-off points stems from a particular view of humanity, and yet they all share the basic assumption, often coupled with references to personal existence, that the protection due to human life increases *in stages*. Precisely because this development is a continual process, they believe it necessary to divide it up into stages and to determine the moral status of each phase.

Although there has been no broad *interreligious* debate in Germany about the permissibility of stem cell research, where the religious standpoints were consulted they were often surprising. The mere realization that not all religions are fundamentally opposed to the notion of human life meriting increasing protection as it grows was confusing to those who had always thought of religious faiths as "uncompromising" protectors of life. Judaism, for example, holds the view that human beings do not merit full protection until birth. The fertilized egg cell certainly merits respect and protection, and – with few exceptions – abortion is still morally reprehensible, and yet the embryo is deemed to be part of the mother and not a life in its own right until a newborn baby.

Whereas advocates of Group 1 (protection of life from the start) could only agree to stem cell research on cells from umbilical cord blood (Option 1) or adults (Option 2), advocates of the (extremely heterogenous) Group 2 (protection of life in stages) went further and could have no fundamental objections to research on surplus embryos from IVF treatments (Option 4).

F. Position (3): Weighing up Different Goods and Compromising

It will come as no surprise that, even with intense debate, the advocates of the two groups discussed above were unable to connect, let alone reach an agreement. Their views of humanity were just too different. The politicians attempted to find a compromise, which of course was not going to satisfy everyone. What the advocates of protection of life from the start (Position 1) had categorically ruled out was exactly what the various *proposed compromises* brought back into the discussion, in a way "putting society to the test". Whilst fundamentally acknowledging *protection of life from the start*, the politicians asked whether it would not be possible to permit research on embryonic stem cells within the restrictions of a numeric and maybe also temporal framework. They argued that it could be justifiable, taking into account the lofty goals (of healing) envisaged, to weigh up the value of life against these other goods. Society should be capable of recognizing the peculiarity and the threshhold value of this measure and of ensuring that respect for life *per se* is not lost through this restricted form of stem cell research, that it would not become a case of life itself being viewed with disparagement.

There are many indications today which suggest that this undertaking has failed. At the end of January 2002, for example, a bill was passed by the German Parliament fundamentally amounting to a *prohibition of embryonic stem cell research*. Since the wording permitted one exception (research on surplus embryos harvested prior to January 1, 2002), however, the public received the entire bill as a *permit for stem cell research* and lamented it as an opening of the floodgates.

G. Conclusion

The debate about stem cell research assumed a whole new dimension in Germany from the moment the DFG spoke up in favor of this research and called for a Parliamentary decision. No other medical ethical debate in Germany over the past few years has ever taken up so much space – especially in the print media. The only dispute which was comparably dramatic was the one surrounding the transplantation law (until November 1997 Germany had no special legislation for this area). The difference to that debate and its connected issue of brain death, where individuals can ultimately choose their own personal consequences and sign a written declaration (organ donor card) to this effect (or not), is that this dispute about embryonic stem cell research forces us to make decisions about others who cannot be consulted, as well as about those who could possibly profit in the form of therapy from the research findings in the future. The stem cell debate thus also potentially represents a change of course for medical ethical debate in the new millennium: reflecting the possibilities and limitations of the principle of autonomy – dominant in the past few years – in conjunction with medical ethical policy.

III. Summary

Although the international debate about embryo research and therapeutic cloning hit the headlines in Germany too, for a long time it appeared that the discussion would not have any *practical* consequences for Germany as a research location. The unconditional protection of embryonic life, guarded in Germany by one of the most stringent laws worldwide, just seemed too established.[10] And even though individual researchers repeatedly pleaded for the Embryo Protection Law to be relaxed, arguing that Germany's standing as a research location was in danger, not least because genetic researchers were leaving the country, the German Research Community (DFG) issued a statement to the effect that research on embryonic stem cells should not be permitted and work with ethically unproblematic adult stem cells encouraged instead. For many this directive was both clear and comforting. When two leading researchers in this field, Oliver Brüstle and Ottmar Wiestler from the University of Bonn, demanded that the DFG change its position and permit research with embryonic stem cells, their calls and the discussions in their wake still seemed to be of no practical relevance. The DFG repeatedly reinforced its position that research should only be permitted on adult stem cells, even if this meant that German researchers lost their advantage in the race for scientific know-how.

With this background in mind, it is possible to appreciate the weight of an announcement – which took the public completely by surprise – made by the DFG on May 21, 2001 *in favor of* research on *embryonic stem cells* and its repercussions. The DFG was still of the opinion that the use of adult stem cells would always be preferable, and yet believed science had now reached a point where "neither potential patients nor scientists in Germany should be excluded from these developments any longer". The DFG spoke of a "process of weighing up the embryo protection legislation on the one hand against the freedom of research legislation on the other". In other words, the DFG had changed direction, provoking a debate which had to lead to practical consequences. The advocates of unconditional protection for human life and the research advocates were no longer in the same boat. Suddenly they were opponents, and in this difficult situation politicians were forced into having to find a consensus. This was to prove extremely difficult, best shown by the fact that the decision expected of the German Parliament to permit embryonic research was repeatedly postponed until it finally came into being on January 31, 2002. These debates in the German Lower House, especially the last ones towards the end of January, were unanimously heralded by political observers as great parliamentary moments. Considering the import of this issue, it is actually amazing that a decision was reached within just six months. They were, after all, discussing no less than the appropriate handling of human life. The fact that the proposal which was finally accepted was drawn up *jointly* by politicians across the whole party political spectrum (whether Greens, Social Democrats or Conservatives, whether left-wing, liberal or right-wing), and that this process interestingly occurred under the overall supervision of women, characterizes the special situation (Gesetzentwurf, 2002). It will come as no surprise, however, that everybody was forced to give and take from their original standpoints. One of the key points:

> It is decreed that the import and use of human embryonic stem cells is fundamentally forbidden. (...) Only stem cells already in existence on January 1st, 2002 may be imported and used. Import and use of these cells must be

for research purposes and only in pursuit of high-ranking research-related endeavors. It must be impossible to achieve equally good results with animal or other human cells. The stem cells must be harvested from embryos which were created for the purposes of pregnancy, but which for reasons unrelated to these embryos were never implanted (Gesetzentwurf, 2002).

This resolution amounted to no less than an order to march across the Rubicon. And even though in this case it did not lead to a "civil war", some Germans were overcome by a melancholy certainty that in crossing the Rubicon they had become *moral strangers* in their own country.

Notes

* Translated into English by Sarah C. Kirkby, B.A. Hons. Exon.
1. Towards the end (prior to a decision being reached by the German Parliament), the wealth of articles and reports in the daily press was complemented by a number of articles providing overviews, helping readers through the thicket of different ethical standpoints (Stollarz & Prüfer, 2002; Schmidt, 2002).
2. In early May, delegates of the FDP party conference followed a motion by the executive to permit research on embryonic stem cells and alter the embryo protection law. This made the FDP the first Party in Germany to advocate embryonic stem cell research.
3. A collaboration of all the Associations for the Disabled in Germany, representing a total of 2.5 million members.
4. DFG is the central public funding organization for academic research in Germany. DFG is thus comparable to a (national) Research Foundation.
5. The ban on consumptive embryo research should be maintained, likewise those on PID and euthanasia.
6. Their position regarding PID remained open. It was telling, however, that the German medical convention turned down all proposals aimed at a total rejection of PID with a clear majority.
7. Between the two, in mid-November, the European Parliament voted in favor (317 to 190 votes, 28 abstainers) of supporting embryo research on surplus embryos with EU funds.
8. *Rubicon* is the ancient name of a river in northern Italy, forming the border between Italy and the Province of Gaul. In January of the year 49 BC, before Julius Caesar became Emperor, he crossed this river with his troops and started the Roman Civil War. The crossing of this boundary signifies irrevocable commitment, the point of no return.
9. It was very noticeable in the German debate that whilst Protestant and Catholic standpoints were aired freely, Muslim and Jewish positions were barely acknowledged. This was partly due to the fact that Germany is currently also in the middle of a domestic political debate about coexistence with Islam, stemming from the "headscarf conflict" (Must a Muslim teacher in a religiously neutral country like Germany cease to wear her headscarf with all its symbolic religious import?), the permissibility of animal slaughter for religious reasons and a great deal of uncertainty following September 11th, 2001.
10. The situation is similar with physician-assisted suicide: this has been and still is heatedly debated in Germany and yet, with German history in mind, nobody seriously expects legislation to change.

Bibliography

Arens, C. 2001. *Ethische Fragen in der Medizin. Die Entwicklung im Jahr 2001.* Bonn: Katholische Nachrichten-Agentur.

Bülow, D.v. 2001. Verantwortete Wissenschaft – rechtliche und ethische Grenzen der Stammzellenforschung. In: Bundesministerium für Bildung und Forschung (ed.), *Humane Stammzellen. Perspektiven und Grenzen in der regenerativen Medizin* (pp. 39-54). Schattauer: Stuttgart.

Bündnis Menschenwürde. 2001. Aufruf [On-line]. Available: <http://www.buendnismenschen-wuerde.de>.

Deutsche Forschungsgemeinschaft (DFG). (2001a). *Empfehlung der Deutschen Forschungsgemeinschaft zur Forschung mit menschlichen Stammzellen*, 3 May. [On-line] Available: <http://www.dfg.de/aktuell/stellungnahmen/lebenswissenschaften/empfehlungen_stammzellen_03_05_01.htm>.

Deutsche Forschungsgemeinschaft (DFG). (2001b). *Vorschlag des Präsidiums der Deutschen Forschungsgemeinschaft an den Hauptausschuß, die Entscheidung über Verwendung menschlicher embryonaler Stammzellen zu verschieben*, June. [On-line] Available: <http://www.dfg.de/aktuell/ stellungnahmen/dokumentation_1.html#vorschlag>.

Gemeinschaftswerk der Evangelischen Publizistik. (ed.) 2002. *"Zum Bilde Gottes geschaffen:" Bioethik in evangelischer Perspektive. Vorträge eines Kongresses der Evangelischen Kirche in Deutschland am 28./29. Januar in der Französischen Friedrichstadtkirche zu Berlin.* Frankfurt: Evangelischer Pressedienst.

Gesetzentwurf der Abgeordneten Böhmer, von Renesse, Fischer, Seehofer, et al. (2002). *Entwurf eines Gesetzes zur Sicherstellung des Embryonenschutzes im Zusammenhang mit der Einfuhr und Verwendung menschlicher embryonaler Stammzellen (Stammzellgesetz – StZG).* Berlin, 28 February.

Jachertz, N. 2001. 104. Deutscher Ärztetag: Gespanntes Abwarten. *Deutsches Ärzteblatt 98* 22: 01. June, A-1429.

Klinkhammer, G. 2001. TOP I: Ethik – Die Unverfügbarkeit menschlichen Lebens. *Deutsches Ärzteblatt 98* 22: 01. June, A-1440.

Markl, H. 2001. *Liberty, responsibility, human dignity: why there is more to life science than just biology.* Speech by President on the occasion of the 52nd Regular General Meeting of the Max Planck Society for the Advancement of Science. Berlin, Plenary Assembly, June 22. [On-line]. Available: <http://www.mpg.de/reden/2001/hv/markl_e.htm>.

Nida-Rümelin, J. (ed.) 1996. *Angewandte Ethik. Die Bereichsethiken und ihre theoretische Fundierung.* Stuttgart: Kröner.

Rau, J. 2001. *Will everything turn out well? For progress befitting humanity.* Berlin Address by Federal President Johannes Rau in the Otto-Braun-Saal of the Berlin State Library, 18 May. [On-line]. Available: <http://eng.bundespraesident.de> (speeches / Fr 05/18/2001).

Schmidt, K.W. 2002. Konsequenz und Kompromiss. Zum Einfluß der Menschenbilder auf die ethische Beurteilung der Stammzellenforschung. Eine Analyse. *Frankfurter Rundschau*, 22, 26. January 6.

Stollarz, V. & Prüfer, T. 2002. Widersprüche verstehen – ein Ethikbausatz für die Embryonendebatte. *Frankfurter Allgemeine Sonntagszeitung*, 13 January, 2: 66-67.

Wolfrum, R. 2001. Welche Möglichkeiten und Grenzen bestehen für die Gewinnung und Verwendung humaner embryonaler Stammzellen aus juristischer Sicht? In: Bundesministerium für Gesundheit (ed.), *Fortpflanzungsmedizin in Deutschland: Wissenschaftliches Symposium des Bundesministeriums für Gesundheit in Zusammenarbeit mit dem Robert-Koch-Institut vom 24. bis 26. Mai 2000 in Berlin* (pp. 235–242). Nomos: Baden-Baden.

Zentrale Ethikkommission bei der Bundesärztekammer. 2001. Stellungnahme der Zentralen Ethikkommission zur Stammzellenforschung, 23. November. *Deutsches Ärzteblatt 98* 49: C-2553.

8 Bioethics in Switzerland

Fabrice Jotterand

I. Introduction

Over the past fifteen years, the field of bioethics has dramatically evolved and developed in Switzerland for reasons I map in the present paper.[1] From the creation, in 1979, of a Central Ethics Committee (CEC) – appointed by the Swiss Academy of Medical Sciences (SAMS) – to the foundation of the Swiss Society of Biomedical Ethics (1989) and the newly created International Master in Medical Humanities[2] in 2002, with its headquarter in Lugano (Switzerland), bioethics has come to the center of attention in the media, public opinion, politics and academia. As this overview shows, bioethics in Switzerland began in the mid-1980s as a response to a "social protest" by which various groups and organizations (particularly pro-life organizations) demanded more accountability in relation to certain medical practices (e.g., abortion, biotechnology, genetic research, and so forth). To give an adequate reply to the public and to provide academic credentials to bioethical reflections, the Swiss Society of Biomedical Ethics (*Schweizerische Gesellschaft für Biomedizinische Ethik*, SGBE; *Société Suisse d'Ethique Biomédicale*, SSEB) was created in 1989, a date that can be considered the birth of bioethics as a recognized field in Switzerland.

In what follows, I outline the major stages of the development of bioethics in Switzerland. I first examine the socio-cultural context, which is important for understanding the development of bioethics in this country. I then turn to the different stages of its development, in which I distinguish two distinct periods. The first period precedes the "bioethics era": from the foundation of the Swiss Academy of Medical Sciences in 1943 until 1988. The second period begins with the creation of the Swiss Society of Biomedical Ethics in 1989 and continues to the current situation.

II. Socio-cultural Context of Switzerland

The socio-cultural context of Switzerland is characterized by its linguistic, cultural, and religious diversity. On the linguistic level, three majors groups constitute the Swiss population: (Swiss)-German (63.3%), (Swiss)-French (19.2%), and (Swiss)-Italian (7.6%). The remaining population is either part of the fourth national group (the Romansch – less than 1-0.6%) or belongs to various other linguistic groups (8.9%) (Office Fédéral de la Statistique, 1997). Further data on the ethnic constitution of the Swiss population reveals even more diversity. The permanent resident population by nationality shows that almost 20% (19.8% – more or less 1.45 million people of a population of 7.28 million) are actually foreigners. Of the 19.8%, 5.1% are from Asia, 3.5% from North America, 2.6% from Africa, and 0.2% from Australia/Oceania. The remaining foreigners belong to other European countries (Swiss Federal Statistical Office, 2001). In terms of religion, Roman Catholics and Protestants, the two primary religious denominations, share almost the same percentage of nominal believers (Roman Catholics 46% and Protestants 40%) (Office Fédéral de la Statistique, 1997a).[3]

The above statistics reveal the eclectic composition of Swiss society, which is also clear when we look at how each ethnic and religious group diverges in its moral and political orientations. One clear example is the 1977 vote on the issue of abortion-on-demand in the first trimester of pregnancy: Protestant Swiss-French cantons favored its liberalization, whereas cantons with a majority of Catholic Swiss-Germans rejected the initiative (Schoene-Seifert, et al., 1995, p. 1585). There is also a tendency for each ethnic group to refer to the scholarship in other European countries of the same linguistic background. For instance, Swiss-French look at France and Quebec, Swiss-Germans to Germany and Swiss-Italians to Italy.[4]

Interestingly, Catholic theologian Alberto Bondolfi notes that the relationship between the diverse linguistic parts of Switzerland and its "linguistic representatives" (i.e., France/Quebec, Germany, and Italy) is not exclusively due to linguistic influences but also to the fact that many professors and scholars are invited to teach or lecture in Switzerland. For instance, French speaking Swiss universities maintain strong connections with France, although scholars from Quebec seem to have particular influence. Professors Jean-François Malherbe (University of Sherbrooke) and Hubert Doucet (University of Montreal) are often invited to lecture and give talks on medical ethics at the University of Lausanne and the University of Geneva. The German influence on Swiss-German universities likewise cannot be restricted simply to linguistic influences but is also due to the fact that many professors teaching bioethics in Swiss-German speaking universities are Germans. Two good examples are Professor Johannes Fischer of the University of Zurich and Professor Stella Reiter-Theil of the University of Basel. Finally, the connection between Ticino (the Swiss-Italian canton of Switzerland) and Italy is the result of the numerous publications of Alberto Bondolfi in Italian (Bondolfi, 2001).

Besides the linguistic/cultural influences, there is another consideration to take into account is how particular legal systems shape (bio)ethical issues. Jean-François Malherbe remarks that the "juridical culture" of Anglo-bioethics and French-speaking bioethics diverges dramatically. He points out that the French tradition, commonly called Roman Law, is *deductive* in essence. This means that law and ethics preserve autonomous spheres of influence as to how they interact with each other. Law and ethics remain separate and aim at the protection of the ethical values of citizens and not at the resolution of bioethical issues, as is the case in the Anglo-Saxon tradition. On the other hand, the Anglo-Saxon tradition is characterized by a system of "common law" which reflects an *inductive method*. In this case, legal and ethical considerations are taken into account in order to resolve what Malherbe calls "medical suits" (Malherbe, 1996, p. 120).

The legal system of Switzerland retains essentially the "Roman Law" tradition in which the relation between law and ethics is mediated through the legislative process. Contrary to a country like the United States, in which the legal system provides the conditions for new laws involving bioethical issues (the most notorious case is the *Roe v. Wade* Supreme

Court case that legalized abortion on demand) to be implemented, the Swiss court remains very vague as far as ethical issues are concerned. The increasing necessity to regulate biomedical procedures, however, suggests that legal aspects will be dealt with through the creation of governmental commissions, as is already the case in Switzerland (Commission nationale d'éthique pour la médecine humaine and Commission fédérale d'éthique pour le génie génétique dans le domaine non-humain) and Europe (*The Convention of Human Rights and Biomedicine*).

III. The Two Periods of the Development of Swiss Bioethics

As noted in the introductory comments, I distinguish between two distinctive periods in the development of bioethics in Switzerland. The first is what I call the "pre-bioethics period", which encompasses the period from the foundation of the Swiss Academy of Medical Sciences in 1943 until 1988. The second period corresponds with the creation of the Swiss Society of Biomedical Ethics in 1989 and other national commissions (mentioned herein above). It also includes the reform of the teaching of medicine in Swiss medical schools and the creation, in 2002, of a International Masters degree in Medical Humanities.

A. *The Pre-Bioethics Period: Bioethical Reflection within the Medical Community (1943-1988)*

One important aspect of this period, as compared to the subsequent era, is the fact that bioethical issues were not part of public concerns or addressed in the media. Reflection concerning the moral aspects of the practice of medicine was limited to the medical profession. It was only when medicine underwent a crisis[5] that people outside the medical field became involved in the moral dimension of medicine. Hence, bioethics developed in Switzerland somewhat late compared to other countries. Many reasons can be attributed to this situation: first, it is important to note that a civil rights movement that would defend patients' rights was absent in Switzerland; second, the medical profession was used to counting on its strong tradition of medical paternalism to justify its practices; third, the structure of the health care system (general access to medical care) did not raise questions concerning the allocations of resources; and finally, medicine relied on professional organizations to regulate its professional etiquette (Schoene-Seifert et al., 1995, p. 1579; Sass, 1992, pp. 211-212).

This last point is crucial because it shows a certain reticence from the medical profession to embrace the field of bioethics. As a matter of fact in the second half of the 20th century, the regulation of medicine occurred under the supervision of the Swiss Academy of Medical Sciences (SAMS). The Academy was founded in 1943 as the conjoint effort of the deans of five medical and two veterinary faculties and the Swiss Medical Association (*Foederatio Medicorum Helveticorum*, FMH). It is worth noting that the creation of the Academy occurred during a troubled time for medicine, since it coincides with the "Nazi era". Some commentators have pointed out that the Academy's foundation was not fortuitous. Jean-Marie Thévoz, for instance, asserts that the Swiss medical profession purposively created the Academy in order to distinguish itself from Nazi "medicine" (Thévoz, 1992, p. 42).

Currently, the primordial goals of the Academy are to promote the development of medical research (Thévoz, 1992, p. 42) and the professional training of future generations of physicians (SAMS, 2001b). It also aims at reflecting on ethical issues related to medical practice. In 1969, it published its first guidelines concerning the diagnosis and the definition of death. In the 1970s, it issued recommendations on abortion as well as regarding the care of newborns and dying patients.

The ethical dimensions of medicine, however, did not come to the attention of ethicists at that period, as is the case nowadays. Reflecting the paternalistic tradition of the medical establishment, physicians took moral questions into their own hands allowing outsiders to give their opinions only later. Two figures – both theologians – began the opening of medicine to outsiders and helped the Academy to formulate the first guidelines: Father Albert Ziegler who was a chaplain at the University of Zurich and Professor Hermann Ringeling who was a Protestant theologian and professor at the University of Bern.

By 1979, the Academy appointed a Central Ethics Committee (CEC) to respond to the increasingly challenging issues raised by new technologies and practices in medicine. The Committee was responsible (and still is) for the establishment of working-groups – constituted of people from diverse professional backgrounds, such as the medical and nursing professions, the legal profession, and ethics – charged with ensuring the protection of patients and society through reflections and discussions of problems raised by contemporary medicine. Furthermore, it elaborates guidelines that do not possess legal force but are considered to have considerable moral force.[6]

Current research of the Academy includes reflections on the future developments of medicine, potential problems it may encounter, and how it may impact human life, health, and society. The Academy has the central task of researching and reflecting on three specific areas, as formulated by the Academy:

(1) Training – Research:
    a) promotion of the professional training of the coming generation of physicians, especially in clinical research;
    b) support of the high quality of research in biomedical and clinical research;
    c) acquisition of knowledge from basic research and from practical clinical research, taking into account, in particular, the needs of the basic providers.
(2) Bioethics – Social Accountability:
    a) identification of new ethical questions arising from top biomedical research and from the development of new technologies, and the drawing up of ethical and procedural instructions;
    b) clarification of continual ethical questions relating to medical developments and their impact on society;
    c) development of information for the public about the contentious aspects of medical developments and their consequences for society.
(3) Future Perspectives:
    a) reflection on the future of medicine;
    b) identification of perspectives for the future development of medical science and the assessment of the impact of such developments on the provision of health care to the population (SAMW, 2001a, 2001b).

Although members of the Academy represent experts from various fields of research, it is important to note that the first non-physician member of the Central Ethical Commission was Catholic theologian Alberto Bondolfi who was nominated in 1988 (1988-2000). The creation of two other commissions (The Committee on Scientific Integrity in Medicine and Biomedicine, and the Ethics Committee for Animal Studies) besides the Central Ethical Commission, reflected the willingness of the Academy to take ethical issues seriously, but such concerns remained within the context of medical institutions and under the control of physicians. In short, medical ethics was mostly formulated *by* physicians, *for* physicians.

B. The Birth of Bioethics: The Creation of the Swiss Society of Biomedical Ethics (1989-future)

The need to create an institution outside of the constraints of the medical community, which would be able to tackle moral controversies in biomedical research and in the clinical setting, occurred within the parameters of two events. First, the process of the deprofessionalization of medicine resulted in the social questioning of the status of the medical establishment itself. Under the pressure of public opinion, medicine felt obliged to become more accountable regarding certain of its practices (as already mentioned, abortion, new biotechnological procedures, and so forth). The second event is the increasing and rapid enhancement of genetic research. In 1989, the first intervention on the human genetic make-up took place and one year later the first gene therapy attempt occurred. This period corresponded with the initial steps toward the idea of the mapping of the human genome (1985) and the sequencing of its genes was the concerns of biologist Robert Sinsheimer. The combination of these various scientific advances raised worries in the public opinion. As a result, a public initiative for the protection of life and the environment with regards to genetic manipulations (*Initiative populaire pour la protection de la vie et de l'environnement contre les manipulations génétiques*, Confédération Suisse, 1992) was promoted. It addressed issues concerning the ethical implications of genetic manipulation and subsequently was transformed into a new article (formerly Article 24 novies which is now Article 119) of the Swiss Constitution which asserts that "the genetic endowment of a person cannot be analyzed, registered, or revealed without that person's consent or else on the basis of legal prescription" (Confédération Suisse, 2001; Sass, 1995, pp. 250-251). Following the legal system, the Swiss Academy of Medical Sciences likewise issued medical-ethical guidelines with regards to genetic research and gene therapy (Swiss Academy of Medical Sciences, 1993, 1998). According to the bioethicist Christophe Rehmann-Sutter, it is this particular setting of biotechnological progress and its potential applications that allowed further bioethical reflections in genetic research and interventions (Rehmann-Sutter, 1999, pp. 15-16).

In response to the worries and criticisms of public opinion, some scholars concluded that an institution had to be created in order to maintain a high standard of ethical reflection. They were persuaded that "themes and problems in medical ethics [should not] be (mis)understood as the 'hunting privilege' of fundamentalist groups."[7] Hence, two scholars, Bernard Courvoisier, former president of the Swiss Academy of Medical Sciences from 1985 to 1990, and Protestant theologian Eric Fuchs, professor of ethics at the University of Geneva, undertook the task of creating, in 1989, the Swiss Society of Biomedical Ethics (*Schweizerische Gesellschaft für Biomedizinische Ethik*, SGBE; *Société Suisse d'Ethique Biomédicale*, SSEB) to address bioethical issues, especially in medicine and in biotechnology.

The absence of structures within the context of Swiss universities for rich ethical reflection concerning moral issues demanded the development of an institution with strong academic bases. Thus far the discipline of ethics had not been recognized as a field of research worthy of much attention in academia. The only chairs in ethics existing at that time were found in theology faculties, with the exception of the University of Fribourg (a Catholic University) that held a chair in moral philosophy, in the Neo-Thomist tradition. The lack of attention to the discipline of moral philosophy can be traced historically. The Swiss government is embedded in the Judeo-Christian heritage of Western culture. Hence the primary source for moral guidance has been fundamentally Christian in its outlook (after all, the preamble of the Swiss Constitution begins with: "In the name of God Almighty!"). This means that prior to the process of secularization and the rejection of Christian values, the Swiss government had looked to the clergy for guidelines and moral insight, reflecting the bi-confessional character (Catholic or Protestant) of Swiss society.

Nowadays, the clergy does not have the influence it used to have but the early development of bioethics and the founding steps of the SSEB had been shaped by numerous theologians, whether Catholic or Protestant. Alberto Bondolfi (first president of the SSEB from 1990 to 1996) remarks that the presence of numerous theologians in the early stages of the creation of the SSEB did not reflect a "logic of proselytism or confessional indoctrination", that is, an effort to promote a particular moral teaching derived from Christian principles, either Protestant or Catholic. The absence of institutions either in philosophy or in medicine with a particular interest in bioethical issues can explain this state of affairs (Bondolfi, 1999, p. 19). Furthermore, it appears more and more obvious that moral reflection on biomedical issues in a pluralistic Switzerland is grounded on a humanistic tradition.[8] As a post-Enlightenment society, Switzerland accepts moral pluralism so that the government reflects the plurality of *Weltanschauungen*.

The focus of the Swiss Society of Biomedical Ethics is to create a place for reflection and open discussion concerning bioethical issues without any particular ideological, political, and religious perspective, while taking into account the particularities of each main ethnic group represented in Swiss society (SSEB, 2001). Its range of action varies from the promotion of interdisciplinary research and teaching in the field of biomedical ethics to the encouragement of a dialogue between people and groups of diverse professional training and moral convictions (SSEB, 1999, p. 6).[9] Particularly, it exercises its "influence" through the publication of the journal *Bioethica Forum* and by the organization, every two years, of seminars with the purpose of educating those confronted in their professional activities with bioethical issues. As such, the SSEB compensates for the lack of specific teaching of bioethics in medical schools (Bondolfi, 1999, p. 19).

IV. The Institutionalization of Bioethics

The move towards the institutionalization of bioethics has been apparent in the last few years. In two reports, the Swiss Academy of Medical Sciences assessed the future of medicine in Switzerland (ASSM, 2000 and ASSM, 2001). The outcome of these two documents reflected the need for a new orientation of medicine. It was established that currently medicine faces a cluster of challenges: improving the relationship of medicine, patient and society, containing the cost of health care, improving society's level of scientific knowledge, assessing biotechnological progress, and coming to terms with societal mores, etc. Particularly, the current organization of the health care system does not appear to meet the specific needs of Swiss society. The efforts by public collectivities, health care companies, and political powers to provide broad-based solutions remain below a satisfactory level and, therefore, it has become necessary to rethink what medicine entails (ASSM, 2000, p. 4).

But most importantly in relation to the development of bioethics in Switzerland, the report pointed out that the education of medical students appears one-sided because of its strong emphasis on "objective knowledge" – curative medicine to the detriment of the development of the physician as person with his or her personality ("*Le développement de la personalité et du sens de l'orientation – par opposition au savoir objectif – sont sous-estimés dans les études.*") (ASSM, 2001, p. 36). The committee that issued the report identified a key aspect for the enhancement of medical practice: medicine requires the acquisition of better scientific data based on natural sciences and it must take into account knowledge obtained by the humanities and social sciences (ASSM, 2001, p. 37).

The so-called Commission Fleiner II represents the early stages of the reform of medicine and the training of medical students. This expert commission, headed by Professor Fleiner, met between 1997 and October 1998, and issued a draft for a preliminary project on basic medical training (LPMéd basic training). The document stipulated recommendations, which came in the form of proposed legislation and was combined with previously proposed legislation on postgraduate and specialized post-academic training in the medical professions (LPMéd of 1996). It was presented to the Federal Council and to the Parliament for approval in 2001 and should be implemented by 2003.

The reform of medicine in Switzerland aims at an integration of a body of knowledge that is not limited to scientific knowledge but also includes the medical humanities. Hence, the recent creation of an International Master in Medical Humanities, with its headquarter in Lugano, reflects the increasing need of interdisciplinary research. Among the multiple dimensions examined within the medical humanities, an eclectic range of themes is considered. To the ethical, deontological, juridical, anthropological, sociological, ecological, and economical dimensions, cultural features such as literature, visual art – particularly cinema – music, history, and philosophy are integrated in the reflection about medicine. According to the originators of the program, such a broad perspective does not constitute a "cultural ornament of bio-medicine but the necessary instrument for a better qualification of the actions of preservation of the health of mankind and the environment" (my translation).[10] (Master Internazionale in Medical Humanities, 2002).

The reform of medicine focuses on the training of health care professionals with the main objective being "to maintain and promote quality health care by warranting the best possible education for academically trained medical professionals" (Swiss Department of Home Affairs, 1999). More precisely, it is a reform of the *approach* of medical education in which the training of doctors will not be limited to a specialty but rather will encompass various medical disciplines (urology, cardiology, etc.). This approach will deal with specific problems (*Problemorientierten Unterricht* – problem based learning) in which other important fields of specialization are considered for their relevance to the issue at stake. The second aspect of the reform concerns the *content* of medical education. To the traditional fields of study, new areas will be added, such as the sociology of medicine, preventive medicine, and bioethics/medical ethics.

The LPMéd will become regulative in 2003 and consequently classes in medical ethics are not mandatory in the current curriculum of medical training in Swiss universities. There is, however, one exception that is worth noting. At the University of Geneva, medical students are required to take classes in medical ethics. Since 1995, the *Unité de Recherche et d'Enseignement en Bioéthique* has provided instruction in bioethics through Alex Mauron who is one of the two people with full professorship teaching in a medical schools in Switzerland. The second position has been created at the University of Basel where Professor Stella Reiter-Theil is Anne Frank-Stiftungsprofessur at the medical school and is in charge of an interdisciplinary institute for bioethics (*Institut für Angewandte Ethik und Medizinethik*).

The development of bioethics has likewise impacted political authorities. At the federal level two commissions have been created in order to reflect on the moral issues raised by medicine and biotechnology. The first commission was formed in 1998 and is concerned with research on genetic engineering in non-human areas (*Commission fédérale d'éthique pour le génie génétique dans le domaine non-humain*). Its main concern is to examine and evaluate ethically the evolution and applications of new technologies. The other commission (*Commission nationale d'éthique pour la médecine humaine*) was appointed by governmental authorities in 2001 and is composed of 21 members (including medical professionals, lawyers, ethicists, biologists, etc). Its primary task is interdisciplinary reflection on the future of medicine and the development of the medical sciences as well as to discern potential social, legal, and ethical questions pertaining to the field of medicine.

V. Concluding Remarks

Rather than reiterating the different stages of the development of bioethics in Switzerland, I wish, in these concluding remarks to reflect on the importance and necessity of the field of bioethics. Although bioethics in Switzerland is relatively new compared to the birth of the field in the United States,[11] systematic reflection on moral issues has always been part of the field of medicine as this brief presentation has demonstrated. Before the advent of bioethics, however, ethical issues were part of an internal reflection on the intrinsic nature of medicine. Under the pressure of social and political forces ethical issues have moved outside the sphere of medicine – for complex reasons that are beyond the scope of this paper. To some extent this move is important and significant as to the status of medicine. It is important because medicine is in crisis and seems unable to generate the values necessary to sustain its practice. The creation and development of bioethics attests to a growing concern with moral issues that appear to have been ignored, or at least not seriously considered, within medicine. On the other hand, this move is unfortunate because it has created a loss of identity within the medical profession (the deprofessionalization of medicine).[12] What used to be considered a profession with high ethical standards is now one whose moral foundations are questioned. This creates a multitude of moral understandings pertaining to the practice of medicine. Hence, the development of bioethics is, to some extent, a positive move. But a reconsideration of the philosophical foundations of medicine should also come to the center of attention. By looking at the ends and goals of medicine, one can derive constructive elements concerning bioethical issues. Bioethics must be a continuous endeavour in Switzerland but should remain bound to reflection within the philosophy of medicine.[13]

Notes

1. The present essay is a recasting of a previous essay entitled "Development and Identity of Swiss Bioethics" in H. Tristram Engelhardt, Jr. and L.M. Rasmussen (eds) *Bioethics and Moral Content: National Traditions of Health Care Morality*. Boston: Kluwer (2002).

2. For an overview of this new degree in Medical Humanities go to <http://www.medical-humanities.ch>.

3. These numbers do not represent a clear picture of the religious identity of the Swiss people. I use specifically the terminology *nominal* believers in order to demark them from churchgoers. What I mean by *nominal* is the denominational affiliation of Swiss citizens to a state church whether Protestant or Catholic. This affiliation does not signify necessarily a religious commitment, but rather, is a way for the state to collect taxes in order to meet the financial needs of parishes belonging to the state churches.

4. An outline of the different traditions in bioethics in France, Germany, and Italy can be found in Dell'Oro & Viafora (1996). For an overview of the German-speaking world see Alberto Bondolfi (1996, pp. 199-227) and Hans-Martin Sass (1992, pp. 211-231; 1995, pp. 247-268). Jean-François Malherbe has examined the situation in the French-speaking world, (1996, pp. 119-154) and for an outline of Italian Bioethics see Adriano Bompiani (1996, pp. 229-286).

5. The reasons for such crisis can be traced in different ways: (1) moral pluralism that characterizes our post-modern Western societies; (2) the development of new technologies without supervision generates worries within the medical community as well as within the institutions that manage care. The creation of the International Master in Medical Humanities is in part a response to these concerns.

6. Here are some of the latest issues covered by these guidelines:

   (1) Medical-ethical guidelines for genetic investigations in humans (1993)
   (2) Medical-ethical guidelines for the medical care of dying persons and the severely brain-damaged patients (1995)
   (3) Medical-ethical guidelines for organ transplantation (1995)
   (4) Medical-ethical guidelines on the definition and determination of death with a view to organ transplantations (1996)
   (5) Medical-ethical guidelines for the transplantation of human fetal tissue (1998)
   (6) Medical guidelines for somatic gene therapy in humans (1998)
   (7) Medical-ethical guidelines on borderline questions in intensive-care medicine (1999)

   Other guidelines (e.g., medical-ethical guidelines for assisted reproduction technologies (1990), and medical-ethical guidelines for xenotransplantation (2000), etc.), are also available in French or German. For further details on the content of these recommendations see SAMW (2001c).
   Recently, the Academy extended the scope of its regulative task. To deal with the question of scientific integrity in scientific research (false data, plagiarism, etc.) the Academy appointed, in 1999, another committee (The Committee on Scientific Integrity in Medicine and Biomedicine – CIS) specifically charged to oversee and ensure appropriate scientific behavior. It also commissioned an Ethics Committee for Animal Studies as a regulative agency overseeing the use of animals in biomedical research. For more details see SAMS: Ethics (SAMS, 2001a).

7. Bondolfi, (1999, p. 19, translation mine): "Beide [Courvoisier and Fuchs] waren schnell darin übereingekommen, dass Themen und Probleme der Medizin-ethik nicht als 'Jagdreservat' für fundamentalistische Gruppierungen (miss-)verstanden werden dürfen."

8. In the presentation of the newly created International Master in Medical Humanities, the originators of the degree specifically assert that the medical humanities should reflect humanistic knowledge: "Les Medical Humanities, perçues comme un instrument d'analyse des causes et des

consequences de cette crise de la médecine moderne, pourraient être définies comme une interaction de savoirs humanistes capables d'analyser les grands et les petits problèmes générés par la bio-médecine moderne ..." ("The Medical Humanities, conceived as an instrument of analysis of the causes and the consequences of the crisis of modern medicine, could be defined as an inter-action of the [various sources of] humanistic knowledge able to analyze the great and small problems generated by modern bio-medicine ...")

9. Article 2 stipulates: "La SSEB a pour buts: (a) de promouvoir la recherche et l'enseignement interdisciplinaires dans le domaine de l'éthique biomédicale; (b) de promouvoir l'ouverture et le dialogue entre personnes et groupes de formation et de convictions différentes ..." ["The SSEB has as its goals: (a) to promote interdisciplinary research and teaching in the field of biomedical ethics; (b) to promote the openness and the dialogue between people and groups of different edu-cation and conviction ...," (translation mine).]

10. "Les Medical Humanities ne constituent pas un ornement culturel de la bio-médecine, mais l'instrument nécessaire en vue d'une meilleure qualification des actions de préservation de la santé de l'être humain et de l'environnement."

11. For an overview of the "birth of bioethics", see Jonsen (1998).

12. For development on the issue of the deprofessionalization of medicine see Engelhardt (2002).

13. For more on the relation between bioethics and the philosophy of medicine see Thomasma & Pellegrino (1981), Pellegrino (1998), Khushf (1997). For a critical assessment see Caplan (1992).

Acknowledgment

I would like to thank Ana Smith Iltis for her comments on a previous draft of this essay.

Bibliography

Académie Suisse des Sciences Médicales. 2000. *Nouvelle orientation de la médecine: Rapport intermédiaire de la 1ère Séance de réflexion*, 25/26 août. Bienne: Académie Suisse des Sciences Médicales.

Académie Suisse des Sciences Médicales. 2001. *Nouvelle orientation de la médecine: Rapport intermédiaire de la 2ème Séance de réflexion*, 19/20 janvier. Bienne: Académie Suisse des Sciences Médicales.

Bompiani, A. 1996. The outlines of Italian bioethics. In: R. Dell'Oro & C. Viafora (eds). *History of bioethics: international perspectives* (pp. 229-286). San Francisco: International Scholars Publications.

Bondolfi, A. 1996. Orientations and tendencies of bioethics in the German-speaking world. In: R. Dell'Oro. and C. Viafora (eds), *History of bioethics: international perspectives* (pp. 199-227). San Francisco: International Scholars Publications.

Bondolfi, A. 1999. Zur Lage der Medizinethik in der Schweiz. 10 Jahre SBGE. *Bioethica Forum* 29: 17-20.

Bondolfi, A. 2001. Personal interview, University of Zurich, June.

Caplan, A.L. 1992. Does the philosophy of medicine exist? *Theoretical Medicine* 13: 67-77.

Confédération Suisse. 2001. *Constitution fédérale de la Confédération suisse*. [On-line]. Available: ⟨http://www.admin.ch/ch/f/rs/101/⟩.

Confédération Suisse, Initiative populaire fédérale. 1992. *Initiative populaire fédérale pour la protection de la vie et de l'environnement contre les manipulations génétiques (initiative pour la protection génétique)*. [On-line]. Available: <http://www.admin.ch/ch/f/pore/vi/vi240t.html>.

Dell'Oro, R. & Viafora, C. (eds) 1996. *History of bioethics: international perspectives*. San Francisco: International Scholars Publications.

Engelhardt, H.T., Jr. 2002. Managed care and the deprofessionalization of medicine (pp. 93-107). In: W.B. Bondeson (ed.), *The ethics of managed care: professional integrity and patient rights*. Dordrecht: Kluwer Academic Publishers.

Jonsen, A.R. 1998. *The birth of bioethics*. New York: Oxford University Press.

Khushf, G. 1997. Why bioethics needs the philosophy of medicine: some implications of reflection on concepts of health and disease. *Theoretical Medicine and Bioethics* 18: 145-163.

Malherbe, J.-F. 1996. Orientations and tendencies of bioethics in the French-speaking world (pp. 119-154). In: R. Dell'Oro & C. Viafora (eds), *History of bioethics: international perspectives*. San Francisco: International Scholars Publications.

Master Internazionale in Medical Humanities. 2002. Présentation. [On-line]. Available: <www.medical-humanities.ch>.

Office Fédéral de la Statistique. 1997a. *Le paysage religieux helvétique: des tendances nouvelles*. Berne: Office Fédéral de la Statistique. [On-line]. Available: <http://www.statistik.admin.ch/news/ archiv97/fp97063.htm>.

Office Fédéral de la Statistique. 1997b. *Les frontières linguistiques en Suisse sont pratiquement stables*. Berne: Office Fédéral de la Statistique. Available on-line: <http://www.statistik.admin.ch/news/archiv97/fp97104.htm>.

Pellegrino, E.D. 1998. What the philosophy of medicine is. *Theoretical Medicine and Bioethics* 19: 315-336.

Rehmann-Sutter, C. 1999. *Zur Aufgabe der Schweizerischen Gesellschaft für biomedizinische Ethik*. *Bioethica Forum* 29: 15-17.

Sass, H.M. 1992. Bioethics in German-speaking western European countries: Austria, Germany, and Switzerland. In: B.A. Lustig, B.A. Brody, H.T. Engelhardt, Jr. & L.B. McCullough (eds), *Bioethics yearbook Vol. 2: regional developments in bioethics 1989-1991* (pp. 211-231). Dordrecht: Kluwer Academic Publishers.

Sass, H.M. 1995. Bioethics in German-speaking western European countries: Austria, Germany, and Switzerland: 1991-1993. In: B.A. Lustig, B.A. Brody, H.T. Engelhardt, Jr. & L. B. McCullough (eds), *Bioethics yearbook Vol. 4: regional development in bioethics 1992-1993* (pp. 247-268). Dordrecht: Kluwer Academic Publishers.

Schoene-Seifert, B. 1995. History of medical ethics: Europe. In: Warren T. Reich (ed.), *Encyclopedia of bioethics*. New York: Macmillan Pub. Co.

Societé suisse d'éthique biomédicale. 1999. Status de la SSEB. *Bioethica Forum* 29 (November).

Société suisse d'éthique biomédicale. 2001. *Présentation*. [On-line]. Available: <http://bioethics.ch/presentation.htm>.

Swiss Academy of Medical Sciences. 2001a. *Ethics*. [On-line]. Available: <http://www.samw.ch/content/e_Ethik.htm>.

Swiss Academy of Medical Sciences. 2001b. *SAMS at a glance*. [On-line]. Available: <http://www.samw.ch/content/e_Samw.htm>.

Swiss Academy of Medical Sciences. 2001c. *Medical-ethical guidelines*. [On-line]. Available: <http://www.samw.ch/content/e_Richt.htm>.

Swiss Department of Home Affairs. 1999. The medical professions. *EDI/FDI-themen-e-Die Medizinalberufe*. [On-line]. Available: <http://www.edi.admin.ch/e/themen/medizin.htm>.

Swiss Federal Statistical Office. 2001. Population: permanent resident population by nationality. Neuchâtel: Swiss Federal Statistical Office. [On-line]. Available: <http://www.statistik.admin.ch/stat_ch/ber01/eufr01.htm>.

Thévoz, J.M. 1992. Research and hospital ethics committees in Switzerland. *HEC Forum* 4(1): 41-47.

Thomasma, D.C. & Pellegrino, E.D. 1981. Philosophy of medicine as the source of medical ethics. *Metamedicine* 2: 5-11.

9 Bioethics in Greece: A Regional Approach

T. Garanis-Papadatos and P. Dalla-Vorgia

I. Introduction

Bioethics in Greece has been intertwined with the Hippocratic tradition, a tradition which, incorporated in the famous Hippocratic Oath, permeated Western culture for many centuries. Hippocrates, who, according to historical sources, was said to possess very acute judgment, appreciated the importance of the relationship between doctor and patient, a relationship that was codified into the brilliant Hippocratic Oath. This Oath was adopted by the Medical School of Baghdad and was disseminated into Europe by the Arabs. It was forgotten for many centuries but was rediscovered in Europe during the Enlightenment era of the seventeenth century (Granitsas, 1991). Enriched by the Christian humanitarian spirit and the necessary legal framework, the Oath became the foundation of the medical profession for many centuries (Merikas, 1987, pp. 39-48).

Traditionally, physicians exercised significant paternalistic authority over their patients and society. Following the liberation of the Greek state from Ottoman dominance and the foundation of the first Medical Faculty in Athens, for many decades, nothing important was done or written in Greece regarding medical ethics (Ioannidis & Epivatianos, 1990, pp. 119-127). However, recent historical and sociopolitical developments have led to considerable changes in medical ethics and understandings of medical authority.

Following a narrow interpretation of the Hippocratic Oath, medical practice in Greece has been shaped in a paternalistic framework, which is not surprising if one takes into consideration the features that form the picture of the Greek societal context: living traditions, strong family bonds, vertical structure of families (three generations living under the same roof), and strong religious feelings. Although these characteristics do not exist to the same extent as in the past, especially in large urban centers, they have nevertheless formed the axis around which the doctor/patient relationship has been understood. This traditional framework, although derived from benevolent customs, has been strict and one-sided, based on the absolute authority and the high social status of the physician. It has, therefore, left no room for the expansion of other values and notions, such as the concept of autonomy.

The notion of autonomy is central in the evolution of secular bioethics. In the past few decades, autonomy has been internationally recognized as a fundamental right, which can be overridden only under exceptional circumstances. This sensitization is not accidental; it can be explained both from the social and the legal point of view because the development of the notion of autonomy did not take place *in vacuo*. It is the result of a social evolution which is being reflected in the judicial systems of many countries. In the American and Western European world, the evolution of autonomy has moved in parallel with social and technological progress. According to Veatch (1985), the evolution of autonomy presupposes abundance of resources as well as the existence of technological skepticism and liberal individualism. Although the United States does possess these characteristics to a degree that contributed considerably to the expansion of bioethics, the situation is not the same in European countries, especially southern European countries, such as Greece.

Autonomy is not of course an unknown notion in Greek jurisprudence. The Greek Constitution of 1975 provides fundamental directions regarding respect for human beings and self-determination. According to Section 2 paragraph 1, respect and protection of the value of a human being constitute the primary obligation of the State. According to Section 5 paragraph 1, a person's right to develop freely his or her personality, insofar as this does not infringe upon the rights of others or violate the constitution or public morality, is also protected. Moreover, Section 21 paragraph 3 refers to the obligation of the state to care for citizens' health and to adopt all special measures that are deemed necessary for the protection of youth, old age, disability, and the relief of the needy. For example, recent legislation – namely Act 2071 of 1992 and Act 2517 of 1997 – regarding the National Health Service, includes specific provisions aiming at the protection of patients' rights.

Differences among American, European, and Greek perceptions concerning bioethics is reflective of significantly different social realities. Discrepancies, however, also derive from the nature of the varying legal systems. In the United States, the notion of autonomy is viewed through the prism of human rights. Justification for respecting individual autonomy is sought in the theory of philosophical individualism and in the theoretical framework of constitutional rights, especially rights to liberty and privacy. In the European context, the situation has not followed the same pattern. Here, courts typically reach decisions according to the particularities of each case and avoid extracting generalized conclusions. In the last decade, however, a certain convergence of the American and the European approaches has been observed, in large measure because the European Declaration of Human Rights is acting as a common framework for those European jurisdictions that have signed and ratified the Declaration. Moreover, the existence of the European Union has had a unifying impact on the legislation of member states. While it is true that the history and the tradition of each country dictates approaches that cannot be easily comprehended by those who come from different social and judicial systems, many have appreciated a need for unity. According to Morgan, for example:

> Ethical relativism, cultural heterogeneity and legal specificity are jealously guarded ideals. Yet, in each country of Europe, including Eastern Europe, similar questions arise with respect to law, medicine and bioethics. There exist, however, differences of a philosophical, economic, social, political and even geographical nature which are not easily (even if desirably) bridged (2001).

The need for a unified approach also appears in the fields of medicine, bioethics and law.

Bioethics in Greece should be seen through the prism of the historical and social traditions that have shaped the development of this country at all levels. International experience and international bibliography constitute the most valuable tools for those who work in the field of bioethics. Nevertheless, the use of foreign bibliography in the teaching of bioethics is often criticized as being one-sided, and educators are reprimanded for using examples in bioethical theory that are not usual in the Greek societal context. Rapid developments in biomedicine and biotechnology, especially in the fields of reproductive technology and human genetics, however, have amplified such criticisms. The emerging dilemmas have acquired a more universal character, going beyond traditional approaches to the doctor–patient relationship, seeking the ramifications of the intrinsic value and meaning of the existence of a human being. It is towards this universal approach that bioethics in Greece should be headed, while simultaneously respecting the cultural characteristics of the living Greek social environment.

II. Central Issues

A. Professionalism

The basis for a successful practice of medicine on a personal level is the trust between health care professionals and patients. It is necessary that this trust exist throughout the duration of the relationship, since its lack at any phase makes it impossible to function.

The Hippocratic tradition, as has already been mentioned, has influenced bioethics deeply in Greece and the main concern of doctors, even today, is to benefit their patients and not to harm them. Traditionally, however, the notion of benefit did not emphasize respect of patients' rights, nor did it appreciate autonomy as important. Greek doctors traditionally acted paternalistically, which today is not always accepted in the same way, as it used to be. The image of the family doctor, who has the time and interest to take care of his patients, no longer exists. However, one could say that the doctor–patient relationship is still a matter of sentiment rather than contract in Greece, and this could partly explain the very few malpractice cases that come to court. Although Greek doctors continue to reflect a rather paternalistic attitude, this does not mean that patients' rights are not protected in Greece. Relevant legislation does exist and "modern" patients who understand their healthcare and their rights have started to make relevant claims.

1. *Patients' rights.* Specific legislation on patients' rights was introduced in 1992 (Law 2071/1992). Until then, general legislation, as well as legislation on specific issues, like transplantation, protection of childhood, research on human beings, and so forth, covered the issue. Greece has also signed and ratified the "Convention for the Protection of Human Rights and Dignity of the Human Being with regard to the Application of Biology and Medicine" (1997), which provides patients with better protection of their rights.

2. *Medical confidentiality.* Medical confidentiality has always been respected in Greece. It is one of the few issues on which most of the interested parties agree (Dalla-Vorgia & Garanis, 1991). The Hippocratic Oath has a specific section concerning confidentiality: "All that may come to my knowledge in the exercise of my profession or outside of my profession or in daily commerce with men, which ought not to be spread abroad, I will keep secret and will never reveal." The Greek Penal Code (Section 371) punishes infringement of medical confidentiality, unless the doctor is fulfilling a duty to protect a legal or otherwise justifiable interest of his own or of other concerned parties. Even in court doctors are not obliged to testify about what has been confided to them during the practice of their profession, unless a specific license is granted from the local Medical Association. Furthermore, the

1939 Code of Practice of the Medical Profession imposes a duty to keep absolutely secret everything that has come to the doctor's attention during the practice of his profession and which constitutes a secret of the patient or the patient's family. The Code of Medical Deontology of 1955 states that the doctor must take every possible precaution to protect medical confidentiality in his professional records and scientific publications. In practice, there exist potential problems, such as hospital situations where a great number of people have access to medical records or where there may exist conflicts of interest, as is often the case with regard to AIDS patients where there may exist conflicts of interests. Law 2472 of 1997 on Data Protection, provides for the processing of personal data.

   3. *Consent to medical treatment or research*. The issue of informed consent has not been given much attention in Greece. The Greek Constitution states that due respect should be paid to the person and that the autonomy of the individual should be respected. Also, doctors who act without consent might be accused of offending or infringing on personal freedom. However, despite the existence of the patients' rights law, which requires consent, patients are not always informed, nor is their individual consent necessarily sought (especially in minor interventions). Decisions are often made by doctors in cooperation with relatives. This situation can be attributed to several underlying factors: (a) the paternalistic attitude of Greek doctors leads to a feeling of their being the most appropriate persons to make decisions; (b) there have been very few cases of malpractice in Greece and this makes doctors feel "safe" in their decision-making; (c) very often patients themselves waive their rights to decide by saying that "the doctor knows best"; (d) the issue of consent is very closely related to the truth-telling issue and Greek doctors still often feel that, by not telling the truth, they are protecting their patients. As familial bonds remain comparatively strong in Greece, physicians prefer to inform the patient's family and proceed to joint decision-making. Nevertheless, as people become more aware of their rights, as medical law expands and as insurance systems develop further, the number of malpractice cases will increase and patients will expect a different attitude from their doctor.

B. Reproduction

Reproduction in Greece, which is a country with a population-aging problem, is an important issue. Officially, family, marriage, motherhood and childhood are under the protection of the State according to the Greek Constitution, however, in practice, much remains to be achieved.

   Abortion is legal in Greece and, although contraception is well supported, the number of legal and illegal abortions is very high. Law No. 1609 of 1986 permits abortion under certain circumstances: it must be performed with the consent of the woman by an obstetrician-gynecologist, with the participation of an anesthesiologist, in a health care establishment. One of the following conditions must also be met: (a) the duration of the pregnancy is less than 12 weeks, (b) there are indications of serious disorders of the embryo (up to 24 weeks), (c) there is an unavoidable risk to the life of the woman, or to her physical or mental health, (d) the pregnancy is a result of rape, seduction of a minor, incest or abuse of a woman unable to resist (up to 19 weeks). However, not only now (even in absence of its prerequisites), but even before the enactment of this law, thousands of abortions were being and still are performed by obstetricians. It should be noted that the Greek Orthodox Church has always opposed abortion.

In the area of medically assisted reproduction, lack of a legal framework and the relevant infrastructure have been the main problems, although various methods and especially homologous and heterologous insemination have been performed in this country for more than 40 years now. Today Greece is very close to establishing a law regarding the regulation and functioning of Assisted Reproduction Units. The problem, however, is twofold. First, it concerns the existing "freedom" of professionals to act in the way they think best, following their integrity and conscience and general rules of medical conduct. This fact has nurtured the expansion of the private market, the size of which presents a considerable threat to any regulating attempt. Second, the issue has an inner dimension as well, which concerns how the law is created in a societal context as the result of the ethical attitudes of this society towards certain practices and technological developments.

The first regulating attempts took place in 1987 and were motivated by the relevant report of the Council of Europe, which referred to some basic principles concerning, among other things: the responsibility of society to future generations; the presumption of family as the basic cell of society, which has a right to full protection by the State; the importance of the family environment; the need to avoid exploitation of women and to protect embryos and children (Decision No. 7 of the Plenary of the Central Council of Health, 1987; Committee of Experts on Progress in the Biomedical Sciences, 1989).

The Central Council of Health in Greece endorsed these principles and emphasized the need for any kind of future legislation in this field to abide by them. In 1988, with a following decision (Decision No. 9 of the 56th Plenary of the Central Council of Health, 1988) it incorporated the more specific and technical principles of the above-mentioned Report.

In the years that followed no particular progress was made. Law 2071 of 1992, regarding the modernization and organization of the National Health Service, in section 59 stipulates that a presidential decree will determine the terms and conditions for the establishment and function of units of human artificial fertilization. The same decree will determine all details related to the ethical, professional, legal, and financial regulation of such units. Assisted Reproduction Units are to function only in specifically equipped and structured public or private hospitals, or in specifically equipped and structured private clinics. Various committees were consequently established whose terms of reference were to create the necessary legal framework. Their efforts, however, were abortive as their reports and proposals never became law for political or other reasons.

The most recent *ad hoc* committee was established in 1997 and submitted its proposals in 1999. The main points of these proposals were the following:

- *Place of treatment*: Methods of medically assisted reproduction must be carried out in public hospitals, private clinics or day-care centers according to the requirements of the law.
- *Central authority*: The members of the Committee proposed the establishment of an Authority (similar to the Human Fertilization and Embryology Authority of the United Kingdom) which will grant or suspend treatment and research licenses for these Units and control their operation.
- *On whom the methods shall be performed*: Methods of medically assisted reproduction can be applied to married or non-married couples who live together.
- *Gamete donation*: Donation is to be carried out under conditions of anonymity. Financial profit is forbidden.

- *Embryo research*: Such research is permitted only on surplus embryos, which have been donated for this purpose, or on frozen embryos. Research is permitted only during the first 14 days after conception.
- *Filiation*: According to existing Greek legislation, especially Article 1463 of the Civil Law, the relationship of the child with the mother is established at birth. According to Law 3089 of 2002, regarding Medical Assistance to Human Reproduction, partial surrogacy is permitted by permission of the Court. The woman to whom permission is granted is considered the legal mother a presumption which can be rebutted if the surrogate proves the child is genetically hers. Post-mortem insemination with the husband's sperm is also permitted with Court permission.
- *Preimplantation diagnosis*: As a diagnostic technique which is still in the research stage, and as it concerns couples who may carry defective genes but who do not suffer from a sterility problem, its application should require a research license and special approval by the Central Authority.

Finally, it should be noted that regulation and legislation should also be in line with the Convention on Human Rights and Biomedicine of the Council of Europe which Greece has signed and ratified. Thus, informed consent of the parties involved is absolutely necessary, individual privacy should be respected, sex selection is forbidden except when sex-linked genetic diseases are concerned, creation of human embryos for research purposes is forbidden, and reproductive cloning is forbidden.

C. Death and Dying

Every culture faces death in a different way and there exist many discrepancies regarding perceptions of death, attitudes in the clinical context, and even death rituals. As in many Western countries, physicians in Greece often consider the death of a patient a professional defeat. Their medical education has not adequately prepared them to deal closely with life's most certain phenomenon. This is beautifully described in the words of a psychologist working with dying children:

> She turned to the people with whom she worked: her teammates. They were all faced with something in common: the threat of death … For members of the medical team to be confronted with a new threat that is more tangible and less powerful than the threat of death, is often an easy way of displacing the real problem and letting it remain unsolved. Sometimes a team's dysfunctioning is the reflection of a larger institution that avoids and denies death (Papadatou, 1991).

The introduction of sophisticated technology into the clinical context, however, is generating a wide variety of ethical dilemmas that physicians are facing every day. Such dilemmas are causing changes in the way death in the hospital is perceived. More and more people are realizing that prolonging the life of a hopelessly ill patient is not always the best course of action and, moreover, does not always constitute the best interpretation of the notion of the "physician's duty". End-of-life decisions in relation to the specific issue of euthanasia are one of the most important dilemmas which medicine is facing today.

Similar questions often arise in the Greek medical context and issues such as "death with dignity" and the "right to die" are increasingly being discussed in the public forum. Issues, however, like "Do-Not-Resuscitate Orders" or withdrawal of artificial nutrition and hydration are not being discussed except in professional circles.

Although the traditional approach favors the preservation of life at any cost, the reasoning behind this attitude is under pressure today. Thus, despite the official position held by the Greek Medical Association, the dilemmas of end-of-life-decisions, namely withholding and withdrawing life-prolonging treatment that is of no health benefit to the patient in question, constitute a burning issue and often appear in the mass media.

The prevailing attitude of medical professionals in Greece is that helping the dying person with compassion and respect is a fundamental duty of the doctor. Nevertheless, such assistance, which can be given in order to alleviate physical and mental distress, may in no way lead to the direct termination of treatment.

An important characteristic in Greek culture is the role of the family. Family bonds are tight and although this situation has started to change in large urban areas, the family still remains the strongest support mechanism of the terminally ill patient. In the last stages of illness, Greeks continue to show respect for human life, as well as endurance, hope and self-sacrifice. The majority of Greeks are also religious people and the Orthodox Church vehemently opposes euthanasia. The doctrine of the sanctity of life is closely related to the beliefs of the Greek Orthodox Church, whose views on the issue of euthanasia could be summarized as follows: "The Church does not acknowledge the term euthanasia. In order to understand this view one should have previously understood the preaching of the Church regarding human life, to have understood the depth of the spirituality of Church" (Round Table, 1991).

In Greek legislation, a distinction is made according to the criterion of whether the patient has expressed a request to die or not. Euthanasia is deemed to be the situation where the death of a patient is hastened without his explicit request, whereas when this request exists, the legal situation falls under the term "homicide by consent". Euthanasia, therefore, corresponds to mercy killing without the patient's consent and is thus illegal. The term "euthanasia" is nowhere to be found in the Greek Penal Code; it exists only in different pieces of legislation concerning domestic animals. The Greek Penal Code, on the other hand, in Section 300, refers to homicide by consent:

> Whoever decided on and committed homicide after the serious and persistent request of the deceased who was suffering from an incurable disease, because of mercy towards him, shall be punished by imprisonment.

(Critics of this legislation believe that it should rather be called homicide by mercy, which equals mercy killing). Homicide by consent is a penal offense that satisfies the following three conditions:

- Untreatable disease or situation that derives from serious physical harm. The knowledge of this situation constitutes the justification for the feeling of mercy.
- Persistent request by the patient, expressed by himself (and not by a proxy) and reflecting his real will. "Request" is not synonymous with "consent". It possesses a much stronger connotation; expressing a persistent, repeated demand by the patient, who must be in a position to understand his condition.
- Mercy as the sole motive which leads the perpetrator to the act of homicide.

According to Section 300 of the Penal Code, homicide by consent is punished with imprisonment. This is perceived as a quite lenient approach, due to the fact that the legislators acknowledge that the real motive for this act was the feeling of mercy, but still do not wish to leave this act, which is deemed to be a homicide, unpunished. The Greek Medical Association has repeatedly stated its opposition to any form of euthanasia, as human life is absolutely protected under Greek legislation and jurisprudence, sometimes even contrary to the patient's will, and the Code of Medical Ethics instills an obligation in physicians to protect and save human life.

Section 301 of the Penal Code refers to assisting another to commit suicide; such assistance is punished in the same way as homicide by consent. It should be pointed out that the Greek Penal Code was enacted in 1950 and, therefore, the regulations it contains express views about life which were dominant half a century ago. Many legal scholars believe that Section 300 is obsolete and should be amended according to the needs of modern society, i.e., in a way which acknowledges personal dignity. Nevertheless, this critique does not mean that euthanasia should be legalized.

In Greece, various debates regarding the issue of medical decisions at the end of life reveal the bipolarization of existing attitudes and opinions – a bipolarization based on the conflict between the doctrine of the sanctity of life and the physician's duty to preserve life, on the one hand, and on the notion of the quality of life and of the individual's right to decide about his or her own life, on the other hand. Approaching this issue from "a right to die" perspective leads to a legal framework based on patients' rights. In the past decade, Greece has experienced an increasing interest regarding patients' rights. In 1992, Act 2071/1992 directly addressed the rights of patients for the first time, following the model of the European Charter of Hospital Patients' Rights of 1979. Section 47 of Act 2071 stipulates, *inter alia*, that patients possess the right to consent but also to refuse any diagnostic or therapeutic act proposed. Although the Greek Constitution safeguards the right of all persons freely to develop their personality, protecting and promoting autonomy (article 5.1), in the medical context the absolute and traditionally interpreted duty of beneficence makes attitudes more conservative. Taking into consideration the traces of paternalism which still exist in the Greek medical setting, it is doubtful whether a physician would accept easily – or even at all – the expression of the right to refuse treatment by a patient, without trying very hard to change the patient's or his relatives' decision. Moreover, when in doubt, traditional views favoring preservation of life still prevail. It should be also noted that cases and disputes concerning end-of-life decisions have never reached the Courts, as medical litigation regarding medical ethical dilemmas is almost non-existent in Greece.

D. Access to Health Care

Transformation in health services started in Europe after the Second World War. The public health sector was continuously reorganized and expanded, and the notion of health as a good to which all citizens should have equal access became part of the European democratic constitutions. In Greece, however, the situation was different: the civil war that followed the Second World War and the period of dictatorship (1967-1974) prevented the development of the health sector. The main characteristics of this transitional period included unequal access to health services and health personnel, as well as unequal allocation of financial resources between urban centers and rural areas.

As a result, it was only in 1974 that Greece managed to enter its transitional phase as far as health was concerned (Report of a Committee of Experts regarding the Planning and Organization of Health Care Services, 1994). The introduction of the National Health Service (NHS) in 1983 (Law 1397/1983) marked the most important transformation to have ever taken place in the Greek health system. Article 1 of the above mentioned law stipulated the basic principles of the new health care system: (1) state responsibility for the provision of services, (2) equal distribution of health care services, (3) sufficient coverage of the needs of every citizen irrespective of age, gender or ability to pay, (4) decentralization of services, and (5) emphasis on primary care and improvement of the quality of health care services (Report of a Committee of Experts regarding the Planning and Organization of Health Care Services, 1994). Although the first law for the Greek NHS was providing for almost all organizational aspects and employment issues, the provisions regarding the funding of health care services were very inadequate. Thus, although the NHS was aiming at major transformations in the system of health care provision, the link between planning and funding remained weak (Sissouras, 1990). The main sources of funding of the Greek health care sector are the state budget, social funds, and private expenditure. The Greek population enjoys universal coverage without additional out-of-pocket expenses. Nevertheless, despite the fact that equity and free access to health care are the fundamental principles of the Greek health care sector, there still exist regional inequalities in the distribution of health care resources as well as in the provision of health care among the various social insurance funds.

During the 1980s, emphasis was given to the development of services and equity, whereas, during the 1990s, the focus was on efficiency and cost containment. According to recent studies, the main problem is that inequity in the allocation of resources in per capita health spending and in health indices, still remains high (Economou, Karalis, & Kyriopoulos, 1999; Yfantopoulos, 2000). The most important problems today also include high side-payments, low user satisfaction, and inequities in the distribution of health care resources and access to services (Kyriopoulos, 2001). It is estimated that the actual level of private spending amounts to 42% of the total spending on health, a figure which is among the highest in the European Union and OECD countries (Kyriopoulos, 2001). The real level of health expenditure in Greece, remains however a point of disagreement.

Many efforts to reform the existing system have taken place since the establishment of the NHS, the latest focused on the regionalization of health care services, efficiency, management, and hidden-economy activities. It should be noted that a number of endogenous factors, such as the cultural environment, social beliefs about illness and the family structure, play an important role in the shaping of health services' consumption. Moreover, the aging of the population and the rapid technological biomedical progress have also affected the health care system (Gitona et al., 1992).

The existing socio-political and legal system in Greece recognizes the existence of a right to health care, a right that derives from the establishment of the state's responsibility to provide health care to its citizens. It is thus reasonable to accept the existence of a respective right, although the definition of its content is a very difficult task as this is undergoing continuous changes. The nature of this right is said to be, according to legal scholars, twofold: social and individual. The Greek NHS was built on the notion that health is a social good, but a more careful reflection of the existing laws reveals the

individualistic dimension of health as well. The Greek health care system reflects the combination of these two dominant positions: the liberal and the socialist, the former focusing on the individual's integrity, the latter connecting health with the general notion of
social well-being (Kremalis, 1987).

E. Ethics Consultation and Ethics Committees

The first attempt to establish an Ethics Committee in Greece took place in 1965 in the
Institute of Child Health by the late Professor S. Doxiadis, an eminent pediatrician and
pioneer in medical ethics. Political turmoil led this committee to cease functioning in
1981, but it was started again in 1990. Other attempts to establish ethics committees were
also made, including a Legislative Decree (No. 97/1973), which mainly concerned the
approval of clinical drug research by the Central Committee on the Control of Drugs, and
a Ministerial Circular (A2/oik3061/5.6.78) issued in 1978 (when Professor Doxiadis
was Minister of Health), which imposed the establishment of ethics committees at the
local level.

Although these attempts were quite ambitious, they did not meet with general acceptance, which was necessary for the establishment of local ethics committees. The necessity
of ethics committees may today be acknowledged by many people, but this is not a feeling shared by the majority of practitioners. The traditional approach to medical practice,
deeply rooted in paternalistic attitudes, has not completely disappeared from the Greek
health context, and this may constitute one of the reasons for a certain distrust towards
ethics committees in the hospitals (Garanis-Papadatos & Dalla-Vorgia, 2000). In ancient
times, for the Hippocratic physician, the opinion of his peers was of primary importance
in the medical family. Today, although physicians discuss difficult cases as a team, they
do not hold a very positive stance towards the existence of a clinical ethics committee, as
they believe that such a practice would threaten independent clinical decision-making.
Physicians in Greece, and probably in other countries, state that they want to be autonomous in their decision-making, and very few consider ethics committees an ally, which
could be of considerable help during a crisis. The role of clinical ethics committees, however, does not justify such fears; the existence of a committee does not entail the abolish-
ment of the notion of personal responsibility. In Greece, the role of the committee would
and should be only advisory, shifting the physician's responsibility is not legally or ethically acceptable. The role of the committee should also be educational, as it can provide a
more organized way of thinking and make possible the expression of opinions from other
specialists as well.

For the above-mentioned reasons it is not surprising that there exists very few local
hospital ethics committees and that attitudes are more favorable towards research ethics
committees. Actually, in the Greek hospital setting, the task of evaluating research protocols and their ethical ramifications is carried out by the scientific committees that review
research projects. Scientific committees, whose establishment in state hospitals is compulsory, were set up by Law 1397/1983 and, according to it, they may appoint various subcommittees such as an ethics committee, an education committee, a public relations
committee, and so forth. However, not all scientific committees have such subcommittees.

For a while, it looked as if all the efforts towards establishing ethics committees had
been completely aborted. Interest in this area, however, was recently renewed because of

problems and dilemmas caused by rapid developments in biomedical technology and changes in the societal context, which seem to require different approaches toward protecting individual health. Act 2071 of 1992 regarding the "Modernization and Organization of the National Health Service" provides, for the first time, for the establishment of a National Council of Medical Ethics and Deontology, which was recently renamed to the National Ethics and Deontology Committee by Law 2519/1997. Section 61 paragraph 4 of the above-mentioned Act posits that local ethics committees must be established in public and private hospitals and clinics. Their task will consist not only of informing the public but also in adopting prohibitive attitudes towards new scientific possibilities that have not been adequately explored. These efforts, however, are mainly focused on research concerns. The tasks of such committees include consultation on issues of medical ethics to the Governing Board of the hospital or the clinic, as well as an application of basic rules and bioethical principles. It is clear that the role of these committees is only advisory. Nevertheless, very few have been established in hospitals and, those that do exist function mainly as research ethics committees; their establishment has constituted a part of the effort to abide by international rules regarding proper research conduct (such as the Declaration of Helsinki).

At the national level, there exist two other committees: the Hellenic Committee on Bioethics of the General Secretariat for Research and Development (Ministerial Decision 3455/488/11.4.1997) and the Greek Orthodox Church Bioethics Committee. The former plays an advisory role to governmental and state organizations on the ethical, legal and socio-economic aspects of biotechnology. It also ensures that the public is properly informed on relevant matters and that the proper studies be promoted. The latter was established in Athens in 1998 and has focused so far on the issue of transplantation.

Recently, two new committees were founded at the national level: the National Committee on Human Rights and the National Committee on Bioethics (Law 2667/ 17.12.1998 FEK 281). Both answer directly to the Prime Minister.

Note, however, ethics committees should not be regarded as a panacea since their function has certain drawbacks. One such drawback, on which many commentators agree, is the feeling on the part of the medical staff that the burden of responsible decision making has shifted to such committees. Although clinical ethics committees have been known to be used in this way, this does not necessarily have to be true. Physicians should be aware that their personal responsibility does not cease to exist. Committees, therefore, should not be seen as an ethical and legal cover for the physicians' team but rather as a discussion forum. For this, basic rules and guidelines would be necessary in Greece, too.

It should be pointed out that, despite various reactions to the establishment of ethics committees, as Greece has signed and ratified the European Convention for the Protection of Human Rights and Dignity of the Human Being with regard to the application of biology and medicine (Convention on Human Rights and Biomedicine of the Council of Europe, 1997) according to which research ethics committees are a requirement, their establishment will have to be more seriously dealt with. It is, however, also a matter of political will, as the medical *status quo* is very powerful.

Moreover, international developments regarding the role of autonomy in the clinical setting as well as in medical decision-making, have had an impact on the existing situation in Greece, and it seems that paternalism as a way of thought and practice has started to lose ground in Greece, as has happened in other countries. Individuals are becoming aware of their rights and are demanding that their autonomy be respected. The rapid progress of technology has made ethical issues more perplexing in the hospital setting and physicians themselves are increasingly realizing the need for guidance. The effectiveness of clinical ethics committees and the experience that other countries have gained should be examined so that it may be applied in this country as well.

Efforts to establish clinical committees in Greece should focus around the following points:

- *Terms of reference*: The aims of the committee should be clearly defined in order to avoid internal conflicts between the staff.
- *Membership*: The committees should be multidisciplinary, have no less than nine and no more than eleven members and should include in their composition members distinguished in medical practice, psychology, law, philosophy, theology, sociology or health administrators. International experience has proven the usefulness of including lay members as well.
- *Independence of the committee*: This is a very important prerequisite, although it is difficult to achieve, if the committee functions in a hospital setting and answers to the hospital. It has been suggested that such committees should answer directly to the Ministry of Health, but this approach presents its own drawbacks.
- *Access*: Different approaches exist regarding who should have access to the hospital ethics committee: physicians, nurses, family members, or all of the above.
- *Education of the members of the committee*: Some training is usually considered necessary for the members of the committee. Two main approaches have been reported here: training in ethical theory and training in the process of ethical deliberation (Slowther, Hope, & Ashcroft, 2001).
- *Role of the committee*: Clinical ethics committees are needed in Greece because, by education in biomedical ethics, the contribution in the generation of guidelines for good ethical practice as well as the analysis and discussion of cases may promote ethical thought in the clinical setting and may help eliminate paternalism and the authoritative practice of medicine from it.
- *Confidentiality*: The introduction of a case to a clinical ethics committee seriously challenges the confidentiality surrounding this case. The members of the committee will have access to the records of the patient in question, a fact that raises ethical problems. Safeguards are, therefore, needed, which will protect the rights of this patient and which will create an ethical framework for the workings of the committee. Another issue concerns the involvement of family members in the discussions taking place.

F. Transplantation

The modern history of transplantations in Greece started in 1936 when the first cornea transplantation was achieved. In 1968, the first kidney transplantation from a cadaveric donor and the first one from a living and genetically related donor were successfully performed. The first pancreas transplantation took place in 1989; liver transplantation followed in 1990; and lung transplantation in 1992 (Varka-Adami, 1993).

Until 1968, there existed in Greece no relevant legal framework. Act 445 of 1968 allowed for the first time the use of cadavers in the laboratories of the Medical Faculty of the University of Athens. Act 821 of 1978 on "Removal and Transplantation of

Biological Substances from Humans" did not manage to promote the issue of transplantations as was expected. This piece of legislation was replaced by Act 1383 of 1983, which remained active for 16 years, until it was replaced by Act 2737 of 1999. A very important aim of all these pieces of legislation was not only to create an infrastructure for transplantation in Greece but also to avoid any commercialization of human tissues and organs.

The new law (2737/1999) does not differ very much from the previous one; however, it has taken into account the relevant articles of the Convention on Human Rights and Biomedicine of the Council of Europe (1997), as Greece was one of the first member states to sign and ratify the Convention. Nevertheless it has created numerous controversies: although its aim was to clarify the legal position of doctors regarding the certification of brain death as well as to resolve certain scientific and organizational issues, which would generally enhance transplantations in Greece, it has generated vivid discussions mainly concentrated on the following points:

First, removal of tissues and organs from a *living* person is allowed only when the transplantation is for the spouse of the donor or a blood relative up to the second degree. This restriction does not apply to bone marrow transplantation. Although this article is considered too restrictive, the reasoning behind it concerned the prevention of commercialization as well as better protection of donors and recipients.

Second, there exists significant controversy regarding removal of organs and tissues from *cadaveric* donors. The key notion here is brain death: the present law connects removal of organs and tissues from deceased persons with brain death, as was the case with the previous law.

In 1985, the Central Council of Health in Greece issued a report which adopted the criteria of brain death accepted in Europe, i.e., the criteria defining brain stem death. According to Greek legislation, when the attending physician diagnoses death of the brain stem and, if the function of certain organs is maintained with technical support, the physician is obliged to write the death certificate in collaboration with an anesthesiologist, a neurologist and a neurosurgeon. Physicians who are members of the transplantation team are not allowed to participate in the procedure regarding the diagnosis and certification of brain death. The attending physician must immediately inform the National Transplantation Organization, and together they inform the spouse or the relatives of the deceased about the possibility of organ donation.

The Greek Orthodox Church, despite its hesitations regarding the issue of brain death, considers transplantation an action of love and altruism (Christodoulos, 1992).

The problems associated with the difficulties in the acceptance of the notion of brain death by lay people as well as by physicians are already well known. Suffice it to say, that also in Greece the percentage of ignorance regarding the concept of brain death is not at all negligible and sometimes creates adverse feelings towards the prospect of organ removal. A survey among a sample population of medical doctors, nurses and medical students in the two largest Greek cities (Athens and Thessaloniki) has revealed that there is a low rate of awareness regarding the definition and the diagnosis criteria of cerebral death, a fact which leads to a small percentage of people finally becoming organ donors (Dardavessis, 1989).

Third, another controversial issue of the present law concerns consent for the removal of organs or tissue from deceased persons. The Committee preparing the bill, which later became law, accepted, under great pressure, the doctrine of "presumed consent". Although it was acknowledged that "presumed consent" would certainly promote transplantation in Greece, it was also generally believed that, for reasons regarding the danger of overriding the autonomy of the individual, the Greek state could not undertake the burden of a publicity campaign on as wide scale as would be necessary, if presumed consent were to be incorporated in the legislation. So, according to the current law, the removal can be carried out if the potential donor has given written consent. If, on the contrary, he or she has, with a written statement, expressed opposition to the prospect of organ donation, the removal cannot take place.

This law has been very innovating in adopting a new system according to which citizens can express their will to become donors: in every general census of the population, every adult is asked to declare in writing if he or she consents or refuses consent to the removal of tissues and organs from his or her body in case of death. If such a declaration has not been made, insurance organizations and municipal authorities may undertake the gathering of these declarations. Consent or refusal may always be withdrawn. If the potential donor had not previously expressed consent or refusal, the removal is carried out only if the husband or wife, adult children, parents or siblings of the deceased do not dissent.

Despite the various legislative acts, and the efforts of individual physicians, the rate of transplantation in Greece has never been as high as it could be, taking into account the medical facilities and the population of this country. The low rate is, in part, due to lack of resources and lack of coordination between the various hospital departments, as well as lack of public awareness. In an effort to increase the availability of organ donors, the Hellenic Transplant Service (HTS) initiated in 1989 educational programs addressed to the public and health professionals. Professional education programs were focused on Intensive Care and Neurosurgical units' staff. Representatives of the HTS, responsible for the coordination of transplants in Greek hospitals, offered continuous support and advice to the staff of these units. As a result, two years after the beginning of the program, it was determined that donor referral had increased (96.2%), medical reasons for not using donors had decreased (22.3%), and the percentage of donors had also increased (27.4%) (Varla-Leftherioti, Catsani, Sarris, Zarmakoupi, Mitsaki, Stavropoulou-Gioka et al., 1991).

The most negative factor, however, is considered to be the problem of substructure and coordination. In the years 1980-1990, the major factors which influenced organ transplantation were, first, the extreme helplessness of renal failure patients (in relation to transplant access) and, second, the stiffness and practical immobility of health authorities to act in elaborating the necessary budgets and arrangements for the organization of a national transplantation service (Koniavitou Hatzdiyiannaki, Protogerou, Dracopoulos, Siakotos, Sigounas, Syrakos et al., 1991). This led the renal failure patients' community to establish contact with transplant centers abroad and to sign agreements, which had many drawbacks regarding the scientific prerequisites, while the health authorities were absent from the process.

At present a great effort is being made by the National Transplantation Organization for the promotion of transplantations by organizing a system which can guarantee transparency, protection of patients' rights and, at the same time, quick response to a transplantation call.

III. Conclusions

The future cannot exist without a present and a past. And in the country where philosophy and the Hippocratic tradition were born, the recent past and the present of bioethics are not especially encouraging.

During the last decade, there have been many attempts to promote this field, some based on individual initiatives, others taking place on the legislative level (e.g., establishment of ethics committees and legislation on patients' rights); nonetheless, they have not been sufficient. In general, the field of bioethics has not been adequately supported by the state or by successive authorities who have the power to really enhance education and interest in bioethics. The reasons for this are manifold: the Greek National Health Service is constantly facing serious organizational and financial problems, and bioethics is by some considered to be a luxury. Moreover, the traditional paternalistic approach to the doctor–patient relationship, as described above, has prevented relevant efforts from materializing.

In the future, attention should mostly be paid to the establishment of local ethics committees and to wide-spread education. Education is of paramount importance, as it can promote new ways of communicating with patients as well as training in ethical deliberation. Although in the Greek academic environment there exist many nuclei of ethical and philosophical discourse regarding health issues, they do not suffice and, most importantly, they do not aim to cover a broader need for education in bioethics. The need for this sort of education has been acknowledged by the majority of developed European countries, who do not follow the same pattern as the United States. In Greece, bioethics is not being taught in a systematic way and education in this subject could be described as rather scarce. Students, during their years in the Faculty of Medicine, as for example in the Medical School of the University of Athens, do not follow strictly scheduled courses in bioethics. Instead, they attend various lectures concerning issues incorporated into different subjects: e.g., lectures about the ethical dimensions of research incorporated in the teaching of epidemiology, ethical problems within preventive medicine incorporated in community medicine, and so forth. Many of these lectures are offered on an optional basis. The Department of Forensic Medicine offers an elective course on issues of medical responsibility and deontology. Another more systematic course in bioethics is offered at the National School of Public Health. Teaching bioethics in Greece, except in strictly philosophical classes, should comprise elements of medical law as well. This would prove to be very important for the practice of good medicine, which raises both medical and legal issues.

A final observation regarding Greece is that bioethics should focus not only on dramatic issues, such as life and death or genetics, but should also concentrate on issues that seem to have a minor importance but which are vital for everyday practice.

Bibliography

Christodoulos, Archbiship of Greece. 1992. *Religious review of transplantations*. Iatriko Vima, May, 32–39.
Committee of Experts on Progress in the Biomedical Sciences (CAHBI). 1989. *Human artificial procreation*. Strasbourg: Council of Europe.

Convention for the Protection of Human Rights and Dignity of the Human Being with regard to the Application of Biology and Medicine. 1997. *Convention on human rights and biomedicine.* Oviedo 4.IV.1997. European Treaty Series No. 164.

Dalla-Vorgia, P. & Garanis, T. 1991. Hippocrates is dead, long live Hippocrates. *Bulletin of Medical Ethics* 66: 28-31.

Dardavessis, T. et al. 1989. Publicity on matters concerning cerebral death and transplantation. *He ll Iatr* 55: 142–149.

Economou, C., Karalis, G. & Kyriopoulos, J. 1999. Complementary insurance and managed health care schemes in Greece; eighth meeting of health and health policy forum, Kalamata, 28-30 May (in Greek).

Garanis-Papadatos, T. & Dalla-Vorgia, P. 2000. Clinical trials in Greece: ethical review proceedings. *European Journal of Health Law* 7: 441-447.

Gitana, M., Androutsopoulos, D., Drizi, B., Kyriopoulos, J. 1992. Private health care consumption: measurement and trends, 1957–1988, *Primary Health Care* 4(2): 63–68

Granitsas 1991. Medical deontology. *Iatriko Vima*, December 1991 [1st part], February 1992 [2nd part].

Ioannidis, I.A. & Epivatianos, P. 1990. The need for teaching of medical ethics in medical schools. *IATRIKI* 58(2): 119-127.

Koniavitou Hatzdiyiannaki, K. et al. 1991. The ugly head of commercialism in organ transplantation in Greece. In: Land, W. and Dossetor, J. (eds), *Organ Replacement Therapy: Ethics, Justice, and Commerce.* Berlin: Springer-Verlag.

Kremalis, K. 1987. *The right to the protection of health.* Athens (in Greek).

Kyriopoulos, J., Economou, C. & Dolgeras, A. 2001. Side payments in the Greek health sector: the dilemma of equity and efficiency. In J. Kyriopoulos, T. Beazoglou & D. Heffley (eds), *Health economics in the new era.* Athens: Exandas.

Merikas, G. 1987. Today's physician. *IATRIKI* 51: 39-48.

Morgan, D. 2001. *Issues in medical law and ethics.* London-Sydney: Cavendish.

Papadatou, D. 1991. Working with dying children: a professional's personal journey. In D. Papadatou & C. Papadatos (eds), *Children and death.* New York: Hemisphere.

Round Table 1991. Dilemmas in the provision of health services to severely ill subjects. *IATRIKI* 59(6): 576-590.

Sissouras, A. 1990. Backgrounds and development in health care in Greece. In: A.F. Casparie, et al. (eds), *Competitive health care in Europe: future prospects.* Dartmouth: Grover Publishing Company.

Slowther, A., Hope, T. & Ashcroft, R. 2001. Clinical ethics committees: a worldwide development. *Journal of Medical Ethics* 27: (supplement), i-ii.

Varka-Adami, A. 1993, *The law of transplantations.* Athens-Komotini: A.N. Sakkoulas Editions.

Varla-Leftherioti, M. et al. 1991. The effectiveness of the Hellenic transplant service program for intensive care units' health professional on donors' report. *Transplant* 2(1): 14–20.

Veatch R. 1985. The ethics of critical care in cross-cultural perspective. In J.C. Moskop & L. Kopelman (eds), *Ethics and critical care medicine.* Dordrecht: D. Reidel Company.

Yfantopoulos, J. 2000. Health inequalities: some of the issues and evidence from Greece. In: A. Ritsatakis, J. Levett & J. Kyriopoulos (eds), *Neighbours in the Balkans: initiating a dialogue for health.* Athens: World Health Organization.

10 Bioethics in Italy since 1997

Maurizio Mori

I. Introduction

The watershed year for Italian bioethics was 1997. The birth of Dolly the sheep in Scotland at the end of February 1997 caused such cultural turmoil that bioethics was given a new social status. Before Dolly's birth, bioethics was already a growing discipline that increasingly attracted attention from educated people, but it was still a field restricted to a few specialists.[1] Dolly's birth radically changed the level and magnitude of the interest in these topics: bioethics became a matter of public debate and a source of political concern. The media has been so deeply involved in this issue, for such a length of time, that the word "bioethics" itself has become popular and has gained a place in common usage.

The "Dolly affair" likely would have been sufficient to start this new "bioethics blooming", because cloning has a deep symbolic meaning in Western culture and incites strong feelings. However, in Italy several factors contributed to such a new atmosphere and, in one sense, prepared it. On Saturday, February 1, 1997, just before the annual "Pro-life Day" celebrated by the Roman Catholic Church, four well-known Italian intellectuals supported a new bill, presented by the Italian Pro-Life Movement and signed by over a million citizens, that would modify article one of the civil code. According to the present law, a human being acquires "legal capacity" – i.e., full acquisition of a person's rights – at birth: according to the proposal, "legal capacity" would be acquired immediately "at conception".[2] Since two of these intellectuals were Professor Francesco D'Agostino, the president of the National Committee for Bioethics, and Professor Giuliano Amato, the Minister of Treasury, their public Pro-Life declaration started a great deal of polemical discussion.

On February 10, the Constitutional Court decided against the proposal of a referendum on abortion promoted by the Radical party and signed by about another million citizens. Opposed to the Pro-Life bill, this proposed referendum was aimed at increasing the availability of abortion, so that (among other things) abortion would have been permissible even in private clinics (not only in public hospitals as it is now) and for young women under the age of 16 without their parents' consent. According to the Court, this referendum could not take place because it was informed by a perspective that considers motherhood to be only a woman's "private affair". The Court held that this view was in contrast with the Constitution, in which motherhood is a "social matter" deserving public consideration. While the current law allows abortion to support motherhood, the referendum's proposal moved in the opposite direction. It is not difficult to imagine that this decision raised significant new controversies.[3]

A few days later, the team of Professor Carlo Flamigni (in Bologna) announced the birth of Elena, the first baby born by means of a brand new technique. The progenitor cell of the oocyte had been frozen and kept for some time. It was defrosted and matured *in vitro*, and finally fertilized *in vitro*. This new procedure allows women to store their gametes, which earlier could not be frozen without permanent damage. Elena was a healthy baby, but such an "extraordinary birth" attracted much attention: Cardinal Biffi, bishop of Bologna, declared that it was *"un evento bestiale"* ("a bestial event"). Debate over reproductive issues and limits to be established on science started again, receiving front-page news stories for days.

As one can see, the whole month of February 1997 was full of bioethical controversy. At the end of February, Italian newspapers broke the usual informational embargo to report about Dolly's birth, which was a real blow. Besides a few rare voices inviting a more cautious attitude and claiming that further reflection was needed, the reaction to Dolly's birth was of absolute and irrevocable condemnation.[4] Some scholars appeared to be furious and really worried for the advancement of science, saying that Pandora's box had been opened and that from now on humanity was in real danger. Harsh criticism and heavy words continued for days, so that afterwards one could no longer ignore bioethical issues or even the word "bioetica" itself. Only a decade ago, scholars politely scoffed at the idea of being involved in bioethical reflection, claiming that it dealt with issues that could easily be managed through traditional disciplines; now, bioethics receives public recognition, social sanction, and academic standing.

II. The Field of Bioethics in Italy

In an amazingly short time, controversies on Dolly's birth changed the status of bioethics in Italy, bringing it from the margin to the center of cultural debate. Such a sudden and unexpected "explosion" of the field had various side effects, one of which is that a number of people became "bioethics experts" in a day. Apart from this, scholarly bioethics bene-fited from the situation, because publishers became more interested in offering bioethical works, and many important books were translated into Italian. (See, for example, Harris, 1997; Jonas, 1997; Singer, 1997, 2000, 2001; Engelhardt, 1999; Beauchamp & Childress, 1999; Callahan, 2000; Ford, 1997; Kuhse, 2000; Dworkin, Frey, & Bok, 2001.)

Moreover, some Italian secular scholars produced significant contributions on various issues: C.A. Defanti (1999) wrote a unique contribution that is possibly the first history of the concept of death from the Renaissance to contemporary times, examining also many issues related to this topic. Death is the topic of B. Morcavallo's interesting book (1999), which focused on how the concept of whole brain death is related to the concept of person, and has far-reaching effects on the traditional sanctity of life doctrine. P. Borsellino (1999) boldly defended a view of autonomy that holds that the patient-physician relationship has already changed significantly and that it will continue to change, especially from a legal viewpoint. A. Santosuosso (2001) wrote a thoughtful history of the relationship between medicine and law, and M. Barni (1999) provided a connection between traditional medical deontology and bioethics. Fucci G. Ferrando (1999b, 2002) wrote possibly the most complete and informed legal analysis of assisted reproduction according to Italian law; feminists and psychoanalysts also presented their views on the matter.[5] D. Neri (2001) presented the issues of stem cells and cloning, and G.F. Azzone (1997, 2000, 2003) explored some bioethical issues assuming a wider evolutionary perspective and a liberal standpoint. S. Fucci (1998) contributed to nursing ethics, a field that has received additional attention since the importance of nurses within health care is increasing, even though – unfortunately and for unknown reasons – nursing ethics is not blooming as one would have expected (see also Cattorini & Sala, 1998; Spinsanti, 2001; and a special 1998 issue of *Bioetica. Rivista Interdisciplinare*, *IV*[3]). Proceedings of interdisciplinary and pluralistic conferences on death and birth as well as on autonomy provided a variety of positions on such issues (Cattorini, D'Orazio, & Pocar, 1999; Istituto Veneto di Scienze, Lettere ed Arti, 1999, 2001). Two important books deserve special mention: the first is the collection of papers on bioethics written by Uberto Scarpelli (1998), who was a pioneer of the new discipline in Italy and who died an untimely death in 1993. The other is a book by E. Lecaldano (1999) that is certainly one of the best articulated and mature contributions provided from a secular perspective followed by a "Dictionary of Bioethics" (Lecaldano, 2002). G. Berlinguer (2000) wrote a comprehensive book presenting his views on "everyday bioethics", which is focused not on crucial and exceptional cases but on "everyday practice"; and L. Battaglia (1999) argued for a different perspective relying on the paradigm of "complexity" as a basis for bioethics. Finally, debate has been increasing about the role of non-human animals, which in the last several years has grown. Besides translations of P. Singer's (1997, 2000, 2001) and T. Regan's (1976, 1987, 1989, 1990) books, Italian scholars have published their own contributions to this growing debate (Battaglia, 1997; Pocar, 1998; Cavalieri, 1999; Marchesini, 1999, 2001).

Catholics have been even more active and, since 1997, a veritable flood of books has been published. Here I can mention only a few of the many important contributions. Msg. E. Sgreccia (1999) expanded his textbook, which provides the basis of a general view called "ontologically grounded personalism". Cardinal D. Tettamanzi (2000) did the same with another general book (see also Sgreccia, Spagnolo, & Di Pietro, 1999; Spagnolo, 1997; Spagnolo & Gambino, 2002). A. Pessina (1999) considers foundational aspects of such a view, pointing out the paradoxes of "techno-sciences" and focusing his analysis on a few basic normative issues as exemplary of former problems. L. Ciccone (2000) and M. Aramini (2001) provided a general overview of a Catholic position. F. D'Agostino (1998) presented a Catholic perspective starting from the viewpoint of the philosophy of law, holding that the European legal tradition can provide clues for solving bioethical issues (see also Dalla Torre, 1997; Tarantino, 1998). A. Bompiani (1997) and others focused their attention on the growing European legislation concerning bioethics, which (according to them) is informed with "personalistic criteria" and is respectful of an interpretation of "human rights" (see also Bompiani, Lorete Beghè, & Marini, 2001).[6] G. Angelini (1998), P. Cattorini (1997), G. Piana (2002), F. Viola (1997, 2000) and C. Zuccaro (2000, 2002) (in various ways) defend a Catholic view, relying on a phenomenologically oriented approach, which leads to a sort of "relational personalism": most of this approach's practical conclusions are equivalent to those reached by "ontologically grounded personalism", but on some issues there are significant differences. While most of these books are skeptical about a future increasingly dominated by biological techniques, a recent work by S. Spinsanti (1998) welcomed and examined new challenges to the physician–patient relationship.

Apart from books on such diverse topics, the most discussed issues have been reproduction (specifically on the so-called "status of the human embryo") and death issues.[7]
More recently, a corpus of literature on food biotechnology is growing.[8] As I said, this list
is far from being complete, but I hope that it gives an idea of the current range of Italian
publications in the field.[9]

A remark should be made concerning bioethics textbooks for high school students. In
recent years, some bioethical issues (abortion, euthanasia, and so forth) have been a
favorite topic of discussion with students: this trend was favored by an agreement signed
by the Ministry of Education and the President of the National Committee for Bioethics
in 1999 (see below, section 4), and a consequence of this new interest was an impulse to
create new publications devoted to teaching bioethics.[10]

Since 1997, no major changes have occurred regarding journals devoted to bioethical
matters. Italian bioethics has four major publications: *Medicina e Morale*, which is the
oldest (founded in 1951), is published by the Catholic University and presents a strictly
Vatican-based perspective. *Bioetica. Rivista Interdisciplinare* was established in 1993 and
is the only journal open to ethical pluralism. Being specifically devoted to bioethics and
published by the *Consulta di bioetica* (see below, section 5), in a sense, *Bioetica* is the
complement of (or perhaps the opposite to) *Medicina e Morale*: both are wholly devoted
to bioethical issues but from two different perspectives. *Bioetica* promotes ethical pluralism, and its only limiting criteria is scholarly excellence, while *Medicina e Morale* also
requires agreement with Catholic doctrine.

Another important journal, *Notizie di Politeia*, founded in 1985, deals with any topic
of applied ethics from a pluralistic perspective. While regular attention is devoted to
bioethical issues, the journal's interests are not limited to bioethics. Similar remarks can
be made about the last journal, *L'arco di Giano*, a journal of medical humanities, which
was founded by Sandro Spinsanti in 1993: being devoted to medical humanities, it has a
wider concern than the others mentioned here. In 2000, Spinanti left *L'arco di Giano* and,
in 2001, started *Janus, Medicina: Cultura, Culture*, a new quarterly that continues and
develops his medical humanities perspective. The only really new journal is *Etica delle
Professioni*, a biannual that has been published since 1999 by the Lanza Foundation of
Padua, a Catholic institution interested in various branches of ethics: accordingly, the
journal is devoted to different professional ethics, including medical ethics.[11]

In concluding this general overview of the Italian intellectual *milieu*, the last remark is
about the academic situation: in November 1997, Demetrio Neri became professor of
bioethics at the University of Messina. Neri was professor of history of philosophy and,
being a well-known bioethicist, officially moved to bioethics, breaking the monopoly held
by Catholics in the field. Before then, only two professors taught bioethics, and both were
Catholics: Mgs. E. Sgreccia, who received tenure at the Catholic University in Rome in
1990, and P. Cattorini, a physician and philosopher, who was associate professor in
Florence (now he is at the University of Varese). Neri's new position was a further interesting sign of the new cultural relevance of bioethics and propelled new hopes for a more
pluralistic discussion within the University. However, in 1999, a significant reform of university professorships took place and, since then, new openings have been available: the
number of bioethics professors increased, both in the humanities and in medical schools.
Most of them are Catholics, but there is a group of secular scholars. It is too early to evaluate the impact of the reform on this specific aspect of a complex cultural system.

Looking backwards with the aim of seeing in one glance the situation of scholarly bioethics, one must say that although some important books have been published in the English speaking tradition, most bioethical publications have been produced within a continental framework. It is always difficult to determine the influence of academic debates on public opinion, but there is a sense in which the predominance of continental philosophy contributes to a cultural *milieu* unfavorable to the ongoing "bio-medical revolution". Some of these difficulties will be sorted out in the following pages.

III. Italian Legislation Concerning Assisted Reproduction

Apart from changing bioethics' public importance, Dolly's birth also had two further immediate and more practical effects on Italian society. The first was a general precautionary and temporary ban of any sort of cloning (even for soya) issued immediately on March 7, 1997. One interesting consequences of this ban will be considered later on (in section 7).

The second practical effect of Dolly's birth was much more important and direct for bioethics. Its impact was so strong that it created a political realization that Italy urgently needed new legislation on assisted reproduction. On March 12, 1997, Ms. Marida Bolognesi, chairwoman of the Commission for Social Affairs, presented to the lower Chamber a program to reach a "unified bill" on this matter. About 40 bills were at the Parliament, and the Commission began to examine them in order to reach a new proposal to be agreed upon by the majority. Controversies on this issue will occupy the largest part of the narrative, because they are of the utmost relevance for Italian bioethics. There is a sense in which debates on this issue determine the stream of the whole cultural reflection, conditioning social *milieu* and all the other discussions. Insofar as this discussion is intertwined with politics and political equilibria, it will be useful to present a brief history concerning the Italian political situation.[12]

After the public announcement, the Bolognesi Commission worked quietly for the whole of 1997. In January 1998, a first draft of the new unified bill was presented to the public and fueled the controversy. The Bolognesi bill was what Linda Nielsen calls a "half-way model" of regulation, i.e., a bill allowing some interventions and forbidding others. So it permits assisted reproduction only as a therapy for infertile couples, excluding any single or post-menopausal woman. To prevent commercial trade of gametes and possible abuses in the area, gametes could be collected and stored only within the National Health Service, which would then provide and distribute them to private licensed fertility clinics (both public and private). Donor insemination was permitted only for married couples or stable heterosexual couples who declared that they had lived together for at least two years. The number of embryos created *in vitro* had to be kept to a minimum and could not exceed four. Experimentation on embryos – as well as cloning – was strictly prohibited (Proposta Bolognesi, 1998).

Ms. Bolognesi was convinced that the bill's framework was adequate, even though she admitted that it was encumbered by too many restrictions and heavy penalties. However, this was the unavoidable price that had to be paid in quite difficult political bargaining for regulating assisted reproduction: she claimed that the Italian political situation did not allow more than what was reached. As soon as the draft was released, a new stage of public debate opened: quite spontaneously, various social groups published their own manifestos stating their various positions on the issue. The first one was published in the *Corriere della sera* on February 10, 1998, supporting procreative liberty; it was promoted by two active secular centers, *Politeia* and the *Consulta di Bioetica*. Afterwards, other organizations stated their cases in the public arena, representing the entire spectrum of views.[13]

Apart from various details (such as the request for a couple to self-certify their two years of cohabitation, or limiting the number of gametes to bank at the NHS, which likely will be a source of endless litigation), liberal critics of the bill (like myself) pointed out that the bill was poorly framed, because it pointed in the wrong direction. It assumed that assisted reproduction is a kind of therapy, while it is actually a new form of reproduction. Moreover, even if donor insemination is permitted, in practice access to such techniques is discouraged in various ways, as if assisted reproduction was a sort of "dangerous treatment" to be approached with great care. Finally, it is wrong to forbid experimentation on spare embryos and ridiculous to include a cloning ban in such a bill, since cloning is a totally different issue.

Conservative critics attacked the bill mainly on the issue of artificial insemination by donor (AID), stressing that it would have been a source of the destruction of the family as well as a real danger for newborns' welfare. They remarked that the article on the *in vitro* creation of embryos was loose and ambiguous, since embryo freezing was not clearly banned. Interestingly enough, however, the issue of the embryo's "right to life" was not heavily stressed in the public debate – or at least not as much as one would expect. The greatest emphasis was placed on AID as a practice that would disrupt the family. In any case, critics insisted that protection of the right to life in *in vitro* situations was quite different from its protection in the case of abortion and, therefore, that a ban on embryo freezing and experimentation would not have any *immediate* effect on current abortion law. This left open the possibility that such a new protection of *in vitro* procedure would have favored a cultural change leading to a more restrictive form of the abortion law.[14]

On June 3, 1998, the Catholic newspaper *Avvenire* published a letter in which Carlo Casini, the president of the Italian Pro-Life Movement and an influential member of the Federation of European Popular Parties (EPP) offered his support for Mr. Berlusconi to join the EPP, if Berlusconi committed himself to policies in defense of life and of the family. The next day (June 4), Berlusconi answered that he had always been in favor of protecting life and the family, and his "liberalism" had always been consistent with policies defended by EPP. At the end of June, Berlusconi joined the EPP.

This exchange of letters, however, went almost unnoticed, because on June 3, the Commission for Constitutional Affairs stated that the Bolognesi bill was acceptable under the Italian constitution and could be presented for Parliament's examination. On June 4, the media's attention was devoted to this decision, with interviews of the Commission's chairwoman, Ms. Rosa Russo Jervolino, a well known Catholic politician of the PPI (Italian Popular Party). On the same day, the *Osservatore Romano* – the Vatican's newspaper – harshly attacked the Commission's decision, stating that the bill was an attempt to "violate God's plans for human beings" and could not receive any sort of support (even throughout "abstention") from Catholic politicians. A prompt and polemic answer by the leader of the PPI fueled the controversy, and bioethics immediately became an issue of "hard politics". For days, bioethics was on the front pages, becoming a subject of popular interest, even though the analyses of the issues lost the required precision and attention (see Mori, 2003).

After the early June eruption, bioethical debate continued at its usual pace until September 26, 1998, when a decision of the Constitutional Court on assisted reproduction was published. It stated that a husband who had given his consent to artificial insemination by donor cannot change his mind and disown the child.[15] This decision was warmly approved, but it became the matter for new debate. Further attention was given to another new case decided by a court of Palermo in December 1998 that allowed the request of a wife to be implanted with frozen embryos inseminated with her deceased husband's sperm.[16]

In January 1999, the Bolognesi bill was included in the agenda of the lower Chamber. Some criticized such a step, observing that the cultural atmosphere was not favorable to the bill and that the left-wing coalition was not sufficiently unified on the issue: the item was not included in the political agreement of the ruling majority and, therefore, it was covered by the "conscience clause", allowing any member of Parliament (MP) to vote according to his or her own personal views. However, the prospect was that some left-wing MPs would vote against the bill while a number of liberal and secular right-wing MPs would support it. Therefore, a positive decision was made, and the Bolognesi bill was included in the agenda. But as soon as the bill arrived in the Chamber in early February, it was clear that it would not have had an easy *iter*. The original formulation of article one was rather anodyne, stating that assisted reproduction was a sort of therapy that needed regulation to protect "the rights of all the subjects involved". A new formulation that was completely different in tone was approved, stating that access to assisted reproduction is allowed only in the conditions specified by this law, which protects "the rights of all the subjects involved, *in particular of the conceptus*". Even if in quite general terms, this is the first time that a legislative text ascribed "full rights" to the *conceptus*. Moreover, on February 4, article four (concerning donor insemination) was quashed and Ms. Bolognesi resigned her direction of the bill, since it was clear that all previous prospects had failed. The direction of the bill was taken by Mr. Alessandro Cè, who succeeded in securing the approval of a text that was significantly different from the one prepared by the Bolognesi Commission (which took over one year of hard work to complete). The new text was approved on May 26, 1999, by a vote of 266 to 153, indicating that all liberal and secular MPs of the right-wing had voted against the bill.[17] One wonders whether this was the price paid for Berlusconi's entry in the EPP.

According to the text approved by the Chamber, donor insemination was prohibited, as well as any embryo freezing. Homologous insemination was permitted not only for married couples but also for stable, unmarried ones – a clause that raised the criticism of the Catholic Church. Moreover, a transitory norm allows what is called the "embryo preadoption"; i.e., the possibility for a woman to ask that a frozen embryo that is stored in a fertility clinic be implanted in her womb. However, some Catholics opposed such a proposal, saying that "pre-adoption" is a sort of surrogacy, which should never be permitted. So cardinals and bishops have been quibbling among themselves regarding whether allowing "pre-adoption" is tantamount to an implicit admission of surrogacy's morality, and if so whether such a practice was permissible in this case. This controversy would have presented some amusing aspects, if only it did not have important consequences for the lives of many women and couples. Finally, the temporary "pre-adoption" clause was approved, and the MPs' enthusiasm was such that at the last minute the Chamber approved a recommendation inviting the government to revise the abortion law according to the new perspective assumed by the text just approved.

This final recommendation appeared to be a direct attack on the abortion law, again raising many controversies. The next day the leader of DS (the left's Democratic Party, the major ruling party), Mr. Walter Veltroni, declared that the bill would never become a law. Since in the Senate the left-wing coalition was stronger than in the Chamber, this statement was charged with being a sort of threat to the Parliament's sovereignty. However, the new transversal majority appeared to be strong and willing to pass the law, even though it was rather dissonant with other Italian legislation on the issue.

This judgment is confirmed by two different facts which attracted some attention. The first is a decision of Judge Letizia Schettini in Rome permitting a case of "surrogate pregnancy" (February 14, 2000). A married couple, who were infertile, and the wife's friend were willing to have a surrogate pregnancy, so that the couple could have their own child. Judge Schettini's decision created a tremendous mess. At the very beginning almost all comments were negative, but later some defended the decision. This demonstrates that current Italian legislation does not necessarily forbid surrogate pregnancies.[18]

The other fact supporting my thesis is a well-argued decision (March 16, 1999) of the Supreme Court (*Corte di cassazione*) on donor insemination that not only confirmed what the Constitutional court already stated more briefly in the case of a husband consenting to AID, but also remarked that AID could not be considered an "immoral issue".[19]

When the Senate Commission, chaired by Francesco Carella, received the bill from the Chamber, it reframed it anew, introducing a few significant changes. If the Carella bill had to be approved, then the whole discussion would have started over again. In early September 1999, however, even right-wing senators did not appear determined to examine the issue, which was not included in the agenda. However, in October, something changed: the Carella bill was considered by the Commission and immediately rejected. Even the Senate majority appeared to think that the Chamber's text was a sound basis for discussion. Once again, the situation was very odd, because the ruling coalition – which enjoyed significant support for the bill – saw their version of the bill rejected by a transversal majority.

By the end of January 2000, senators of the "ruling minority" presented more than 1800 amendments but, at the beginning of March, they were immediately rejected. Even some amendments suggested by the Senate "justice commission" that aimed at more proportional penalties for these "crimes" (in some cases heavier than for murder) were not accepted. In mid-March – while in the Senate the discussion of the bill was going on – Cardinal Camillo Ruini, President of the Italian Bishops' Conference, stated that "it is necessary to approve as soon as possible the law on medically assisted reproduction ..., even though we cannot ignore some grave ethical perplexities raised by the text approved by the Chamber ... It is to be avoided ... both further postponements and any modification which had to make it worse, especially if donor insemination had to be permitted" (Ruini, 2000, p. 16; see also 2001, p. 340).

After a few days of discussion, the Senate decided to suspend the vote and postpone it until after the then-imminent regional election of April 16. Results of this mid-term vote were so dim for the ruling left-wing coalition that Prime Minister Massimo D'Alema had to resign. The newly formed cabinet was led by Giuliano Amato, who, in 1997, had supported a Pro-Life proposal to modify article one of the civil code, but no political program was established for the assisted procreation law.

At the end of May, the bill was included in the agenda of the Senate, and discussion started again. Voting was scheduled for June 7, 2000, and the prospects were that Italy would have the much-awaited new law. But on the morning of June 7, a large number of right-wing Senators did not show up on time. From 9:30 a.m. to approximately 11:30 a.m., the Senate approved two crucial amendments: the first erasing the "rights of the embryo", and the other allowing AID. After that, the session was suspended for some time and at about noon most Senators arrived. They justified the delay in various ways: some had been trapped in Rome's traffic jam, others could not find a taxi, and so forth. Voting continued on other articles and, at the end of June, the bill was sent back to the lower chamber. But at this point no one was interested in pressing for a new debate. No bill was passed in the legislature.

The official excuses clearly being unbelievable, we are left with the problem of explaining the right-wing Senators' behavior: why, after having strenuously defended the bill, did not they arrive to vote on it? There have been several conjectures on the matter. One is the following: considering that the absent Senators came mainly from Catholic parties who joined the right-wing coalition and since the bill came from the center-left ruling coalition, they did not show up because the merit of the new law would have been ascribed to the effect of Catholic party's joining the ruling coalition, which would have received the Church's approval. In other words, right-wing Catholic senators did not show up in order to prevent the left-wing Catholic party from gaining the Church's gratitude from the new law.

Such strategic behavior was long-sighted. In the political election during the Spring of 2001, the Church encouraged it members to vote for those parties that had given particular attention to the protection of human life and the promotion of the traditional family. This encouragement had a role in the final result of the election: the right-wing coalition won the election by a few votes, and possibly the weight of the Church was decisive. Since electoral mechanisms guarantee a solid majority to the ruling coalition, the new political situation strongly influences the cultural *milieu*.

Given this new cultural situation, debates on assisted reproduction received renewed attention in early February 2002. On Saturday, February 2, some professors of gynecology at the University of Rome signed a declaration on "The embryo as a patient" and presented it to Cardinal Ruini.[20] However, it was the Pope's Sunday speech that attracted the media's attention: he praised the declaration and explicitly approved the initiative of the Italian Pro-Life Movement, leading it to present again the bill for modifying article one of the civil code. This bill was presented to the President of the Chamber on March 26, signed by over 550,000 people and supported by new statements signed by over 400 academics.

On March 27, 2002, the Chamber started to discuss the bill on assisted reproduction that was approved by the Chamber in the last legislative session. After a few sessions, it was approved on June 18 with 268 votes in favor, 144 against and 10 abstaining. Once again, the *conceptus* was endowed with legal rights, AID was banned, embryo creation was strictly restricted and spare embryos are not permitted (a further decree will decide what to do with existing abandoned spare embryos).[21] Once again, MPs had the freedom to vote, which explains the existence of such a large "transversal majority".

Setting aside the controversies over the "*conceptus*'s rights" (which concern questions regarding the right to life), it is worthwhile to observe that never before were long provisions of a bill justified by appeals to "natural law" and "respect for natural procreation". Another recurrent justification is that the law will put an end to the current "procreative Far West" due to the absence of regulation on gynecologists of fertility clinics. For example, when, in early July 2002, newspapers reported that two black twins were born to a white couple in the UK; this mistake was seen as a confirmation of a restrictive law forbidding AID.

The bill is now scheduled for a vote in the Senate before Summer 2003, but a first delay seems to show that, once again, the route will not be easy. However, thus far the ruling majority appears to be determined to pass the new law. The most plausible prospects are that, in 2003 Italy will have a new restrictive law on assisted reproduction.

It is too early to predict reactions to the possible new legislation. At the political level, some parties announced the intention to start the process for having a public referendum to abrogate the law, which is seen as a violation of people's basic rights to reproductive freedom. At the legal level, the new law will change the balance of the Italian system, and it is not clear what the consequences will be and how the old rules will be interpreted. At the social level, certainly the new law will favor what is already called "reproductive tourism"; i.e., the practice of people going abroad for assisted reproduction. Some Italian physicians already have established (or are going to establish) fertility clinics in nearby countries (Malta, Switzerland, and so forth) in order to provide efficient service. Moreover, the new law will certainly resurrect a new anti-clericalism.

At the cultural level, finally, the new law is a clear defeat for secular culture as well as for ethical pluralism. For over a decade, secular culture considered bioethics to be a secondary and marginal topic, while Catholics invested resources and energies in the field. The effects of these investments are now becoming visible. Vatican Catholics are harvesting the fruits of their cultural supremacy in the media. On the one hand, they silenced a few liberal Catholics who supported liberal legislation; on the other hand, this job was not too difficult because even a great deal (if not the majority) of secularists are in favor of setting strict limits on such practices. The neat majority emerging in the Parliament seems to be a sign of this cultural supremacy, which conditions Italian reflection in the field.

One may wonder whether this situation is real or simply apparent: are Italians (who have a very liberal law on abortion as well as a very secularized way of life) really against AID, and so forth, or is such an opposition the result of a political and cultural situation dominated by Catholic lobbying? It is difficult to give a precise answer, since public opinion polls go in opposite directions, depending on the source commissioning the survey.

My opinion is that the current situation is a contingent stage of a wider process and that Italians will opt for liberal and secularized legislation. The main reason for such a view is the following: in order to have a bill discouraging any assisted reproduction, Catholics had to focus their criticism mainly on the (alleged) disruptive consequences of AID and on the "right to life" of the embryo. They did not criticize artificial insemination as such, and now most Italians (even most Catholics) are convinced that AIH is an ethical practice that encounters no moral objection. When Cardinal Ruini spoke of some "ethical perplexities" raised by the bill approved by the Chamber, these words were interpreted as referring to the access it granted to non-married couples to use artificial insemination. This means that the Church has stepped back from declaring artificial insemination strictly immoral, because this prohibition would be incomprehensible to most Italians (as is the Church's prohibition on contraception). Most Catholic criticisms of AID depend either on traditional considerations or on merely consequentialist arguments. So far this strategy appeared to be convincing, but it may be that in the future people will understand that the social consequences of assisted reproduction are not as bad as is currently depicted. At that point, all current worries and prohibitions will be dissolved.

Having stated the reasons for my propensity that the present situation manifests a sort of "moral appearance" supported by strong Catholic lobbying instead of a "moral reality", I have to admit that my views could be a form of wishful thinking. It might also be that, in the future, other considerations could be discovered that perpetuate current prohibitions and that moral change in Italy will be much slower than I would reckon. In this sense, I think that we should be very careful not to undervalue this historical situation. Any further future development is difficult to predict at this stage.

IV. Ethics Committees

Debates on assisted reproduction certainly had a prominent impact on Italian bioethical debates, and solutions in this field seem to provide the keynote for the whole of bioethical reflection in the country. Another issue that had significant influence is that of the National Committee for Bioethics, which has existed since 1990 as a board to advise the President of the government. Controversies began immediately when the first National Committee was established; however, it became more inflamed when Mr. Silvio Berlusconi (ruling a center-right coalition) in December 1994 nominated what was immediately called the "Bishops' committee" because of the overwhelming majority of Catholics on the Committee. As a matter of fact, three secular members resigned the appointment, but the Committee was very active, producing 23 reports in four years. Of course there was an inflexible condemnation of cloning, but most of these reports had practically no impact on public opinion, except for *Identity and Statute of the Human Embryo* (June, 1996), whose basic idea was epitomized in the expression: "an embryo is one of us". This report was quite influential and helped to frame cultural background for discussion on assisted reproduction.[22]

This Committee expired at the end of 1998 and a new Committee was appointed on March 23, 1999, by Mr. Massimo D'Alema, ruling a center-left coalition. It was chaired by Giovanni Berlinguer, who was one of the three who resigned from the former Committee. This Committee lasted until the end of 2001 and it was the most balanced Committee ever appointed. It included a larger number of women and the most pluralistic set of members since the Committee was established in 1990: 35% of its members were non-Catholic.

President Berlinguer tried to establish a National Committee to respond to a new idea of the Committee and of bioethics itself not as a discipline dealing with the controversial issues of life and death, but as one more concerned with "everyday medical issues" that normal people have to face in common life. Instead of being a board devoted to releasing reports on difficult topics from the top of the "experts' tower", a National Committee should be open to an interactive dialogue with society on more "normal problems". This general view was pursued in two main directions.

The first concerned a program for teaching bioethics in high school. An agreement with the Ministry of Education was signed in November 1999, stating that bioethics was a discipline to be included in the school curriculum. As noted earlier, teachers often already utilized bioethical issues for cultural discussions with students. This agreement aimed at establishing a more formal framework for pluralistic teaching of the subject matter. Even though it was unanimously approved by the National Committee, this proposal was immediately criticized by *Avvenire*, the newspaper of the Italian bishops. Cardinal

Ersilio Tonini expressed his deep concern and anxiety, observing that now professors with a secular worldview had the opportunity to teach on such delicate issues.[23] To overcome these new troubles, a special Commission was appointed with the task of specifying procedures and solving possible new controversies. But this Commission was slow and no further official program was issued. The only goal reached by the agreement was to provide a sort of legitimization for teachers' programs in bioethics.

The second direction is well represented by a report for the reform of the system of Local Ethics Committees, which was prepared by a working group coordinated by Demetrio Neri. This report appeared important, because, since March 18, 1998, Local Ethics Committees are mandatory by law.[24] This means that every hospital now has an ethics committee, with many people involved in the process. However, the roles and functions of what is called "*Comitato Etico Locale*" are not yet perfectly clear.

Certainly they must evaluate protocols for clinical trials and this new function will change the practice of clinical experimentation. For instance, when the Lipobay case came to the fore in Summer 2001, it was discovered that two Committees did not accept the protocol for that drug, which attracted significant new attention to the system of ethics committees. However, what is still unclear is the function of ethics committees in crucial clinical cases. In some hospitals, there are requests for ethical advice regarding clinical practice, but, in most institutions, such a function is completely disregarded. Some interesting institutional arrangements have been set in order to satisfy both the different roles and functions, especially in Tuscany, where ethics committees are particularly active. (For a brief discussion on the "Tuscany model" see Immacolato, 1999).

But a clarification of the issue was needed, and the National Committee's Report provided such an answer. The crucial idea was to make a neat distinction between the two major functions and to set up two different institutions: on the one hand, a committee for experimentation (what in the United States is called an "IRB") and, on the other hand, a committee for ethical advice regarding clinical practice (that in the United States is called an "ethics committee" in the strict sense).

This proposal is neither new nor original, but what was new was the working methodology used by the National Committee: when, in April 2000, a first draft of the report was ready, it was sent for examination to all Italian local ECs for comments, criticisms, and suggestions. Moreover, two different national conferences were organized in 2001 to discuss such proposals.[25] A lot of good work was done, but so far all such efforts appear useless because no reform is in view – unless the European Union requires it.

Berlinguer's Committee instituted a new working style, and, from this viewpoint, it was fresh air for Italian culture. However, it was too slow or reluctant to face crucial and controversial issues, such as treatment of individuals in a permanent vegetative state (PVS) or euthanasia (see below, section 6). Another example of this is provided by the issue of experimentation on stem cells. A first draft of a report on the issue was almost ready by May 2000. It included some controversial proposals, such as the possibility of using embryonic stem cells for research, but the working group wanted it discussed in the plenary session before the Summer. Discussion was delayed and, in mid-August 2000, the Donaldson Report in the United Kingdom was announced by international press. Immediately the issue of stem cell experimentation became an urgent topic to be examined.

In early September, Minister of Health Umberto Veronesi appointed an *ad hoc* Commission chaired by Nobel Prize winner Renato Dulbecco to provide scientific and ethical directions on the issue by the end of the year. This was enough to start harsh polemics: the Dulbecco Commission included a majority of secular scientists and bioethicists and was accused of being a sort of devaluation of the National Committee. However, it reported on December 28, 2000, that it had reached two major proposals. First, it suggested a new "Italian way" in stem cell experimentation consisting in creating new totipotent stem cells through cloning, which appeared to be agreed upon unanimously. But at the last minute, just before the press conference, Catholics presented their dissenting opinion, even though it was too late to include it in the published report. Second, a large majority of the Dulbecco Commission suggested that it was permissible to experiment on spare embryos, while the Catholic minority presented a dissenting opinion.[26]

This last conclusion is similar to that reached by an equivalent majority of the National Committee, which approved its report on October 27, 2000. But, while the Dulbecco Report was discussed on the front pages of the newspaper for days, the National Committee Report was hardly known (and was not available in print until August 2002). However, neither report had any practical implementation. Catholics immediately managed to provide financial state funding only for research on stem cells from adults, preventing in this way any state-funded research on embryonic stem cells.

Even though Catholics could avoid any embryo experimentation, both the Dulbecco and National Committee reports showed that, in early 2001, the situation on the issue of embryo experimentation was in flux. Considering that political elections were forthcoming in the Spring, Catholics were afraid that a new center-left government would allow such experiments. To prevent such a possibility, some Catholics succeeded in having the Parliament approve without any debate the European Convention of Bioethics, article 18 of which explicitly forbids any embryo experimentation in the absence of former legislation regulating the practice.[27]

Given such a controversial situation, the fact that the National Committee avoided reexamining the issue of the embryo is taken as an implicit mark of approval conferred on the former position. It could be that such a decision was dependent on the necessity of maintaining an equilibrium within a very pluralistic Committee, but the reluctance and slowness in taking firm stands on crucial as well as controversial issues precluded the Committee from being as incisive as desirable for setting lasting reference points for Italian bioethics.

As already mentioned, the Spring of 2001 political elections were won by a center-right wing coalition lead by Mr. Berlusconi, who, on June 12, 2002, once again appointed a new National Committee, with Francesco D'Agostino as chair. While the Berlinguer Committee was balanced and nuanced, representing many positions, the new D'Agostino Committee was formed by a strong majority of Catholics (a ratio of about 4:1). Moreover, it includes only a few scientists and a large number of jurists and bioethicists, including the President of the Italian Pro-Life Movement and other members of a Pro-Life Task Force. No official program was presented at the beginning and therefore no evaluation of the Committee's future activity is possible. But a glance at the Committee's composition is enough to foresee hard times ahead for ethical pluralism.

V. Patients' Rights

Another issue that was more quietly debated – but that is of the utmost importance – is that of patient autonomy and an individual's right to be informed about his or her health conditions. Several factors contributed to bringing about what has been called "a silent revolution" (Immacolato, 2002), but, in about a decade, Italians' attitudes to truth telling and individual autonomy have completely changed: in the early 1990s, it was "normal" to speak with the family and to withhold information from the patient, now the situation is reversed. The patient is now the center and must be informed of his or her health conditions. Of course, this practice is not yet followed in every case, but a significant change of the general attitude has occurred: recurrent challenges to the patient's right to know are perceived as "old fashioned" or "politically incorrect".

A first factor bringing about this "silent revolution" is to be found in court decisions on the so-called "Florence case", which occurred in the early 1990s: head surgeon Dr. Massimo was condemned for having treated a patient without her informed consent (Santosuosso, 1999). Courts at various levels converged in asserting a patient's right to the truth, and this case deeply changed the background of the physician-patient relationship. Since then, doctors have been careful to obtain a signed informed consent form before beginning any treatment – even if only as a merely "bureaucratic" procedure that must be performed to avoid legal troubles.

A second factor contributing to creating the new attitude is the new code of medical ethics (codice deontologico) issued by the Italian Medical Association in 1989.[28] While the former version stated that relatives should receive health related information, beginning in 1989 any relevant information must be given in any case directly to the patient. Relatives no longer receive any information (unless the patient consents to it). This trend was reinforced by a series of new laws on privacy, which started in 1996. Finally, a role was played by European Union's various directives, including the acceptance of the already mentioned European Convention of Bioethics.[29] As a matter of fact, informed consent is now so relevant that it is one of the major criteria for the quality evaluation of a health care institution: credits for being qualified as a "high quality hospital" are gained according to whether informed consent is regularly provided to patients.

A third factor favoring autonomy has depended on the social actions of various institutions. Groups such as the Consulta di bioetica have spent considerable efforts to promote autonomy.[30] In the early 1990s, the Consulta launched a version of a "living will" – called "Carta dell'autodeterminazione" or "Biocard" – appropriate to the Italian situation. It is rather specific in its formulation and presents several clauses that can be chosen or not. A new updated version of the Biocard was presented in 1998, it immediately attracted the attention of the public, and a few thousand individuals have requested forms, even though the media devoted only marginal attention to it.[31]

The new version of the Biocard was created to be consistent with current Italian legislation, but there are two important problematic issues. The first is about a specific clause concerning voluntary donation of one's bodily remains in case of permanent vegetative state (PVS). The other is a general problem about the validity of being represented by a previously designated person. On this issue, there are two opposite opinions: some lawyers say that it is already valid since it is a will, while others emphasize that it has no force at all, and its inclusion is a sort of "revolutionary turn" in the Italian system. To solve this controversy, the Consulta elaborated a new bill that recognizes the faculty of a citizen to appoint a "surrogate decision maker" for health matters. Supported by about 20 MPs, the bill was presented at the Italian parliament on February 10, 1999, and again in the new 2001 legislature.[32]

Given the general political situation, it is quite unlikely that it will be discussed soon, but at least the "living will" issue abandoned mere intellectual circles and entered the world of legislation. As a matter of fact, the new action was noticed: Professor A. Fiori (of the Catholic University of Rome and vice-president of the National Committee for Bioethics) objected that the Biocard is useless and the bill is quite dangerous because consent given when a person is healthy is invalid, since "nobody can know which reactions the patient will have when he is prey of a disease, given the fact that diseases are usually so fierce as to upset in a short time some former convictions, even religious ones" (Fiori, 1999, p. 356).[33]

If this claim were coherent, then any consent itself would be invalid, because it is always possible to hold that in the next moment the patient will change his or her mind.[34] However, in one sense it is better that a Biocard be signed by a patient who knows about his or her condition and is competent to decide according to his or her views. Therefore, a group is studying new versions of the Biocard aimed at specific diseases such as Alzheimer, ALS, and so forth, so that a person can sign it at the beginning of the process. Possibly, the real reason that justifies the strong Catholic opposition to the Biocard is that it is perceived as a sort of Trojan horse to introduce euthanasia: emphasis on self-determination would be but a preliminary step to smooth the road leading to the acceptance of euthanasia (which will be considered in the next section). So far, however, the current version of Biocard carefully avoids any claim in that direction.

A final factor that contributed to stimulate new attention for autonomy (in a wide sense) was provided by the so-called "Di Bella case", from the name of an 80 year-old physician who claimed to have discovered an effective "multi-therapy" (as he calls it) against cancer. Violent controversies sprung up because this "multi-therapy" had no scientific support and – being quite expensive – it was not included in the treatments paid for by the Italian NHS. However, Di Bella followers claimed to have a right freely to choose one's therapy (paid for by the NHS). In the winter of 1997/98, the Di Bella case was on front pages for months, and the crisis of confidence in medicine was so deep as literally to paralyze the activity of health care institutions for weeks. Di Bella was even invited to present his new "discovery" to the European Parliament in Brussels, where he stated that one and the same "therapy" was effective for cancer as well as for ALS and even for Alzheimer's dementia. Pressures for the "Di Bella therapy" were so strong that the Constitutional court (May 26, 1998) decided that the NHS had to respect patients' free choice and pay for it – at least until the end of a new trial to prove its effectiveness. The results of this clinical trial were unfavorable to the "Di Bella protocol", and, in the fall of 1998, the issue slowly faded away. Unfortunately, only a few of the many ethical issues raised by this case have been discussed, and most interpretations picture the Di Bella case as a protest of cancer patients and their families against insensitive oncologists worried only with scientific protocols. There is some truth in this interpretation, but I think that the protests depend on something deeper, which has to be found in people's inability to understand the ongoing passage from an old style "artisan" medicine to the new trends of an "industrial" medicine, in which therapies are impersonal and standardized.[35]

The Di Bella case was important not only for its influence on the issue of a patient's "freedom of choice", but also because it made clear that not all patients are confident in scientific medicine and that there are many who resort to forms of "alternative medicines" – an issue that was usually disregarded in Italian culture. In the last few years, however, this phenomenon emerged more clearly. The Italian Medical Association published a special report on the issue of "complementary medicine" (as they are called) and, in June 2002, decided that qualified physicians can offer some "complementary therapies". Moreover, a bill was elaborated and discussed in the past legislature, and possibly a new law regulating the whole field of "non-standard practices" could be passed in the near future.[36]

VI. End of Life Issues

The other hotly and frequently debated topic is euthanasia. Reflection concerning the issue changed rapidly in a few years, and we have to consider the different stages and levels of the discussion. It started in the early 1990s, when newspapers referred to the Dutch experience. At that time, Catholics tried to consider euthanasia a sort of unspeakable taboo; i.e., something which is not even worth considering, being self-evidently wrong. The *Consulta*, together with a few scholars, opposed such a trend and succeeded in keeping it an open issue to be carefully discussed. As a matter of fact, now euthanasia is an issue freely and frequently debated.

Even though the *Consulta* defended the morality of voluntary euthanasia from the beginning, such a solution was never urged, because it reckoned that the Italian public opinion would be quite reluctant to accept such a step. However, since 1997, the situation on the issue has changed at both the cultural and institutional levels. Evidence for a change of ethos is provided by a sociological inquiry published in 1999 by a Catholic group that showed that in Rome 13.9% of physicians and nurses have received at least one request for active euthanasia in the last three years, and that such requests were advanced by educated patients, who were well attended by their families (i.e., not just poor and desperate people). Nobody knows how many were accepted, but in any case this shows that attitudes towards "non-natural death" are changing.

In the spring of 1998, Mr. Mario Forzatti, armed with a gun, broke into an intensive care unit where his beloved wife was being treated and disconnected her until he was sure that she was dead. He said that she did not want to be treated and that they had a reciprocal agreement. This case, together with continuous debates, opened a new level of reflection on death issues. These debates were stimulated by different sources, such as various papers published by Indro Montanelli, a well-known old journalist, who was a strenuous defender of voluntary euthanasia: in December 1999, when he was 93 years old, Montanelli declared at a public conference in Milan that he would have chosen how to die by himself. (He died on July 13, 2001.) This statement raised many controversies but also a great deal of consensus. Another source was the reflection of the Waldesian church, which, in 1999, produced a report stating that, in some extreme cases, active euthanasia can be justified by Christian morality. This report was discussed in the media as a religious voice in open dissent with the Roman Catholic Church.[37] A third source was the action of the Italian branch of Exit, which was very able to stimulate the media's interest on the issue. To capture journalists' attention, this group told stories about the help they provided to willing patients. In November 2001, a nationwide newspaper published an interview about the alleged "death voyages" organized by the group to the Netherlands and to Switzerland for patients willing to be euthanized. The President of the Association was immediately charged with cooperation to murder by a judge, and whether the law was really violated or not is still not settled.[38] Exit contributed significantly to the euthanasia debate, even if its inflexible stand could lead to undesirable counter-effects.

These ongoing cultural debates received two prompt and important responses at the institutional level. The first was an explicit prohibition of euthanasia included in the 1998 Code of Medical Ethics. In previous versions, euthanasia certainly was not permitted, but neither was it expressly mentioned. One interpretation is that previously euthanasia appeared so outrageous that any explicit prohibition seemed superfluous. However, now it is expressly forbidden.

The second institutional response was a new 1999 law establishing services of palliative care and hospices throughout Italy. This was a real novelty for Italy, where palliative care had been almost completely disregarded by "official" medicine as well as by medical schools. Only some voluntary associations, such as the *Fondazione Floriani* in Milano, were developing programs to assist the dying. Palliation was taught at the Italian School of Palliative Medicine (*Scuola Italiana di Medicina Palliativa*, or SIMPA), a private school founded and directed by Dr. Michele Gallucci, an able physician who has devoted his life to spreading the new culture of palliation in Italy. More recently, new educational programs for neurologists caring for patients affected by neurological diseases have been offered by the bioethics group of the Italian Society of Neurology in cooperation with the *Fondazione Gilberto Cominetta*. But before 1999, palliative medicine was the Cinderella of Italian healthcare.

The new law, as well as a significant amount of money for new palliative care programs, attracted the attention of many physicians. There is some risk that many "palliative experts" will suddenly show up all at once, but the new law appears to be well framed to avoid gross misuses. In any case, implementation of the new law slowed down since Ms. Rosi Bindi had to resign from the office of Minister of Health in the spring of 2000 – even though Umberto Veronesi wanted a new law that would make it easier to use analgesics. Italy is one of the last countries in the use of analgesics and the hope is that this law will change the current situation.

The new law on palliative care and hospices started an interesting debate. Bindi is a committed Catholic and worked hard on this law, being convinced both that the dying have a right to be assisted and that palliative care is the best antidote to any euthanasia request. If dying patients receive adequate assistance, they may have fewer motives for asking for active euthanasia. In this sense, efficient palliative care programs are the best *alternative* to euthanasia. This thesis was challenged by many palliative care providers, who retorted that the two practices may be *complementary*, in the sense that palliative care is a preliminary treatment, which – in extreme cases – can be complemented by a request for euthanasia.

Debates on euthanasia were recurrent at the cultural level when, on June 14, 2000, at an academic conference in Milano, the special issue of *Bioetica* on the "Englaro case" was presented. Eluana Englaro was a 20 year-old woman when an accident on January 18, 1992, reduced her to PVS. Her father, who is also her legal representative, asked for the suspension of artificial feeding. On December 30, 1999, the court of appeals in Milano decided to reject Eluana's father request. *Bioetica*'s issue included the court decision as well as other relevant documents and some comments.[39] The new Minister of Health, Umberto Veronesi, was invited to the conference: he came and said that a humane solution for PVS had to be found for such cases. Possibly thousands of these cases exist in Italy, and such burdens should not left on the shoulders of families.

According to the media's criteria, this statement was equivalent to a declaration that the minister of health was favorable to euthanasia. Veronesi confirmed that, even though in his long medical career he had never had a request for euthanasia, the issue is serious and should be considered with an open mind and without prejudices. This was enough to start an inflamed debate and some Catholics even asked for the minister's dismissal.

Attention was already very high on this issue when, on June 19, the municipal council of Torino approved a statement in favor of voluntary euthanasia and invited liberal legislation on the issue.[40] Moreover, on June 20, the court of Monza decided that Mr. Forzatti was guilty of having helped his wife to die and condemned him to more than six years in jail. This sentence raised an outburst of protests and letters supporting Forzatti's act of compassion. Because of these events, for days the issue of euthanasia was in the media. Minister Veronesi was interviewed many times on these issues, and he firmly repeated that modern medicine changed the circumstances of death and that new solutions must be found: withdrawing artificial feeding or active euthanasia could be an option in some cases, although he never argued in any detail. However, these calm statements were enough to fuel hot controversies with Catholics.

This was not the only controversy he had with Catholics,[41] the last of which took place just a few days before he left his position. The reason was that Veronesi appointed another *ad hoc* Commission – the Oleari Commission – to give advice on artificial feeding for PVS. The Oleari Report was published in early June 2001, stating that artificial feeding could be withdrawn if some safeguards are complied with. This was enough for titles such as "euthanasia Veronesi style".[42]

As of this writing, Eluana Englaro is still in PVS, waiting for a new court decision, which is expected by the end of 2002. Debates on her case and on Veronesi's statements changed the magnitude of the euthanasia issue in Italy. Before this case, euthanasia was only a cultural debate, while after the case it became a real political option. As a matter of fact, two different bills allowing active euthanasia were elaborated and one of them was presented to the Parliament.[43] It goes without saying that the bill was not even discussed in the past legislature and that it is very unlikely that it will be in the present one. But an important step was made. Further evidence for this new atmosphere is provided by the extensive attention devoted by the media to death issues in April and May of 2002. The first occasion was provided by the final entry of the Dutch law at the beginning of April. In late April, the cases of Miss B. and Ms. Pretty in the U.K. were in the spotlight, immediately followed by the great clamor for the new decision on the Forzatti case by the court of appeals, which discharged him from the former accusation of murder. For over a month, front pages of the major newspapers had been busy in discussing end of life issues. Prudence recommends avoiding any prediction, but in Italy, as in any other Western developed country, euthanasia is an open question. It is unclear when it will be resolved and which answer it will receive.

VII. Organ Transplantation

Three other important events have occurred in Italian bioethics since 1997. The first one is the new law on organ transplantation, approved on April 1, 1999. Since 1972, Italy has accepted the "whole brain death" definition of death and a 1993 law shortened the delay required from the diagnosis of death to organ removal from 24 hours to six hours. But no comprehensive law regulating organ removal had been passed. So the situation was far from being satisfactory for at least two reasons. First, "brain death" is still under attack. In Italy, there is a voluntary association fighting "against organ predation" that is quite active and has an audience in the media. It has no peculiar religious or philosophical ground, but it gives voice to ancestral fears of being prematurely killed. In May 1997, the family of a young "brain dead" man claimed that he was still alive and moving, and for about a week the hospital was paralyzed by people arguing that efforts for resuscitation should continue. This event was in the front pages of the media for days and certainly hindered organ donation.

More important than such recurrent criticism is the obscure situation about who is entitled to consent to organ donation. By tradition, usually the donor's relatives had to give consent and this was a major obstacle to transplants. The new law tried to solve this issue with a requirement that every citizen must decide whether to be a donor or a non-donor. Local health care authorities must register people's decisions on the matter, and those who do not answer the written questionnaire sent to every citizen are assumed to have implicitly consented to donate. This law was applauded by professionals, because it favors organ donation. But it was also criticized by others because it creates a division between donor and non-donor, which may be a dangerous source of societal discrimination.

Even though the new law was approved, underground opposition seems to be quite consistent. Rules stating specific procedures for collecting citizens' consent were to be issued by July 1999, but they have not yet appeared. Minister Bindi sent a letter inviting each citizen to fill out a form consenting to organ donation, but only a minority promptly accepted such an invitation, and in any case the legal value of such forms is still unclear. Even though organ transplants are celebrated as one of the major conquests of contemporary medicine, their practical implementation is not as easy as one would think. Practical problems emerge from time to time because of the short supply of organs. For example, on September 8, 2001, a man on the waiting list for transplantation killed himself. On July 9, 2002 a woman was transplanted with a cancerous organ which started new controversies.[44]

Finally, the issue of organs on the illegal market and commerce emerges occasionally in newspapers. In Italy, there is a deep-rooted taboo concerning the mere possibility of any sort of incentive to facilitate organ transplants; this possibility is perceived as a frightening nightmare, spoiling the good practice of "giving the gift of life".[45] In this positive perspective, some debate was devoted to the new possibility of transplanting hands and external organs. A department of the Monza Hospital (next to Milano) is peculiarly specialized for such interventions. The topic received special attention in the media as well as at the institutional level.[46]

The second event concerned high-level surgery. In May 2000, two Siamese female babies arrived from Peru to a highly specialized surgery center in Palermo: they needed to be separated, and the family was very poor and could not afford to pay for surgery. Surgeon chief Dr. Marcelletti offered the necessary help, and immediately the media launched a campaign in favor of such a great attempt at saving human life. It was a tragic attempt, however, because the death of one of the two babies was certain, but the separation was necessary to give the other twin some chance of life. No one pondered different values in this case, and Catholic theologians promptly supported the separation, arguing that no one would have been directly killed, because this was a case in which the principle of double effect could be correctly applied. Only a few voices manifested a clear dissent or remarked that this was a case of "direct killing": the ethics committee of the hospital approved the surgery with only one dissenting opinion.[47] The Siamese twins were separated: one died during surgery, while the other died a few hours later. Then, quite abruptly, people realized that such a treatment was wrong and unjustified. Some theologians realized that double effect was not applicable to this case, but nevertheless the media's attention faded away quickly, and no trace of this case appears to be left after two years.

The third event was a consequence of the total ban on cloning issued immediately after Dolly's birth (see above, section 3). Minister Bindi's decree forbade not only human and animal cloning, but also vegetable cloning (of soya and other vegetables). This clause irritated some Italian farmers who had already invested in cultivation of genetically modified products, and the ban was soon abrogated to permit such crops. However, the ban of human and animal cloning was reiterated several times prior to December 2001.

A problem occurred in September 1999, when, at the national fair of Cremona, a cloned cattle called "Galileo" was presented to the public. Minister of Health Rosi Bindi immediately ordered that the animal be withdrawn from the exhibition, because it was created against the decree forbidding animal cloning. Dr. Cesare Galli – the biologist who cloned it – was prosecuted for illegal practice and risked serious fines and jail. At the end of April 2000, he was discharged and the affair was closed.[48] Research on cloning was seriously damaged, but this is a different issue. For many Italians, bioethics has to set limits to bio-medical research and, therefore, a delay in the field is not a problem.

The last event also concerns biological research. As in other parts of Europe, various factors (e.g., the spread of BSE or "mad cow disease", and so forth) contributed to a deep concern for food safety. In the winter of 1999/2000, the issue of transgenic food was hotly debated, and some stores were proud to sell only "biological food" (banning any transgenic product). This trend was favored by the Green Party, which joined the then ruling coalition. Within a general policy in support of traditional "biological agriculture" over against the new GMOs, in January 2001, the Minister of Agriculture, Pecoraro Scanio, banned any GMO crop cultivated "in the open field". This was enough for biologists to raise significant protest. Lead by Nobel Laureates Dulbecco and Levi Montalcini on February 13, 2001, about 1500 scientists from all over Italy protested in the streets of Rome against the limitations set on biological research.[49] The protest was mainly against minister Pecoraro Scanio, and it was openly supported by minister Veronesi, who was in favor of biomedical research. This shows the complexity of the Italian situation, where so many diverging souls must live together. Catholics set vetoes any time a human embryo is at stake, while Greens do the same any time uncontaminated nature is in danger. The old war between science and religion is still going on in Italy under new and disguised forms, and the results of this fight are still uncertain.

VIII. Conclusion

My analysis of Italian bioethics since 1997 is certainly incomplete. For instance, I omitted the on-going debate on abortion. But at this point, the reader should have at least an idea of what is going on. Like any industrial and developed Western country, Italy has a secularized lifestyle and a very liberal view of social life. Autonomy and self-determination are undisputed. What I referred to as the "silent revolution" concerning informed consent was certainly enforced by the judiciary but, in this case, judges interpreted an ethos which was already spreading through Italian people. Many physicians as well as a part of society were (and still are) reluctant to accept new directions on "informed consent", but these oppositions are marginal phenomena: they are similar to the rejection of sexual equality, of democracy, and so forth. The judges' directions modified social life, because social background was already ready for such a change. Likely a liberal way of life is deeply rooted in Italian conscience, because anyone has a right to decide on one's "private matters": one can choose about divorce as well as cohabitation, about sexual preferences, and so forth. The right to privacy is going to be widely accepted and enforced. In this sense, there is a solid core of liberal attitudes favoring autonomy about social and personal life.

Given this kernel of deep-rooted autonomy, it is not clear if and how fast this attitude will expand toward the margins and will involve crucial bioethical issues, such as those concerning assisted reproduction and euthanasia. At this point, this process of increasing freedom is not certain, because its establishment largely depends on the role played by culture in such critical historical junctures. Freedom's expansion, as well as people's acceptance of biomedical technologies, require a cultural background that is favorable to such biotechnical novelties. In Italy, it is currently not clear if, when, and how they will be accepted.

These doubts depend on the fact that in Italy there are two opposite "cultural models" or "paradigms" which are in conflict: on the one hand, there is an "analytic" (or "scientific") model, referring to the English-speaking culture, which privileges clarity and exactness, and defends a progressive morality. According to this perspective, biomedical revolution is changing societal conditions, and bioethics must formulate new values for society. It would be a tragedy not to understand what is going on and simply to defend old values unfitting for a new social life. In this sense, liberal legislation allowing assisted reproduction is requested.

On the other hand, there is a "continental" (or "humanistic") model, which refers to German-speaking philosophy. This perspective privileges metaphorical thinking and does not require exactness and precision, because existence's complexity cannot be grasped by logical thinking. Developing a kind of Heideggerian perspective, techno-sciences are seen as an intrinsic violation of nature. In this sense, the task of bioethics is to "set limits" to techno-scientific advancements. This view is held by various trends and is perfectly consonant with the Catholic perspective, which is committed to defending absolute prohibitions and immutable values.

Looking backwards at the intellectual debate, one has the impression that there is no dialogue between the two paradigms and that rational arguments are useless. The solution of the controversy will possibly be provided by practical changes; for instance, the biotechnological industry may become strong enough to condition social life. But any prediction is very risky.

It may be that in the next few years the "silent revolution" that succeeded in firmly establishing autonomy for any health treatment will continue its expansion to invest marginal situations, such as assisted reproduction and euthanasia, with respect for autonomy. But it may also be that scholars following the "continental paradigm" will convince people that marginal situations are outside of human autonomy's appropriate control. Political controversies on bioethical issues presuppose such cultural disagreements.

Another very serious problem is that Catholics are strong enough to control institutions that are devoted to regulating bioethical issues. They can coalesce with some secular factions holding a "continental perspective" and establish strict prohibitions. I dwelled on the issue of assisted reproduction, because it is exemplary of the Italian situation: even if Catholics are a minority and people do not understand Catholic prohibitions concerning artificial reproduction, Catholics could obtain the Chamber's approval of a very restrictive bill on assisted reproduction. If this trend continues and Catholics succeed in their attempt to control Italian moral life through institutional settings, then it is possible that Italy will undergo a sort of new Counter Reformation.

Notes

1. For an examination of the debate before 1997, see Mori (2002b), in which I try to provide some background presuppositions for understanding Italian situation. For other remarks, see Mori, 1998, 1998a.
2. For the text of the proposal see Movimento per la vita (1996).
3. For the ruling of the Constitutional Court and debate, see Corte Costituzionale (1997).
4. Only few dissenting voices were heard at the beginning. See, for example, Neri (1998).
5. Other legal contributions in a liberal fashion are: Baldini (1999), and Corti (2000). For some feminists contributions, see Finzi Vegetti (1997), discussed in (1999) *Bioetica. Rivista interdisciplinare*, VII(3), Boccia and Zuffa (1998), Preta (1999), and Fiumanò (2000). While the former books are in some sense quite critical towards assisted reproduction, a more positive attitude is shown by Botti (2000). For a traditional Roman Catholic view on feminist bioethics, see Mele (1998).
6. There is in Italy an interesting view according to which "human rights" should be a solid basis for bioethics, since they are consistent with natural law (Catholic) morality. The most active philosopher holding this view is Viola (1997, 2000). Other contributions include: Compagnoni and D'Agostino (2001), Massuè and Gerin (2000), and Chieffi (2000). For criticism, see Mori, 2002c.
7. The literature on assisted reproduction and the "embryo issue" is endless. Here I report only a few works, using the crucial distinction between Catholic and non-Catholic: this provides also an idea of the different number of contributions. Non-Catholic: Flamigni (1998, 2001), *Le Scienze Quaderni,* (February 1998), which is devoted to "L'embrione e la vita", and Prodomo (1998). Catholic: Scola (1998), Tre Re (1999), Centro di Bioetica e Dirirri Umani (1995), Sgreccia and De Dios Vial Correa (1998), Aramini (1999), and Garrone (2001).
8. Some interesting titles in this fast-growing literature are the following: Bartolommei (1995, 2003), which presents clear philosophical analysis of the major issues; Poli (2001), which is the best technical presentation of the field; Meldolesi (2002), who is in favor of new GMOs; Pontificia Academia Pro Vita (1999) and Mele (2002) present the Vatican's position on these issues. All the other books are in some way critical toward new biotechnologies: see Celli, Marmiroli and Verga (2000), Tamino and Pratesi (2001), Tamino (2001), Capanna (2002), Carra & Terragni (2001).
9. For a more thorough bibliography and some critical comments, the interested reader may refer to some reviews I have written over the last few years: Mori (1987, 1990, 1995, 1997, 1998, 2000, 2002a) as well as Viafora and Mori (1993).
10. For a debate on the topic, of interest are the following contributions: Deiana and D'Orazio (2001), and the special issue of *Scuole e citte* (2001); and Tugnoli (2002). As for some textbooks, I can mention the following: *Catholic oriented: Ufficio Scuola della Curia Arcivescovile di Milano* (2001) and Doldi (2001). For a pluralistic or secular view, see de Martino (2001) and Mori (2002c).
11. *Medicina e morale* is published by Vita e Pensiero, Largo Gemelli 1, 20123, Milano; *Bioetica* is published by Zadig Editore, via Calzecchi 10, 20129, Milano; *Notizie di Politeia* is published

by Politeia, via C. Del Fante 13, 20121, Milano. *Janus* is published by Zadig Roma, via Monte Cristallo 6, 00141 Roma. *Etica per le professioni* is published by the Fondazione Lanza, via Dante 55, 35139, Padova. There are possibly other journals that I did not mention, because they are mainly local. Only one of these deserves comment: *Bioetica e cultura* is a biannual published since 1992 by the Istituto Siciliano di Bioetica, an institution that is quite active on the isle. They defend a "Mediterranean bioethics", holding that Mediterranean cultures (Jew, Catholic, and Islamic) believe that life ought to be defended, since such a value has a wider and universal as well as rational claim. For a recent presentation of such a view, see Privitera (1999) and Russo (1997). For an early critical analysis of this view, see Neri (1994).

12. In Italy, on February 17, 1992, the judges of Milano began an inquisition called "*Mani pulite*" ("clean hands") involving all major politicians. Italy underwent a time of political turmoil: in a couple of years, most traditional parties dissolved themselves or changed their names. This fate occurred to the Socialist Party, the Republican Party, and the Christian Democracy (DC), the party that had been ruling Italy since the end of the Second World War. DC's departure gave rise to several smaller parties of Christian orientation: one of these (possibly the largest), the Italian Popular Party (*Partito Popolare Itaiano*, PPI), joined the left-wing coalition, while the other parties joined the right-wing coalition. This choice was necessary because in that time Italy modified the electoral system by introducing so-called "bipolarism", in which two coalitions face each other at the elections. In the spring of 1994, Italy had a crucial political election. Mr. Silvio Berlusconi, leading a center-right coalition, won the elections. After a few months, the *Lega Lombarda* left the coalition and joined the center-left (this event is called "*il ribaltone*", i.e., "the big upside down turn"). Berlusconi had to resign at the end of 1994. A "transitory government", led by Mr. Lamberto Dini, ruled until the new elections in the spring of 1996, which were favorable to the center-left wing coalition ruled by Mr. Romano Prodi. Prodi ruled from May 1996 until October 1998, when his government did not receive support on the financial law (only one vote was missing). In this case, the center-left coalition could still count on a majority, and Mr. Massimo D'Alema formed a new government, which lasted until April 2000, when he left the office after mid-term elections, which were quite unfavorable to his policies. From May 1996 to April 2000, the position of Minister of Health was held by Ms. Rosi Bindi, a committed Catholic of the PPI. When Mr. Giuliano Amato formed the new center-left government at the end of April 2000, he gave the ministry of health to professor Umberto Veronesi, a famous oncologist of secular orientation. The Amato government ruled from April 2000 to June 2001. The new elections in the spring of 2001 were won by Mr. Berlusconi's new center-right coalition (which once again included the *Lega*). This time, the center-right coalition appears to be quite solid and – unless something new and unpredictable shows up – it should rule until the end of its mandate in the spring of 2006.

13. For the report of all these manifestos, see *Consulta di Bioetica* (1998a).

14. The reason is related to the fact that the abortion situation involves the clash of two concrete rights (the woman's and the fetus's), while in the case of *in vitro* fertilization, the so-called "right to a child" of the parents is more abstract. On this issue, see Casini (1996), especially pp. 43-50.

15. For the text of the Constitutional Court and a comment, see *Bioetica. Rivista interdisciplinare, VII*(2) (1999c), especially pp. 343-345; Corte costituzionale (1999). This decision was requested by a case of AID that occurred in Neaples.

16. For the text and comments see Tribunale di Palermo (1999). This decision was the final response to the case raised in Cremona in 1984.

17. For the text of the bill, see Disegno di legge n. 4048, 1999.

18. The *ordinanza Schettini* raised a real mess in Italy, as seen by the fact that it occupied the front pages of newspapers for days. Investigations and endless debates had been held: it was a storm for Italians, who realized that a surrogate pregnancy could be accepted by current legislation. For the text of the ruling and some comments see Ferrando (2000), Pagni (2000), and

Documenti sul dossier maternità surrogata (2000). For a critical legal comment, see Busnelli (2001), especially pp. 116-122.

19. For the text of this decision, see Corte costituzionale (1999), with a comment by Ferrando (1999a).

20. For the text of the declaration, some comments and replies, see *Bioetica. Rivista interdisciplinare, X*(1).

21. For the text of the bill and some comments, see *Bioetica. Rivista interdisciplinare, X*(3) (2002c).

22. For criticism to this report, see Mori (1996), Piazza (1996), Viano (1996), and *Iride. Filosofia e discussione pubblica, 19* (settembre-dicembre, 1996), pp. 541-570.

23. For the documents of this controversy, see Avvenire (1999).

24. For relevant decrees of such a reform, see *Bioetica. Rivista interdisciplinare, VI*(3), pp. 447-461 (1998).

25. For a report on the conference held in Massa, see Mancini (2001). For the proceedings, see Immacolato et al. eds, *Notizie di politeia*, 2002, No. 67.

26. The text of the Dulbecco Report is available in English on the Ministry of Health website (2000). For some Italian debates on stem cell research, see *Bioetica. Rivista interdisciplinare, VIII*(3). For a good presentation of stem cells issues, see Neri (2001). On January 10, 2001, Veronesi also appointed another *ad hoc* Commission chaired by Professor Carlo Flamigni, which studied scientific issues concerning human oocyte freezing in order to test whether such a new practice could lead to the "storage" of women's reproductive ability. Moreover, the Flamigni's Commission was asked to enquire into the number of fertility clinics and the number of spare human embryos existing in Italy. The Commission reported in April 2001 with a new protocol for oocyte freezing and stated that in Italy there are about 24,000 spare embryos. Moreover, there are 384 fertility clinics, of which only 323 are actually active. Some of them do only simple insemination (124), 190 perform IVF with embryo transfer, 153 ICSI, and 65 FIVET.

27. For a criticism of Italian acceptance of the European Convention of Bioethics, see the editorial of Mori and Neir (2001). (A transcript of the debate for approval is reported on pp. 397-400.) On the Convention in general, see *Bioetica. Rivista interdisciplinare, VI*(4) (1998).

28. For some comments remarking the novelties of the new 1998 code of medical ethics, see Barni (1999b). Other remarks are in *Bioetica. Rivista interdisciplinare, VIII*(4): 597-610 (2000).

29. For some remarks on the influence of the European Convention about informed consent, see *Bioetica. Rivista interdisciplinare, IX*(2) (2001), especially pp. 235-237, and the papers on the Oleari Report included in the issue.

30. The *Consulta di bioetica* is a private association founded by late Renato Boeri, a well-known Italian neurologist. The *Consulta* is based in Milano but has branches in many Italian cities (Torino, Roma, Firenze, and so forth) and has about 400 members spread all over Italy. Further information can be found in Mori (2002b).

31. For the new formulation of the living will, see Consulta di Bioetica (1997).

32. For the text of the bill, see Consulta di Bioetica (1998b). Also, (2001e). *Bioetica. Rivista interdisciplinare, IX*(2), Supplementary Issue (2001) is devoted to "advance directives". See also Dameno (2002).

33. According to Fiori, any serious disease prevents free choice, because "it is freedom from disease that is lacking to the patients" (Fiori, 1999, p. 356).

34. See Pocar's rejoinder (2000) to Fiori.

35. For some documents and comments on the Di Bella case, see *Bioetica. Rivista interdisciplinare, VI*(2): (1998) and *Bioetica. Rivista interdisciplinare, VII*(2): 291-315 (1999). For an analysis of the literature on this case, see Mori (1999).

36. For the Italian Medical Association's statement and some discussion, see *Bioetica. Rivista interdisciplinare, X*(3) (2002). For an analysis of the bill on "complementary medicine", see *Bioetica. Rivista interdisciplinare, VIII*(1) (2000).

37. For the text of the document, see *Bioetica. Rivista interdisciplinare,* VII(1) (1999). For other statements of the Waldesian group, see Pons (1999). For other interesting views on euthanasia, see Ricca (2002).

38. For the Exit case, see *La Stampa* (2001) and the following days. It was announced that he would be discharged in 2003, but as yet it has not occurred.

39. See *Bioetica. Rivista interdisciplinare,* VIII(1) (2000).

40. For the text of the Turin city council, see Consiglio comunale di Torino (2000) (followed by a criticism of the Cardinal of Turin).

41. Veronesi had at least two other controversies with Catholics on bioethical issues that ought to be mentioned: the first occurred when the Norlevo pill (for emergency contraception) had to become available in Italy as required by European directions. Veronesi not only promptly complied with European requirements but explained that emergency contraception is a serious medical problem and that Norlevo pill was an acceptable way to face it. The other controversy occurred when Veronesi declared at a medical conference that a modern state cannot avoid the regulation of the use of marijuana and other drugs. A minor controversy occurred when he modified the legislation to make the use of morphine easier. When Veronesi left office, a pro-life magazine had the headline: "Go home, Veronesi: never again a minister like you!".

42. For a report of such comments, see Mori and Neri (2001). For the Oleari Report and some comments, see *Bioetica. Rivista interdisciplinare,* IX(2) (2001). Interestingly enough, withdrawal of artificial feeding was performed in other parts of Italy: for a report, see Orsi (2001).

43. For the text of bills on euthanasia, see Proposta di legge della Consulta di Bioetica sui diritti dei malati terminali (2001).

44. On the first issue, see *Corriere della sera,* September 8. (2000) and *Corriere della sera,* September 9, p. 16. (2000). For the response of the Minister of Health, see *La Provincia di Cremona e Crema,* September 9, p. 24 (2000). On the second issue, see *Corriere della sera,* July 9 (2002).

45. For a recent scandal of a man who sold one of his kidneys to pay usurers who were blackmailing him, see *La repubblica,* April 3, p. 24 (2002). For a defense of altruistic donation, see Berlinguer and Garrafa (1996).

46. Regarding this issue, the ethics committee of St. Gerard Hospital of Monza was involved, and an opinion was issued when the first Italian transplant of a hand was performed. For this text and a comment of a physician member of the committee, see *Bioetica. Rivista interdisciplinare,* VIII(4): 735-740 (2000).

47. For the text of the Palermo Ethics Committee, see *Bioetica. Rivista interdisciplinare,* IX(2) 2001, pp. 269–275. Only surgeon Ignazio Marino opposed the splitting, saying that it was a case of direct killing. Interestingly enough, secular bioethicists were perplexed and either asked for a supplement of ethical analysis or remarked that the Catholic stand was inconsistent. See Neri (2000).

48. For documents and a comment on the Galileo affair, see *Bioetica. Rivista interdisciplinare,* X(1) (2002).

49. On this controversy, see the paper by Viano (2001), which stimulated a wider reflection in the special issue of the same *Rivista di filosofia* completely devoted to "*Cultura scientifica e politiche della ricerca*" edited by Viano (2002), n. 2.

Bibliography

_____. 2001. Documenti sul dossier maternità surrogata. *Bioetica. Rivista interdisciplinare* VII(3).

_____. 2001. Proposta di legge della Consulta di Bioetica sui diritti dei malati terminali. *Bioetica. Rivista interdisciplinare* IX(2): 382-388.

_____. 2001. *Scuola e città* LII(4).

Angelini, G. et al. 1998. *La bioetica. Questione civile e problemi teorici sottesi*. Milano: Glossa Editore.

Aramini, M. 1999. *La procreazione assistita. Scoprire il senso di un nuovo modo di nascere*. Milano: Edizioni Paoline.

Aramini, M. 2001. *Introduzione alla bioetica*. Milano: Giuffrè.

Avvenire. 1999. Intervista al Cardinal Tonini. *Bioetica. Rivista interdisciplinare* VII(4): 705-716.

Azzone, G.F. 1997. *I dilemmi della bioetica. Tra evoluzione biologica e riflessione filosofica*. Roma: La Nuova Italia Scientifica.

Azzone, G.F. 2000. *La rivoluzione della medicina. Dall'arte alla scienza*. Milano: McGraw-Hill.

Azzone, G.F. 2003. *L'etica medica nello stato liberale*. Venezia: Istituto Veneto di Cultura, Lettere ed Arti.

Baldini, G. 1999. *Tecnologie riproduttive e problemi giuridici*. Torino: Giappichelli.

Barni, M. 1999a. *Diritti – doveri. Responsabilità del medico. Dalla bioetica al biodiritto*. Milano: Giuffrè editore.

Barni, M. (ed.) 1999b. *Bioetica, deontologia e diritto. Per un nuovo codice professionale del medico*. Milano: Giuffrè Editore.

Barni, M. 1999c. Terzo bilancio dell'attività svolta dal Comitato Nazionale per la Bioetica (Presidenza D'Agostino, 1994-1998. *Bioetica. Rivista interdisciplinare* VII(4): 585-587.

Bartolommei, S. 1995. *Etica e natura*. Roma-Bari: Laterza.

Bartolommei, S. 2003. *Etica e bioculturs*. Pisa: ETS.

Battaglia, L. 1997. *Etica e diritti degli animali*. Roma-Bari: Laterza.

Battaglia, L. 1999. *Dimensioni della bioetica. La filosofia morale dinanzi alle sfide delle scienze della vita*. Genova.

Beauchamp, T.L. & Childress, J.F. 1999. *Princìpi di etica biomedica*. Firenze: Casa Editrice Le Lettere.

Berlinguer, G. & Garrafa, V. 1996. *La merce finale*. Milano: Baldini e Castoldi.

Berlinguer, G. 2000. *Bioetica quotidiana*. Firenze: Giunti.

Boccia, M.L. & Zuffa, G. 1998. *L'eclissi della madre*. Milano: Pratiche Editrice.

Bompiani, A. 1997. *Bioetica ed etica medica nell'Europa occidentale*. Trieste: Proxima Scientific Press.

Bompiani, A., Loreti Beghè, A. & Marini, L. 2001. *Bioetica e diritti dell'uomo nella prospettiva del diritto internazionale e comunitario*. Torino: Giappichelli.

Borsellino, P. 1999. *Bioetica tra autonomia e diritto*. Milano: Zadig.

Botti, C. 2000. *Bioetica ed etica delle donne. Relazioni, affetti e potere*. Milano: Zadig.

Busnelli, F.D. 2001. *Bioetica e diritto privato*. Torino: Giappichelli, Torino.

Callahan, D. 2000. *La medicina impossibile. Le utopie e gli errori della medicina moderna*. Milano: Baldini & Castoldi.

Capanna, M. (ed.) 2002. *L'uomo è più dei suoi geni*. Milano: Rizzoli.

Carra, L. & Terragni, F. 2001. *Il conflitto alimentare. I cibi geneticamente modificati: pro e contro*. Milano: Garzanti.

Cattorini, P., D'Orazio, E. & Pocar, V. (eds). 1999. *Bioetiche in dialogo*. Milano: Zadig Editore.

Casini, C. 1996. *Per un forte Movimento per la Vita nella crisi della società italiana*. Firenze: Centro Documentazione e Solidarietà.

Cavalieri, P. 1999. *La questione animale. Per una teoria allargata dei diritti umani*. Torino: Bollati Boringhieri.

Cattorini, P. 1997. *Bioetica. Metodo ed elementi di base per affrontare problemi clinici*. Milano: Masson.

Cattorini, P. & Sala, R. (eds). 1998. *L'infermiere e il consenso del malato. Questioni di bioetica*. Firenze: Rosini Editrice.

Celli, G., Marmiroli, N. & Verga, I. 2000. *I semi della discordia. Biotecnologie, agricoltura e ambiente*. Milano: Edizioni Ambiente.

Centro di Bioetica e Diritti Umani, Università degli Studi di Lecce. 1995. *I diritti del nascituro e la procreazione artificiale*. Città del Vaticano: Libreria Editrice Vaticana.

Chieffi, L. (ed.) 2000. *Bioetica e diritti dell'uomo*. Milano: Paravia.

Ciccone, L. 2000. *La vita umana*. Milano: Ares.

Compagnoni, F. & D'Agostino, F. (eds). 2001. *Bioetica, diritti umani e multietnicità. Immigrazione e sistema sanitario nazionale*. San Paolo: Cinisello Balsamo.

Consiglio comunale di Torino. 2000. Su eutanasia passiva, eutanasia attiva, assistenza al suicidio e umanizzazione della morte. *Bioetica. Rivista interdisciplinare VIII*(3): 554-556.

Consulta di Bioetica. 1997. Nuovo testo della Carta dell'autodeterminazione. *Bioetica. Rivista interdisciplinare V*(1): 103-107.

Consulta di Bioetica. 1998a. Politeia, Manifesto per la libertà di procreare. *Bioetica. Rivista interdisciplinare VI*(2): 324-336.

Consulta di Bioetica. 1998b. Proposta di legge sul consenso informato e sulle direttive anticipate. *Bioetica. Rivista interdisciplinare VI*(2): 313-323.

Corte Costituzionale. 1997. La sentenza della Corte Costituzionale (n. 35/97) circa l'inammissibilita' del referendum sull'aborto (10/02/97). *Bioetica. Rivista interdisciplinare V*(3): 425-446.

Corte costituzionale. 1999. Sentenza sul disconscimento del figlio nato da fecondazoine eterloga. *Bioetica. Rivista interdisciplinare VII*(2): 343-351.

Corti, I. 2000. *La maternità per sostituzione*. Milano: Giuffrè Editore.

D'Agostino, F. 1998. *Bioetica nella prospettiva della filosofia del diritto*. Torino: Giappichelli.

Dalla Torre, G. 1997. *Le frontiere della vita. Etica, bioetica e diritto*. Roma: Edizioni Studium.

Dameno, R. (ed.) 2002. *Autodeterminarsi nonostante*. Milano: Guerini e Associati Editore.

Defanti, C.A. 1999. *Vivo o morto? La storia della morte nella medicina moderna*. Milano: Editore Zadig.

Deiana, G. & D'Orazio, E. (eds). 2001. *Bioetica ed etica pubblica*. Milano: Edizioni Unicopli.

de Martino, G. (ed.) 2001. *Piccolo manuale di bioetica*. Napoli: Liguori.

Disegno di Legge. 1999. Disciplina della procreazione medicalmente assistita. *Bioetica. Rivista interdisciplinare VII*(3): 531-536.

Doldi, M. 2001. *Bioetica per giovani*. Piemme: Casale Monferrato.

Dworkin, G., Frey, R.G. & Bok, S. 2001. *Eutanasia e suicidio assistito*. Torino: Edizioni di Comunità.

Engelhardt, Jr., H.T. 1999. *Manuale di bioetica. Nuova edizione*. Milano: Il Saggiatore.

Ferrando, G. 1999a. La Corte costituzionale e la Corte di Cassazione si pronunciano sul disconoscimento del figlio nato da inseminazione eterologa. *Bioetica. Rivista interdisciplinare VII*(2): 352-357.

Ferrando, G. 1999b. *Libertà, responsabilità e procreazione*. Padova: Cedam.

Ferrando, G. 2000. Commento all'ordinanza del Tribunale di Rome febbraio 2000. *Bioetica. Rivista interdisciplinare VIII*(3): 471-497.

Ferrando, G. 2002. *Il matrimonio*. Milano: Giuffrè.

Finzi Vegetti, S. 1997. *Volere un figlio. La nuova maternità fra natura e scienza*. Milano: Mondadori.

Fiori, A. 1999. Responsabilità medica e testamento di vita. *Vita e pensiero* 4: 356.

Fiumanò, M. 2000. *A ognuna il suo bambino*. Milano: Pratiche Editrice.

Flamigni, C. 1998. *Il libro della procreazione*. Milano: Mondadori.

Flamigni, C. 2001. *Avere un bambino, come inizia la vita: dal concepimento al parto*. Milano: Mondadori.

Ford, N.M. 1997. *Quando comincio io? Il concepimento nella storia, nella filosofia e nella scienza*. Milano: Baldini e Castoldi.

Fucci, S. 1998. *La responsabilità nella professione infermieristica. Questioni e problemi giuridici*. Milano: Masson.

Garrone, G. (ed.) 2001. *Fecondazione extra corporea: pro o contro l'uomo?* Torino: Gribaudi.

Harris, J. 1997. *Wonderwoman e Superman. Manipolazione genetica e futuro dell'uomo.* Milano: Baldini e Castoldi.

Immacolato, M. 1999. Come incentivare la presenza dei membri dei Comitati Etici Locali? *Bioetica. Rivista interdisciplinare VII*(3): 534-527.

Immacolato, M. 2002. *Il consenso informato in Italia.* In S. De Clementi (ed.), *Cronache di bioetica.* Milano: Zadig Editore.

Istituto Veneto di Scienze, Lettere ed Arti. 1999. *La dignità del morire.* Venezia: Istituto Veneto.

Istituto Veneto di Scienze, Lettere ed Arti. 2001. *La dignità del vivere.* Venezia: Istituto Veneto.

Jonas, H. 1997. *Tecnica, medicina ed etica. Prassi del principio responsabilità.* Torino: Einaudi.

Kuhse, H. 2000. *Prendersi cura. L'etica e la professione di infermiera.* Torino: Edizioni di Comunità.

Lecaldano, E. 1999. *Bioetica. Le scelte morali.* Roma-Bari: Laterza.

Lecaldano, E. 2002. *Dizionario di bioetica.* Rome: Laterza.

Mancini, E. 2001. Comitati etici a confronto a Massa. *Bioetica. Rivista interdisciplinare IX*(4): 745-748.

Marchesini, R. 1999. *La fabbrica delle chimere. Biotecnologie applicate agli animali.* Torino: Bollati Boringhieri.

Marchesini, R. 2001. *Bioetica e scienze veterinarie.* Napoli: Edizioni Scientifiche Italiane.

Massuè, J-P. & Gerin, G. (eds). 2000. *Diritti umani e bioetica.* Roma: Sapere.

Meldolesi, A. 2002. *Organismi geneticamente modificati. Storia di un dibattito truccato.* Torino: Einaudi.

Mele, V. 1998. *La bioetica al femminile.* Milano: Vita e Pensiero.

Mele, V. 2002. *Organismi geneticamente modificati e bioetica.* Siena: Cantagalli.

Ministry of Health. 2000. Dulbecco Report [On-line]. Available: <http://www.ministerosalute.it/>.

Morcavallo, B. 1999. *Morte e persona. Un dialogo fra etica medica, bioetica e filosofia morale.* Napoli: Alfredo Guida Editore.

Mori, M. 1987. Per una bibliografia italiana sulla bioetica. *Prospettive Settanta IX*(1): 145-163.

Mori, M. 1990. Bioetica: una riflessione in corso. *L'informazione bibliografica XVII*(3): (luglio-settembre) 442-452.

Mori, M. 1995. Bioetica: un dibattito in rapida espansione. *L'informazione bibliografica XXI*(3): (luglio-settembre) 343-353.

Mori, M. 1996. Il CNB e lo statuto dell'embrione: un'analisi critica del documento e linee di una prospettiva alternativa. *Bioetica. Rivista interdisciplinare IV*(3).

Mori, M. 1997. Bioetica: la crescita della riflessione laica. *L'informazione bibliografica XXIII*(1): (gennaio-marzo) 38-55.

Mori, M. 1998. Bioetica: le ultime encicliche morali e i commenti. *L'informazione bibliografica XXIV*(2): 182-191.

Mori, M. 1998a. Un primo bilancio della bioetica italiana. In C.M. Mazzoni (ed.), *Un quadro europeo per la bioetica?* (pp. 243-246). Firenze: Leo S. Olschki editore.

Mori, M. 1999. Etica e medicina: il "caso Di Bella". *L'informazione bibliografica XXV*(3): (luglio-settembre) 330-340.

Mori, M. 2000. Sul recente sviluppo della bioetica in Italia. *L'informazione bibliografica XXVI*(4): 516-528.

Mori, M. 2002a. Bioetica: l'emergere delle biotecnologie. *L'informazione bibliografica XXVIII*(4).

Mori, M. 2002b. Bioethics in Italy up to 2002: An overview. In: H.T. Englehardt, Jr. and L.M. Rasmussen (eds), *Bioethics and moral content: national traditions of health care morality. Papers dedicated in tribute to Kazumasa Hoshino* (pp. 97-120). Dordrecht: Kluwer Academic Publishers.

Mori, M. 2002c. *Bioetica. 10 temi per capire e discutere.* Milano: Edizioni Scolastiche Bruno Mondadori.

Mori, M. 2003. Una cronaca delle controversie sulla fecondazione assistita nelle XIII legislatura. *Cronache di bioetica*. Milano: Zadig publishers.

Mori, M. & Neri, D. 2001. Il Rapporto Oleari e la Convenzione di Oviedo. *Bioetica. Rivista interdisciplinare* IX(2).

Movimento per la vita. 1996. *Proposta di legge di iniziativa popolare per il riconoscimento di personalita' giuridica e conseguente modifica dell'art. 1 del codice civile. Bioetica. Rivista interdisciplinare* IV(2): 334-350.

Neri, D. 1994. Nuove vie per la bioetica italiana? *Bioetica. Rivista interdisciplinare* II(2): 311-318.

Neri, D. 2000a. A proposito del vivere e del morire. *L'unità*, May 25.

Neri, D. 2000b. La ricerca sulle cellule staminali: una terza via? Quale terza via? *Bioetica. Rivista interdisciplinare* VIII(3).

Neri, D. 2001. *La bioetica in laboratorio. Cellule staminali, clonazione e salute umana*. Bari-Roma: Laterza.

Neri, D. 2002. Perché tanta fretta? *Bioetica. Rivista interdisciplinare* VI(2): 306-312.

Orsi, L. 2001. Un nuovo passo nel dibattito sulla nutrizione artificiale. *Bioetica. Rivista interdisciplinare* IX(4): 749-757.

Pagni, A. 2000. Il Codice deontologies e la sentenza Schettini. *Bioetica. Rivista interdisciplinare* VIII(4): 674-684.

Pessina, A. 1999. *Bioetica. L'uomo sperimentale*. Milano: Bruno Mondadori.

Piana, G. 2002. *Bioetica*. Milano: Garzanti.

Piazza, A. 1996. L'embrione e' uno di noi? *Bioetica. Rivista interdisciplinare* IV(3).

Pocar, V. 1998. *Gli animali non umani. Per una sociologia dei diritti*. Roma-Bari: Laterza.

Pocar, V. 2000. Perché i cattolici italiani sono contro la Carta dell'autodeterminazione? *Bioetica. Rivista interdisciplinare* VIII(2): 319-329.

Poli, G. 2001. *Biotecnologie. Principi e applicazioni dell'ingegneria genetica*. Torino: UTET.

Pons, G. 1999. *Progresso scientifico e bioetica*. Torino: Claudiana.

Pontificia Academia Pro Vita. 1999. *Biotecnologie animali e vegetali. Nuove frontiere e nuove responsabilità*. Vatican: Libreria Editrice Vaticana.

Preta, L. (ed.) 1999. *Nuove geometrie della mente. Psicoanalisi e bioetica*. Roma-Bari: Laterza.

Privitera, S. 1999. *La questione bioetica. Nodi problematici e spunti risolutivi*. Acireale: Istituto Siciliano di Bioetica.

Prodomo, R. 1998. *L'embrione tra etica e biologia*. Napoli: Edizioni Scientifiche Italiane.

Proposta Bolognesi Bioetica. 1998. *Bioetica. Rivista interdisciplinare* VI(1): 124-135.

Redi, C., Garagna, S. & Zuccotti, M. 2001. Come, da biologi, vediamo il problema dell'embrione. *Bioetica. Rivista interdisciplinare* IX(2): 369-375.

Regan, T. 1989/1990. *I diritti animali*. Milano: Garzanti.

Regan, T. & Singer, P. (eds). 1976/1987. *Animal rights and human obligations*. Torino: Edizioni Gruppo Abele.

Ricca, Paolo (ed.) 2002. *Eutanasia. La legge olandese e commenti*. Torino: Claudiana.

Ruini, C. 2000. Crescere in comunione effettiva e nell'apertura missionaria non perdendo il passo con il rapido evolversi della società. *L'osservatore romano* 20-21 March, 16.

Ruini, C. 2001. *Chiesa del nostro tempo. Vol. 2. Prolusioni 1996-2001*. Casale Monferrato: Piemme.

Russo, G. (ed.) 1997. *Bilancio di 25 anni di bioetica*. Torino: Elle Di Ci.

Santosuosso, A. 1999. *Libertà di cura e libertà di terapia*. Roma: Il Pensiero Scientifico Editore.

Santosuosso, A. 2001. *Corpo e libertà. Una storia tra diritto e scienza*. Milano: Raffaello Cortina.

Scarpelli, U. 1998. *Bioetica laica*. Milano: Baldini e Castoldi.

Scola, A. (ed.) 1998. *Quale vita? La bioetica in questione*. Milano: Mondadori.

Sgreccia, E. 1999. *Manuale di bioetica. Volume I and II. Nuova edizione ampliata e aggiornata*. Milano: Vita e Pensiero.

Sgreccia, E., Spagnolo, A.G. & Di Pietro, M.L. 1999. *Bioetica. Manuale per i Diplomi Universitari della Sanità*. Milano: Vita e Pensiero.

Sgreccia, E. & De Dios Vial Correa, J. (eds). 1998. *Identity and Statute of Human Embryo*. Città del Vaticano: Libreria Editrice Vaticana.

Singer, P. 1997/2000. *Ripensare la vita*. Milano: Il Saggiatore.

Singer, P. 2001. *La vita come si dovrebbe*. Milano: Il Saggiatore.

Spagnolo, A.G. 1997. *Bioetica nella ricerca e nella prassi medica*. Roma: Edizioni Camilliane.

Spagnolo, A.G. & Gambino, G. (eds). 2002. *Human Health Issues*. Roma: Universo Editore.

Spinsanti, S. 1998. *Curare e prendersi cura. L'orizzonte antropologico della nuova medicina*. Roma: Edizioni Cidas.

Spinsanti, S. 1999. *Chi ha potere sul mio corpo? Nuovi rapporti tra medico e paziente*. Milano: Edizioni Paoline.

Spinsanti, S. 2001. *Bioetica e nursing. Pensare, riflettere, agire*. Milano: McGraw-Hill.

Tamino, G. 2001. *Il bivio genetico*. Milano: Edizioni Ambiente.

Tamino, G. & Pratesi, F. 2001. *Ladri di geni*. Roma: Editori Riuniti.

Tarantino, A. 1998. *Il rispetto della vita. Aborto, tutela del minore ed eutanasia*. Napoli: Edizioni Scientifiche Italiane.

Tettamanzi, D. 2000. *Nuova bioetica cristiana*. Casale Monferrato: Piemme.

Tre Re, G. 1999. *Terra di nessuno. Bioetica dei diritti dell'embrione umano*. Palermo: La Zisa.

Tribunale di Palermo. 1999. Il soprawenuto decesso del marito donatore non ostacola fecondazione assistita. *Bioetica. Rivista interdisciplinare VII(2)*: 358-370.

Tugnoli, C. (ed.) 2002. *La bioetica nella scuola*. Milano:Angeli.

Ufficio Scuola della Curia Arcivescovile di Milano (ed.) (2001). *La nuova frontiera della bioetica*. Milano: Centro Ambrosiano.

Viafora, C. & Mori, M. 1993. *Bibliografia sulla bioetica in Italia*. In C. Viafora (ed.), *Centri di bioetica in Italia. Orientamenti a confronto* (pp. 357-386). Padova: Fondazione Lanza and Gregoriana Libreria Editrice.

Viano, C.A. 1996. L'embrione: statuto e regole. *Bioetica. Rivista interdisciplinare IV(3)*.

Viano, C.A. 2001. La protesta degli scienziati. *Rivista di filosofia XCII(2)*: August, 201-217.

Viano, C.A. (ed.) 2002. *Rivista di filosofia* (devoted to "*Cultura scientifica e politiche della ricerca*").

Viola, F. 1997. *Dalla natura ai diritti. I luoghi dell'etica contemporanea*. Roma-Bari: Laterza.

Viola, F. 2000. *Etica e metaetica dei diritti umani*. Torino: Giappichelli.

Zuccaro, C. 2000. *La vita umana nella riflessione etica*. Brescia: Queriniana.

Zuccaro, C. 2002. *Il morire umano. Un'invito alla teologia morale*. Brescoa: Queriniana.

11 Bioethics in the UK

Ruth Chadwick and Michael Parker

I. Bioethics: General

Bioethics[1] is front-page news in the United Kingdom. What is more, it is front-page news virtually every day. Whilst the terms "ethics" and "bioethics" rarely appear in such reports, the high profile of these stories reflects deep public concern about the values underpinning current medical practice and about the ethical and social implications of developments in biotechnology. A scan of the newspapers reveals a very broad range of topics. There is discussion of examples of incompetence within the medical profession and of the most appropriate way to regulate the health care professions. There are stories following up the Alder Hey scandal, in which the organs of children were removed and stored inappropriately without parental consent. There is discussion too about what would constitute an ethical approach to resource allocation and about the need for public involvement in such decisions. There is concern about the impact of poverty on health. These issues are all present alongside the usual headline stories about the ethical implications of developments in reproductive technology and the ethics of reproductive choice; about the ethical implications of genetic testing and of the potential for genetic therapy; about the risks associated with the genetic modification of foods and crops and about the recent parliamentary approval of embryonic stem cell research.

This vast array of issues in the popular newspapers reflects a growing public concern with the ethical implications of developments in health care practice. It reflects too a clamor for public deliberation and debate of the issues and developments that are having a profound effect upon the way we live and on our relations with each other. There is a feeling that such decisions should not be left to the medical profession or to the government and a recognition of the need for public involvement in decision-making.

This reflects broader changes in British society and in our relationship with the professions. There is a desire for more openness, more choice and greater participation. There is also recognition that doctors and other health professionals need to be sensitive to the ethical dimensions of their practice, and this has led to a recognition of the need to ensure, for example, that medical students are adequately educated in ethics. In 1993 the General Medical Council's report "Tomorrow's Doctors" for the first time demanded that ethics be a part of the core curriculum in medical schools (General Medical Council, 1993). This was quickly followed by a national process involving teachers of medical ethics in all UK medical schools in the development of a consensus statement on what ought to be the form of such a core curriculum in medical ethics (Consensus Statement, 1998, pp. 188-192). Medical ethics is now taught as a compulsory subject in all UK medical schools.

It is increasingly expected that health professionals will reflect on the ethical implications of their choices and actions, and this is reflected too at the institutional level. There is, for example, a well-established national system of research ethics committees to which any piece of research involving NHS patients as research subjects must be submitted for review (see below), and there is also a growing number of "clinical ethics committees", which focus on the ethics of clinical practice as opposed to research (see below). There is a small but growing number of clinical ethicists providing ethics support in the clinical setting itself. The recognition of the need for more training has also led to a rapid rise in the demand among those already qualified for short courses, masters degrees and so on, offered on a part-time and full-time basis.

All of this has fuelled the development of a growing number of Centers of Medical Ethics across the UK. Many of these are academic centers within UK medical schools, but some are to be found in other university departments such as law and philosophy. These centers tend to have three roles: providing teaching (in medical schools, short courses for professionals, one-day workshops and so on, as well as in some cases teaching applied philosophy to philosophy students), providing clinical and research ethics support to health care professionals, and carrying out academic research on the ethical implications of health care practice. In this third role, they have been supported by the growth of interest among funding agencies both national and international in funding bioethics research. A range of funding agencies, such as the Wellcome Trust, the European Commission and the Nuffield Trust (among others), have been of major importance for the development of centers of medical ethics in the UK.

There is a recognition too at a national level of the importance of a consideration of the ethical implications of new medical technology, and there has been a range of policy initiatives taken and national bodies established to address these issues, such as the Nuffield Council on Bioethics and the Human Genetics Commission, among others.

To return to the point with which we began this introduction, there is in the UK a growing public interest and indeed a demand for a genuine process of public deliberation and public influence on policy making and science policy-making in relation both to the ethical implications of developments in biotechnology and to those of everyday clinical practice. Attention is now turning in science, public-policy research and bioethics itself to the question of how medical practitioners, policy-makers, scientists, social scientists and the public can be brought together in the public deliberation of these ethical challenges with which we are faced. One initiative among these is the Wellcome Trust's major new initiative to develop an electronic bioethics resource. This resource will be called the "Bioethics Today" and will be launched in 2003.[2]

Having introduced some of the issues very broadly here, we will now go on to look at the way they have arisen and are being dealt with in the UK context.

II. Professional Ethics

The professions most concerned with bioethical issues in the UK are medicine and nursing, although the professions allied to medicine should not be overlooked. Both medicine and nursing have professional bodies that regulate practice and have been involved to a considerable extent in work on ethical issues. The British Medical Association has an active Medical Ethics Committee; the United Kingdom Central Council for Nursing, Midwifery and Health Visiting in its Code of Professional Conduct made it clear that each nurse, midwife and health visitor is accountable for his or her practice and should prioritize the interests of the patient or client, having regard to issues such as confidentiality. The status of nursing as a profession has steadily risen since the UKCC was established and in the light of a number of reforms of nurse education and practice, including taking nursing training into higher education. There is discussion in the UK, as elsewhere, regarding whether nursing ethics is different from medical ethics. The claim that it is might take a number of forms: from the claim that it has a different subject matter to the claim that a different theoretical approach to ethics is appropriate in nursing, such as the ethics of care. It seems to be the case that there is at least a large degree of overlap in subject matter, while there may be differences arising out of the different professional roles. The example of the different history of attitudes to industrial action in the two professions is an interesting case in point: doctors do not have a history of industrial action similar to that of nurses in the UK. Doctors have a long history of being recognized as autonomous professionals – medicine is one of the traditional liberal professions – whereas nursing has only relatively recently been recognized as a neo-profession, less powerful in the political economy of health care. Nurses have had little alternative recourse but to engage in industrial action in order to achieve certain ends. It is no accident that in the medical profession it has been junior doctors who have most notably used the threat of industrial action over workloads. Thus the different history of the two professions has led to different practices, but there is no consensus in the UK that a different ethical approach is appropriate.

Unfortunately, a number of incidents in the UK have shaken public confidence in professional ethics in health care, at least as far as medicine is concerned. The case of Harold Shipman, the general practitioner who was found guilty of murdering patients, surgical incompetence and failure of colleagues to "blow the whistle" have all taken their toll. The medical profession, in particular, has traditionally upheld the view that colleagues do not criticize each other, but public disquiet and governmental pressure has led to the perceived need to review this kind of ethos if the profession is to maintain its autonomous status.

III. Health Care Provider–Patient–Institution Relationship

There is an expectation in the United Kingdom that clinical decision-making and policy making in health care should be open and inclusive and should take seriously the wishes of patients. This is perhaps best captured by the concept of "evidence-based patient choice" (Hope, 1997) which brings together two of the most significant movements in modern medicine. The first of these, "evidence-based medicine" (Evidence-Based Medicine Working Group, 1992, pp. 220-225) is an approach to medicine based on the claim that clinical interventions are to be justified in terms of the existence of evidence for the effectiveness of the intervention rather than on other grounds such as, for example, the authority of the clinician or of tradition. "Patient-centered medicine" too has arisen out of a concern with and a critical response to traditional medical practice and the traditional over-emphasis of the authority of the health care professional. Advocates of patient-centered medicine argue that

the best protection for patients from excessive paternalism is to be guaranteed by emphasizing the point that patients should play the central role in decision-making about their
clinical care (Battista, 1993, pp. 301-304). These two ideas, taken together, have marked a
significant shift in thinking about the relationship between the health care professions and
their patients. Taken seriously, evidence-based patient choice has the potential to enhance the
power of patients and aid the development of an increasingly effective patient-centered
health care (Hope, 1997, p. 1).

The increasing importance of patient autonomy in UK health care practice is a reflection
too of wider social changes which might be seen as broadly "consumerist", conceptualizing
the patient as the ideal consumer (well informed and autonomous) and describing the
conduct of the ethical health care professional in that light. The doctor has the duty to
inform the patient about all reasonable treatments and about their advantages and disad-
vantages. There have, however, long been concerns too in the United Kingdom that this
emphasis on the rights of the patient as consumer and individual has potential harms in
addition to these benefits. An effective and ethical health care system must, in addition to
its responsiveness to the wishes and interests of individual patients, have a concern with
the broader public interest and with the importance of social structures, family networks
and culture in effective health care. Furthermore, there is also a recognition of the dependence
of effective health care provision upon "social solidarity". An important ethical question
then is how one best reconciles respect for individual autonomy with other social values
and the broader public interest (Parker, 1999).

These tensions are also to be found in the professional guidelines and common law by
which health care practice in the UK is governed. Nevertheless, the overriding emphasis in
UK health care practice is on respect for the wishes of the individual patient. The law in
England and Wales, for example, recognizes the importance of consent in the right of the
competent adult patient to refuse even life-saving treatment, and also recognizes the right of
patients to be informed about the various treatment options available to them. The legal
standard in the UK is not, however, that of the "prudent patient" as it is in the US, but that
of the "Bolam Test", which is a professional standard. In the relevant legal case the standard
was expressed as:

> the standard of the ordinary skilled man exercising and professing to have
> that special skill. A man need not possess the highest expert skill; it is well
> established law that it is sufficient if he exercises the ordinary skill of an ordi-
> nary competent man exercising that particular art (Brazier, 1992, p. 119).[3]

In practice, despite being a professional standard, this is becoming ever closer to that of
"informed consent" by virtue of the fact that it is becoming more and more commonly
accepted that patients should be fully informed about the treatments being offered and
their consequences.

Patient involvement in health care provision more broadly is also increasing. Since 1974,
200 Community Health Councils have been established in England and Wales. There are
also equivalents in Scotland and Northern Ireland. Community Health Councils are central
to patient empowerment in the UK. They provide a channel for representation, consultation
and complaint and are an important source of information for the public (Your NHS).
Councils are made up of between 18 to 30 lay members with a chairman, a chief officer

and a variety of other staff. The Chief Officer is a paid employee of the NHS. Half of the committee members are appointed by the local authority, a third are appointed by voluntary organizations and one-sixth by the NHS. The CHC's have a variety of functions but the following are common to all: visiting NHS premises; consultation on the planning and development of local health services; provision of information on local services; monitoring the quality of local services through consumer surveys, etc., and assisting with complaints. In 2000, the UK Government proposed to replace the Community Health Councils with independent advocacy services. However, in 2001, in response to public pressure, the Councils gained at least a temporary reprieve, and it was announced that a patient information advisory group would be established to safeguard patient confidentiality (Kmietowicz, 2001, p. 1199).

In addition to the above, there is lay membership on NHS Trust boards, local and multi-centered research ethics committees and clinical ethics committees.

We shall now turn to specific areas of health care provision.

IV. Reproduction

The issues in reproduction fall into a number of categories. First, there is control of fertility, which includes on the one hand, contraception (including the "morning-after" pill) and abortion and, on the other, access to assisted reproduction. Secondly, there are issues connected with control of the kind of children produced, e.g., with regard to genetic disorders. Abortion, of course, covers both categories insofar as handicap may be one of the grounds on which an abortion is held not to be unlawful.

The key piece of legislation in the sphere of reproduction is the Human Fertilization and Embryology Act 1990, which also amended the 1967 Abortion Act. The law now provides a number of grounds for abortion, which include therapeutic and social grounds relating to the risk of injury to the mental or physical health of the pregnant woman or any existing children of her family. The fourth ground is the most controversial: "that there is a substantial risk that, if the child were born, it would suffer from such physical or mental abnormalities as to be severely handicapped". There is no limit of time for this ground. Disability rights groups, for example, may find this clause problematic as inscribing a eugenic principle into the law.

While abortion remains an issue much discussed in the bioethics literature in general, however, it does not figure large in public debates in the UK. While the "pro-life" lobby is still very active, for example over the availability of the "morning-after" pill, debates about the status of the fetus have to a large extent been replaced by debates about the status of the human embryo, especially in the light of the increasing interest in stem cell research. Discussion leading up to and surrounding the 1990 Act resulted in legislation which countenanced embryo experimentation, licensed by the Human Fertilisation and Embryology Authority (HFEA), up to a 14 day limit for certain purposes. These included the advancement of treatment for infertility, increasing knowledge of the causes of congenital disease, studying the causes of miscarriage, developing methods of contraception, and developing methods of detecting the presence of genetic or chromosomal abnormalities in embryos before implantation. This debate was revived in 2001 in the course of Parliamentary debates about modifying the existing legislation to allow another purpose, namely stem cell research.

The 1990 Human Fertilisation and Embryology Act also established the HFEA as the body entitled to regulate infertility treatments. Debates about infertility treatments cover a number of themes. There is no longer much debate about the ethics of assisted reproduction *per se*, but particular cases or issues have attracted considerable discussion, such as maternal age. Another issue that attracted considerable publicity was the case of Blood (*Regina v. Human Fertilization*, 1997). The issue was whether Diane Blood should be free to be inseminated with the sperm of her deceased husband. Mr. Blood's semen had been removed from him while he was in a terminal coma and subsequently stored. The HFEA held that this was unlawful in the absence of the consent of the sperm donor. The case gave rise to a great deal of public sympathy in the United Kingdom, which demonstrates to some extent that there is support for relief of childlessness, although the circumstances of the particular case must be taken into account.

Where decisions affecting the type of children born are concerned, issues are slightly different. Attempts to control which child is born by, for example, preimplantation genetic diagnosis and embryo selection, are still more controversial, as is sex selection. A small number of facilities have been licensed in the UK to carry out preimplantation diagnosis, but licensed clinics are at present not allowed to offer sex selection except for medical reasons. This is one area where opinion is sharply divided and debate continues.

V. Genetics

Genetics has given rise to more discussion and media interest than perhaps any other issue in the UK. In this field, in particular, there are calls for public involvement in debate, particularly since the birth of Dolly, which happened in the UK at the Roslin Institute. Another important factor has been the anxiety and disquiet over genetically modified food, which has led to worries that a loss of public confidence in science might have a negative impact on human genetics. These concerns were influential in leading the government to revise the regulatory framework for genetics in the UK in 1999. Advisory Committees such as the Advisory Committee on Genetic Testing and the Human Genetics Advisory Commission were disbanded and two new commissions were established: the Human Genetics Commission and the Agriculture and Environment Biotechnology Commission. Other non-governmental bodies also do a great deal of work in this area, such as the Nuffield Council on Bioethics, which has produced reports on genetic screening (1993) and on genetics and mental disorders (1998) and has since worked on genetics and behavior.

In the early 1990s, the main issues were the criteria for introducing genetic screening programs; questions concerning confidentiality and the possibility of non-directiveness in genetic counseling; and the wider issue of "genetic exceptionalism" – does genetics raise issues that are different in kind from other areas of medicine? More specifically, is genetic information essentially different from other kinds of medical information? Much attention has been paid to their practical implications for the insurance industry and employment.

While these questions are still debated, attention has turned to other developments, including genetic databases and pharmacogenetics. Following the international interest in the population database initiative in Iceland, the Medical Research Council and the Wellcome Trust in the UK have undertaken a public consultation on a proposal for a UK national genetic database. This would involve collecting samples from 500,000 adults with informed consent, in order to do research on the genetic factors involved in common diseases such as heart disease. It would seek to incorporate a public-private partnership in order to avoid the concerns about commercial monopoly of the kind that arose in Iceland. The House of Lords Select Committee on Science and Technology also has conducted an inquiry into genetic databases, taking evidence from a wide range of opinion (House of Lords, 2001).

Collection of DNA samples for long-term storage is also important in another major contemporary issue, pharmacogenetics, which involves identifying the genetic variations responsible for differential drug response. It is argued by some that this has the potential to revolutionize not only the practice of medicine, by making possible genetically informed prescribing, but also our disease classifications. The Wellcome Trust's biomedical ethics funding program has placed databases and pharmacogenetics among its priorities for funding as regards the ethical issues. The ethical questions turn on the extent to which informed consent is possible in this context; whether individual research subjects should have access to results; and how confidentiality will be protected – e.g., whether the samples will be coded or anonymized.

In the aftermath of the Dolly experience, there has been much discussion of cloning, with special reference to the moral difference between reproductive and therapeutic cloning. Stem cell research has been debated in both Houses of Parliament and was finally approved on the grounds of its potential to relieve suffering, subject to the establishment of a House of Lords Select Committee to report on the issues.

VI. Organ and Tissue Donation

The situation with regard to organ and tissue donation in the UK is widely regarded as unsatisfactory. Where organ donation is concerned, the Human Tissue Act of 1961 embodied a mixture of an "opting in" and an "opting out" system. Section 1 (1) allows for the situation where an individual has made a request that his body or any specified part be used after his death for therapeutic purposes; while Section 1 (2) provides that the person lawfully in possession of the body may authorize removal if he has no reason to believe "that the deceased had expressed an objection to his body being so dealt with after his death, and had not withdrawn it".

Since the 1980s, a number of developments have led to recognition that this legislation was insufficient in the area of organ transplantation. There were concerns over a market in organs, leading to the rapid introduction of the Human Organ Transplants Act 1989, which made it a criminal offence to attempt to trade in organs.

An ongoing concern, however, is the "shortage" of organs for transplant. The argument from shortage, indeed, has been one of the factors driving the move towards xenotransplantation. That there is a shortage is rarely questioned: it is taken as given in the context of the wider issues of priorities in allocation of scarce health resources. The reasons for it lie partly in unwillingness to donate, from time to time exacerbated by well publicized incidents of medical error or high profile disagreements about criteria for determination of death. Debate about responses to the issue, social or legal, continue.

In 2001, following public concern when it came to light that children's organs had been removed during post-mortems and stored without the knowledge of their parents, the Retained Organs Commission was set up by the Secretary of State for Health. The problem arose partly over different interpretations of what was understood by different parties in consent to the "removal of tissue". The functions of the Retained Organs Commission (Department of Health, 2001) include ensuring that there are accurate records of collections, overseeing the return of tissues and organs to families, and providing advice to Ministers and guidance to the NHS and Universities.

Xenotransplantation has received a substantial amount of attention in the UK, being the subject of two major reports, by the Nuffield Council on Bioethics (1996) and the Advisory Group on the Ethics of Xenotransplantation (1997), chaired by Ian Kennedy. The Kennedy report found the use of pigs as a source of organs for transplantation into humans acceptable; the use of primates unacceptable. Following the Kennedy report the United Kingdom Xenotransplantation Interim Regulatory Authority (UKXIRA) was established to advise the Secretaries of State of the UK Health departments on the action necessary to regulate xenotransplantation, including safety, efficacy and animal welfare.

VII. Death and Dying

In the UK, although competent patients can refuse treatment, including life-prolonging interventions, public policy has remained against active euthanasia, despite public sympathy in particular situations. There have been one or two extremely important cases that have given rise to debate, such as those of Dr. Cox (*Regina v. Cox*, 1992) and Tony Bland (*Airedale NHS v. Bland*, 1993). The distinction between killing and letting die, and the doctrine of double effect, although argued against by some in the philosophical literature, play an important part in policy. So hastening death by administering increasingly large doses of analgesic medication is accepted; deliberately bringing about death is not.

The latter distinction was important in the case of Dr. Cox, who injected a patient with rheumatoid arthritis, suffering from intense pain and expressing a wish to die, with potassium chloride, which is not an analgesic. He was found guilty of attempted murder. In that case, J. Ognall said:

> If a doctor genuinely believes that a certain course is beneficial to his patient, either therapeutically or analgesically, then even though he recognises that that course carries with it a risk to life, he is fully entitled, nonetheless, to pursue it (*Regina v. Cox*, 1992).

The Tony Bland case concerned a patient in persistent vegetative state, which gave rise to different issues again. Tony Bland had been in a persistent vegetative state for over three years when the hospital sought a declaration that they could lawfully withdraw all forms of life support. The case went all the way up to the House of Lords, who relied on the patient's best interests. The argument was not that it was in Tony Bland's best interests to die but that it was not in his best interests to prolong his life in those circumstances. The Bland case has wider implications, for patients who might not be in a persistent vegetative state but for whom further treatment is considered futile.

Physician assisted suicide raises different issues also. The British Medical Association has consistently argued against the legalization of euthanasia but has suggested some reasons for drawing a moral distinction between that and physician assisted suicide, where, while the doctor may help by action or inaction, the patient remains the agent (British Medical Association).

VIII. Mental Health

Are there significant moral differences between psychiatric medicine and medicine of other kinds? Are there also moral differences between different types of psychiatric conditions? If so, what are the implications of these differences for the practice of psychiatric medicine?

Over eighty percent of patients who are treated in a mental hospital or another form of psychiatric unit in the United Kingdom are treated on an informal basis with full agreement between the patient and the care team (British Government Green Paper, 1999). In these cases the primary ethical questions are related to the responsibility to ensure the availability of high quality services for those who need them. Also, psychiatric patients, even when competent, are often particularly vulnerable, often unable to speak up for themselves either because of the nature of their illness itself or because of the attitudes of society towards them. A key question here then must be the provision of means and facilitation for the involvement of service users and service user groups in mental health policy making.

There are also of course people who suffer from psychiatric illnesses who are in fact either unable or unwilling to find access to the support and treatment they need, thereby putting themselves, and perhaps others too, at risk. Such cases raise a range of additional ethical and practical questions. When, for example, is it ethical to treat people without their consent or even against their wishes, either in their own best interest or in the interests of other people? What does it mean to say that a person lacks capacity or is incompetent? How ought one to measure competence? The law in the UK is such that in situations where an adult patient does not have the capacity to consent, he or she should be treated in their "best interest" (Brazier, 1992). There is no proxy consent under UK law. How then ought the best interests of those who lack capacity to be assessed?

The law relating to mental health in England and Wales is currently in the process of significant reform. In the light of a report of the Richardson Committee (1999) in December 2000, the UK Government issued a "white paper" describing a new legal framework to replace the Mental Health Act (1983). Its aim is to reform when and how mentally disordered people can be treated without their consent in their interests or to protect public safety. One key question raised in the consultation is the role of compulsory treatment outside of the hospital setting. Another is the question of what ought to be the criteria for compulsory care and treatment. The Richardson Committee proposed a model that places great importance on the assessment of capacity as the criterion. The Government proposals introduce another model for consideration in addition, which places greater emphasis on the "degree of risk" a person poses to themselves and to others.

Those people who are considered to pose a risk to public safety raise particular ethical issues relating to the best interests of the patient himself or herself and the protection of others, and such cases are sometimes seen to lie on the boundary between the psychiatric services and the judicial system. A case that is particularly difficult, and which has been the subject of much debate in the UK recently, is that of the "dangerous" person with a severe personality disorder. Such disorders are thought by many to be untreatable. What then ought ethically to be done in cases where a person with such a condition is considered dangerous but has not committed any offence? There may be a public interest in detaining such a person, but this conflicts with the underlying legal and ethical principle that a person is innocent until proven guilty.

IX. Research Ethics

The growing importance of "clinical governance" in the National Health Service and the requirement that NHS Trusts monitor the effectiveness of the services they require is leading to a proliferation of clinical audit and health technology assessment. This raises an important ethical question about whether there is a significant moral difference between such audits and medical research. The growth of evidence-based practice too raises questions about the differences or similarities between everyday clinical practice and research. What are the ethical implications of the growth of research-like activities within health care? In relation to research itself, insofar as a distinction can be made, several ethical questions are discussed in the UK context. First, what are the ethical implications of the relationship in research between the healthcare system and pharmaceutical companies? Second, what counts as an effective system of review of such research? Third, there is a whole range of questions relating to the protection of research subjects: what counts as valid consent? Does the payment of research subjects constitute coercion? To what degree of risk ought subjects to be allowed to subject themselves, even if their consent is valid? What counts as an acceptable risk? What other forms of coercion might such subjects be vulnerable to? What are the ethical implications of carrying out research on vulnerable groups (e.g., children, neonates, psychiatric patients and so on). What are the ethical implications of not carrying out such research? What are the ethical implications of research methodology, and who ought to be responsible for the assessment of methodology? How does one balance the requirement for informed consent against the public interest for example in the use of patient records?

Another ethical issue that has received a great deal of attention recently is the question of the ethical implications of research by Western drug companies in the developing world (Bulletin of Medical Ethics, 1999).

There is a well-established statutory system for the review of research on human subjects in the UK. Since 1992, every health district has been required to have a Local Research Ethics Committee to advise NHS bodies on the ethical acceptability of research proposals involving human subjects. More recently, a network of Multi-Center Research Ethics Committees has been established to review research to be carried out in five or more health districts. All research on human subjects taking place "broadly within the NHS", must be submitted to either a Local Research Ethics Committee or a Multi-Center Research Ethics Committee for approval. The effectiveness of the relationship between the two levels of committees has itself been the subject of some debate. In addition to the NHS guidelines establishing research ethics committees, a range of other guidance and legislation is of relevance to the UK context. The World Medical Association's Declaration of Helsinki is one such document. Another is the Guidelines for Good Clinical Practice produced by the International Conference on Harmonization of Technical Requirements for Registration of Pharmaceuticals for Human Use (1996) and subsequently adopted both by the Medical

Research Council and the European Parliament. Another document that will inevitably have an important effect on medical research in the United Kingdom is the recently adopted European Union Directive on Clinical Trials.

Interestingly, despite the sophisticated level of debate in the UK about the ethics of medical research, the most common reason for delay in the approval of research projects continues to be the inadequacy of the patient information sheet.

X. Access to Health Care

Important ethical decisions must inevitably be made about how to use health care resources in any country. Even in very wealthy countries such as the United Kingdom, there are not enough resources for everyone to receive the best possible treatment. Priorities must be set and, within these, priority decisions must be made in the face of growing numbers of reasonable requests for resources and treatment. Such questions have been the subject of debate for a long time but are increasingly so now. The length of time patients spend on waiting lists for treatment and the annual crisis caused by the shortage of intensive care beds each winter, along with high profile discussions about the availability of new drugs, such as Viagra or beta-interferon, mean that resource allocation is more and more the subject of media and hence public speculation. These decisions inevitably have an ethical component. How ought such decisions to be made? By what ethical principles ought they to be judged? What counts as a just distribution of health care resources? Should resources be allocated according to a principle of equality, of medical need, on the basis of first come-first served, or perhaps according to a principle of desert? To what extent ought some perception of responsibility enter into the debate? Should those who refuse or are unable to give up smoking be treated differently than those who do? To what extent ought "age" be a criterion?

In the United Kingdom, most of the major decisions about what and what not to fund are taken locally, by health authorities, primary care groups and general practices (Hope et al., 1998, pp. 1067-1069). Those who make such decisions are increasingly required to justify them to the wider community in ethical terms. This raises a further ethical question concerning the ethical implications of the process by which such decisions are reached over and above the outcome of the decisions themselves (procedural justice). To what extent was the decision making process open, to what extent did it involve patients and the wider community? At what level was their involvement: at the level of setting priorities? Different health authorities have developed their own ways of resolving these questions. One innovative approach has been taken by the Oxfordshire Health Authority, which has established a Priorities Forum whose aim is to "provide a reasonable 'due process' for decision making." The forum brings together general practitioners, medical directors of the local NHS trusts, health authority staff, hospital doctors, ethicists, and non-executive members of the health authority. Members of the local community health council (see above) attend as observers (Hope et al., 1998, pp. 1067-1069). The ethical framework used by the forum focuses on three key areas.[4]

A. *Effectiveness*
Value and efficiency are also considered within effectiveness. "Effectiveness" means the extent to which the treatment (or other healthcare intervention) achieves the desired effect

(notably the proportion of patients who would be expected to show the effect). "Value" means a judgement on how valuable that effect is in the relevant individual(s) relative to the value of other treatments. The impact of a treatment is its value weighted for effectiveness. Efficiency is the impact per unit cost. In making judgements about the value of a treatment, three factors are of particular relevance: the additional length of life that the treatment brings, the contribution that the intervention makes to the patients' well-being, and the level of need of those who benefit from the treatment.

B. Equity

The basic principle of equity is that equals should be treated equally. In making its purchasing decisions, the health authority tries to aim for this ideal. The forum has decided that there should be no discrimination on grounds of employment status, family circumstances, lifestyle, learning disability, age, race, sex, social position, financial status, religion or place of abode.

C. Patient Choice

The authority will not make an exception to a decision simply because a patient chooses an ineffective intervention, since this would deny another patient access to a more effective treatment. However, patients can choose between treatments of similar efficiency. The forum sees it as important, however, that trials testing the effectiveness of treatments should include outcome measures important to patients.

XI. Ethics Consultation and Ethics Committees

Health care professionals and managers are increasingly interested in the ethical dimensions of their work. They are also being called upon more and more to justify the decisions they make in ethical terms. Ethics is now a core subject in the medical curriculum and is taught both to trainee nurses and to medical students. This growing awareness and interest in ethics in clinical practice and the awareness of the need for clinical ethics support has led to the development of a range of different forms of clinical ethics support in the clinical setting in the United Kingdom. This has tended to take one or more of three forms: clinical ethics committees, clinical ethics forums, or the employment of a clinical ethicist.

Clinical ethics committees have already been established in about forty of the four hundred or so NHS Trusts in the country, with many others reporting that they are planning to establish such a committee at the time of writing. The membership of such committees varies from Trust to Trust, but all have members from a variety of clinical and professional backgrounds as well as a number of lay members. Some also have an ethicist as a member and others have access to an ethicist on a consultative basis. Clinical ethics committees tend to play three roles within the Trusts they serve: they engage in the development of policy and guidelines; they provide education and training for trust staff in ethics; and they provide some case consultation – either themselves or by means of a clinical ethicist who plays a linking role between the committee and the clinical centers.

In some Trusts, there has been a certain amount of resistance to the idea of establishing a "committee" as such to deal with ethical issues in clinical practice because of the experience of working with research ethics committees and a perception that such committees are concerned with vetting practice and stopping what is unethical rather than with providing ethics support and guidance and encouraging and facilitating the development of good ethical practice. In some clinical settings, therefore, clinicians and those involved in medical ethics have established "clinical ethics forums" which enable clinicians to meet regularly to discuss ethical issues which arise in their practice, to get some training and so on.

In addition to the above, several trusts make use of the availability of "ethicists" either on the medical school staff or in other university departments such as philosophy or law. In at least one Trust a clinical ethicist is employed as a member of the Trust staff to provide clinical ethics support throughout the Trust, to work in a variety of clinical areas on staff development in ethics, and to establish ethics forums in clinical areas and so on.[5]

Whilst there is no formal or statutory requirement for NHS Trusts to establish clinical ethics committees, they are becoming more common, and a national network of clinical ethics committees was recently established along with an annual conference and a program of regular training workshops for new members of such committees. In 2001, the Nuffield Trust commissioned a survey of clinical ethics support in the United Kingdom. The report of this survey, carried out by Dr. Anne-Marie Slowther, was published by the Nuffield Trust in Spring 2001 (Slowther, Bunch, Woolnough, & Hope, 2001).

XII. Public Health

The ethical issues in public health largely focus on the conflict between the interests of the individual and the interests of society. Good examples include screening and vaccination programs. Public health issues arise also in genetics, with reference to debates about reducing the incidence of genetic disorders in the population. Vaccination has always been a problematic issue from an ethical point of view, insofar as it involves an intervention on a healthy person for the overall good. While it is true that the individual also benefits from the immunity thus produced in the community, the risk to the individual is non-negligible and can be serious for some individuals. Vaccination has been a particularly prominent issue in the UK, in the light of anxieties over the triple vaccine for measles, mumps and rubella. Some have argued that parents should be free to choose single vaccination for their children, citing uncertainties about the safety of the triple vaccine. For those concerned for public health rather than individual choice, however, even raising this issue may have the effect that public confidence in the triple vaccine is reduced, leading to greater reluctance on the part of parents to accept it, thus making more likely the increase in the risk of measles epidemics.

In the area of public health, the ethical ideology of choice competes with ideas about responsibility. This is nowhere more obvious than in the area of diet. The government has set targets for reducing the incidence of certain health problems, including heart disease. There is widespread recognition that patterns of sedentary living and dietary habits are contributing to an extremely high rate of heart disease, and that it is desirable to encourage more awareness of the risks of poor diet and insufficient exercise.

This is one reason why food ethics is becoming an increasingly prominent issue in bioethics in the UK. More significant reasons in terms of trigger factors, however, have been various food-related public health issues, such as BSE. The growing interest in food issues in public policy is shown by the establishment of the Food Standards Agency and the Advisory Committee on Novel Foods and Processes; and in ethics by the establishment of the Food Ethics Council, an independent body on ethical standards in food and agriculture. It seems clear, moreover, that there will be increasing activity in this area of bioethics, in the light of the ever more fuzzy boundary between foods and pharmaceuticals, as products are developed which use foods as a medium for the delivery of health-enhancing or therapeutic agents.

In addition to heart disease, public health targets have also been set for other common diseases such as cancer. In the light of this the proposal, mentioned above, to set up a UK biomedical population collection, which will collect and store DNA samples from 500,000 volunteers with informed consent, is significant. One of the aims of this collection will be to use information gained from the samples and from health care records to investigate the genetic factors involved in these common diseases. This is another example of the way in which the issues in public health, as in other areas of medicine, are increasingly informed by developments in genetics.

Notes

1. Or "biomedical ethics", or "medical ethics" as it is sometimes known (though these terms are both thought to describe an area rather narrower than bioethics, which is also taken to include genetically modified foods and crops).
2. For more information about the Bioethics Today, contact the authors.
3. *Bolam v. Friern Hospital Management Committee* 1 WLR 582, 586, 118 (1957). Quoted and discussed in Brazier (1992).
4. For a fuller discussion, see Brazier (1992).
5. For a full account of the Priorities Forum, see Hope et al. (1998).
6. One of the authors of this paper, Michael Parker, is Honorary Clinical Ethicist for the Oxford Radcliffe Hospitals NHS Trust.

Bibliography

Advisory Group on the Ethics of Xenotransplantation. 1997. *Animal tissue into humans*. London: HMSO.

Airedale NHS Trust v. Bland. 1 All ER 821 (1993), 12 BMLR 64 (1993), Fam D, CA, HL.

Battista, R. 1993. Practice guidelines for preventative care: the Canadian experience. *British Journal of General Practice* 43: 301-304.

Brazier, M. 1992. *Medicine, patients and the law* (2nd ed.). London: Penguin Books.

British Government Green Paper. 1999. *Reform of the Mental Health Act 1983 – Proposal for consultation*. London: HMSO.

British Medical Association. *End of life decisions – Views of the BMA* [On-line]. Available: <http://www.bma.org.uk>.

Department of Health. 2001. *The removal, retention and use of human organs and tissue from post-mortem examination: Advice from the Chief Medical Officer* [On-line]. Available: <http://www.doh.gov.uk/orgretentionadvice/index.htm>.

Evidence-Based Medicine Working Group. 1992. Evidence-based medicine: A new approach to teaching the practice of medicine. *JAMA*. 268, (24): 220-225.

General Medical Council. 1993. *Tomorrow's doctors: recommendations on undergraduate medical education*. London: GMC.

Hope, T. 1997. *Evidence-based patient choice*. London: The King's Fund.

Consensus statement by teachers of medical ethics and law in UK medical schools. 1998. Teaching medical ethics and law within medical education: A model for the UK core curriculum. *Journal of Medical Ethics* 24: 188-192.

Hope, T., Hicks, N., Reynolds, D.J.M., Crisp, R. & Griffiths, S. 1998. Rationing and the health authority. *British Medical Journal* 317: 1067-1069.

House of Lords, Select Committee on Science and Technology. 2001. *Human genetic databases: Challenges and opportunities*. London: House of Lords.

Kmietowicz, Z. 2001. Registries will have to apply for right to collect patients' data without consent. *British Medical Journal* 322: 1199.

Nuffield Council on Bioethics. 1996. *Animal to human transplants: The ethics of xenotransplantation*. London: Nuffield Council on Bioethics.

Parker, M. (ed.) 1999. *Ethics and community*. London and New York: Routledge.

Regina v. Cox. 12 BMLR 38 (1992).

Regina v. Human Fertilisation and Embryology Authority, ex p Blood. 35 BMLR 1, CA (1997) .

Slowther, A., Bunch, C., Woolnough, B. & Hope, T. 2001. *Clinical ethics support in the UK: A review of the current position and likely development*. London: The Nuffield Trust. *Bulletin of Medical Ethics* 150 (August 1999).

Your NHS: How community health councils work [On-line]. Available: <http://www.nhs.uk>.

12 Bioethics in Denmark

Jacob Dahl Rendtorff

I. Introduction

Bioethics in Denmark is characterized by confrontation among utilitarian, Protestant Christian, and egalitarian approaches to moral decision-making. During the last twenty years, there has been constant preoccupation with bioethical issues, and bioethics has moved from a relatively unknown subject to take a central place in public debates. Issues such as new reproductive technology, genetics, organ transplantation, and euthanasia, as well as problems of prioritization in the health care sector, have been extensively debated. In particular, the emergence of new technologies which challenge traditional ethical concepts and recent criticism of the Danish hospital system have driven bioethical discussion.

Close links have been drawn between bioethics and the debate about legal regulation of bioethical issues. The new problems of bioethics have challenged the Danish legal tradition, which is rather positivistic and pragmatic, and based on a rather old Constitution from 1849. Whereas human rights and individual autonomy have become central to the bioethical debate, such concepts do not play a significant role in this legal tradition. Moreover, legal positivism is inconsistent with the moral ideal of protecting human dignity, which has been put forward in bioethical debates as central to legal reform.

Alf Ross, Danish philosopher of law, who had a significant influence on the formation of Danish legal doctrine, refused to recognize medical ethics as a source of law (Ross, 1979). According to Ross, medical ethics can make law more concrete, but it can never replace or shape law (Hybel, 1998, pp. 59 ff.). Focus on the pragmatic, utilitarian aspects of biomedical questions has shaped developments in modern Danish regulation law. This situation has, however, recently changed because of the larger emphasis on ethical questions in the public debate, due to a number of parliamentary reports and the creation of ethics committees and a council of ethics.[1]

The first modern Danish debate on bioethics concerned abortion during the 1960s and early 1970s. This debate resulted in a rather wide-ranging consensus about free access to abortion during the first trimester of pregnancy. Accordingly, abortion legislation in Denmark is very liberal.[2] The legalization of abortion, however, was not conceived in terms of bioethical principles, but rather as a questions regarding a woman's right to make choices over her own body; consequently abortion has been perceived as central to the women's liberation movement. In this context, the embryo has not been considered a person. Only in relation to new debates about reproductive technology has the question of the status of the embryo again become important.

In the Danish welfare state today, however, patient autonomy is widely institutionalized as a basic concept of health law. Concepts of integrity, dignity, and self-determination can be said to play significant roles in the debate on autonomy. Recently, a Bill of Patients Rights was proposed to formalize the concept of informed consent as basic in the Danish health care system (Kemp, Lebech & Rendtorff, 1997). This doctrine of informed consent makes a further contribution to the development of medical ethics in Demark. Even though certain humanistic thinking regarding medical responsibility played a role earlier in the Danish medical world, in practice, the Danish understanding of informed consent includes soft medical paternalism (Jansen, 1991).

Further, the legal rights of persons, or the law of persons, seems to be habilitated in the academic debate and it is no longer reduced to a sub-field of contract law (Dübeck, 1997). This legal thinking concerns the rights to freedom and self-development of the person. The law of persons includes rights to life, freedom from intervention in bodily integrity, and to identity (psychological integrity). The law of persons is based on rights to care and concern, as well as to privacy and protection of personal dignity (Dübeck, 1997).

During the 1990s, a research environment emerged for bioethics in Denmark, which was very important for the development of academic bioethics in the country. Two research programs in bioethics were established by the five Danish Research Councils in 1993. The first, GRAN, explored the foundations and applications of bioethics and collaborated closely with the organizational hearings of the Danish Council of Ethics. Svend Andersen, Professor of theology, of the University of Aarhus, who had also been one of the first members of the Danish National Council of Ethics, directed this research project. The famous Danish philosopher and theologian, Knud Ejler Løgstrup, was the inspiration for Andersen's position on theoretical ethics. However, Svend Andersen also collaborated with Peter Sandøe, a firm consequentialist, who later worked with animal bioethics and was instrumental in the 1998 establishment of a research center for risk evaluation of human and animal biotechnology.

The second project, based in Center for Ethics and Law at the University of Copenhagen, explored the relationship between bioethics and law. It has also collaborated with the Council of Ethics, organizing international conferences about bioethics and biolaw (Kemp, Lebech & Rendtorff, 1997; Rendtorff, 1999). Professor of philosophy Peter Kemp, who was inspired by the French hermeneutic philosopher Paul Ricœur, directed the research. Kemp developed a philosophy of technology in his major work: *The Irreplaceable* (*Det uerstattelige*, 1992). The task of the Center for Ethics and Law was to clarify the relation between bioethics and law, in particular by investigating the concept of biolaw. This research lead to the publication of a book by Peter Kemp, Mette Lebech and Jacob Dahl Rendtorff called *The Bioethical Turn* (*Den bioetiske vending*, 1997). This book presents basic moral principles and a philosophy of the human body in a phenomenological perspective, challenging a positivistic conception of law. Later, Jacob Dahl Rendtorff published *Bioethics and Law, the Body between Person and Thing* (*Bioetik og ret, kroppen mellem person og ting*, 1999), which analyzes the relation between bioethics and law in selected European countries. Moreover, the Center for Ethics and Law became responsible for a European research project, sponsored by the BIOMED II-Program of the European Commission. This project, Basic Ethical Principles in Bioethics and Biolaw, consisting of a collaboration between 22 partners from different European countries, led to the publication of a rather large two-volume research report, *Basic Ethical Principles in European Bioethics and Biolaw* (2000). The report investigates the ideas of autonomy, dignity, integrity and vulnerability in ethics and European law. It proposes that these ideas are fundamental for a future European bioethics and biolaw. Because of the work of the Center for Ethics and Law, these principles for respect and protection of the human person also had some impact on Danish debates on bioethics.[3]

II. Important Bioethics Institutions

Important bioethics institutions in Denmark include a variety of organizations and boards at three levels: central/national, regional/local, and institutional.

A. *Central/National Institutions*

At the central and national level there are (1) The National Board of Health (*Sundhedsstyrelsen*), (2) The Patients' Complaints Board (*Sundhedsvæsenets Patientklagenævn*), (3) The Danish Medicines Agency (*Lægemiddelstyrelsen*), (d) The Danish Council of Ethics (*Det Etiske Råd*), and (4) The Central Scientific Ethical Committee (*Den Centrale Videnskabsetiske Komité*).

1. *The National Board of Health (Sundhedsstyrelsen)* is the leading institution of the health care sector and is responsible to the Ministry of the Interior. Its job is to be aware of health related considerations. It is responsible for orienting the public about health care conditions in Denmark. It controls health care employees, and it can require that employees report on their work in the health care sector. It can withdraw the authorization of a health care worker to practice medicine and has the right to change his or her position, if this person has not followed his or her working duties. Court approval is required for withdrawal of authorization. The National Board of Health has final responsibility for and control of the health care system.

2. *The Patients' Complaints Board (Sundhedsvæsenets Patientklagenævn)* is an independent board that makes decisions regarding patient complaints over maltreatment, and so forth. Complaints regarding the work and actions of health care personnel can also be put to the Patients' Complaints Board. This board states its position of the case, critiques particular health care workers, and can impose sanctions. Before acting on its determinations, however, it reports to the National Board of Health.

3. *The Danish Medicines Agency (Lægemiddelstyrelsen)* is responsible for control and approval of pharmaceuticals and pharmaceutical products. The agency is also responsible to the National Board of Health and the Ministry of the Interior.

4. *The Danish Council of Ethics (Det Etiske Råd)*, established in 1987, was inspired by French developments and contributed to the establishment of ethical debate regarding biomedical problems in Denmark. It is a good indication of Denmark's move from a positivistic and pragmatic legal framework for the regulation of biomedical questions to a higher degree of moralization of law. Many observers argue that the establishment of the Danish Council of Ethics has been important for public understanding of ethical issues, especially when dealing with health care issues in law.

The particularity of the Danish Council of Ethics is that some of the seventeen members must be laypersons, who then contribute to the public debate on bioethics. The establishment of public debate is part of the political advisory functions of the Council. The Council has taken positions on a number of concrete cases. For example, laws on organ transplantation, human medical experimentation, and new reproductive technology, were the result of significant ethical discussions; ethics has become central to the public debate.

Today, the main functions of the Danish Council of Ethics are to advise a parliamentary committee on ethical questions arising from new biomedical technology, to counsel the National Health Service on general ethical matters, and to promote and support public debate on ethical issues. The Danish Council of Ethics has been extremely active formulating papers and reports on nearly all of the main issues of biomedical ethics. The publications and meetings of the Council are very popular, but it is not the case that the parliament always follows the recommendations of the Council. This was, for example, the case concerning its recommendations on organ transplantation.

5. *The Central Scientific Ethical Committee (Den Centrale Videnskabsetiske Komité)* coordinates the work of the regional research and scientific ethics committees. This body sets guidelines for experiments on human beings. It surveys the health care staff's treatment of patients and judges in cases of maltreatment and negligence.

The legal regulation of medical experiments with human beings by a system of research ethics committees, was introduced according to the Helsinki Declaration. Danish physicians, including Poul Riis (the "grand old man" of biomedical ethics in Denmark), were the driving force in the revision of the system of medical ethics. In 1982, the system of research ethics committees was established on voluntary basis. In 1992, it was this system that was legally institutionalized to protect bodily integrity according to the rules of the Helsinki Declaration. Denmark has established seven regional committees, supervised by a central committee. The regional committees consist of members from different groups in society. Each committee has from nine to eleven members, who are elected for four years. The central committee has an appeal function and is responsible for judging all experiments on human beings, embryos and fetuses. The committees ensure the proper procedural functioning of risk evaluation, written information for research subjects, and informed consent. Participation in an ethics committee is without salary, except for the secretariat. The Danish system functions very well and is one of the most developed in Europe.

B. Local/Regional Institutions

The Danish system of ethics at the regional/local level is based on (1) the regional scientific ethical committees (*De regionale Videnskabsetiske Komiteer*), (2) the medical officers of health (*Embedslæge institutionen*), and (3) patient councellors (*Patientvejledere*).

1. *The regional scientific ethical committees (De regionale Videnskabsetiske Komiteer).* As mentioned above, these regional research and scientific ethics committees are controlled by the Central Scientific Ethics Committee, which is responsible for the general evaluation of research. The regional committees evaluate biomedical research projects, including experiments on human beings, deceased human beings, human fertilized eggs, and so forth, from the standpoint of scientific ethical criteria. Biomedical research projects must be submitted to the committees for approval. If there is disagreement in these committees, the proposals for research projects are submitted to the Central Committee on biomedical

research. In the regional research ethics committee system, there are seven regional committees. But, as regional, they are organized in accordance with the political administration (*amterne*) and not in the particular hospitals.

The Danish system of regional research ethics committees is well organized with participation of physicians, other professionals and lay people. The system is based on a judicial understanding of reviewing research protocols, and it follows general legal requirements when considering research proposals. The process integrates ethical considerations and clinical considerations within medical research (Hybel, 1998).[4] The framework of the law contributes to procedural installation of autonomy and informed consent as key terms for clinical ethics. The establishment of a system of research ethics committees has had an important influence on the general protection of informed consent in clinical practice. But it has accomplished little beyond that. The isolation of research ethics committees from clinical reality within the legal system can paradoxically be said to have helped cause the lack of formalized clinical ethics.

2. *The medical officers of health* (*Embedslæge institutionen*) is another institution that has significant importance at the local level. This institution supervises regional health care on behalf of the National Board of Health. It is familiar with regional health conditions and reports to the National Board of health.

3. *Patient counsellors* (*Patientvejledere*) are appointed by the country's authorities and are included in the debate on the ethical treatment of the patients because they work directly with patients within the hospital.

4. *Other organizations.* In addition, the Danish Medical Association (DMA) and the DMA's Medical Ethics Board (*Lægeforeningens Lægeetiske Nævn*) play an important role contributing to the formulation of ethical norms in Denmark. These organizations are important for defining and implementing ethical norms.

III. Issues in Bioethics

The Danish debate on bioethics really began with the report *The Price of Progress* (*Fremskridtets pris*) (Ministry of the Interior, 1984) on reproductive technologies. This report was inspired by British initiatives that lead to the Mary Warnock Committee Report. *The Price of Progress* was the first Danish report concerning such new technology. The report contained a proposal for the creation of the Danish Council of Ethics and argued for the need for ethical reflection on concepts of normality, disease, and health in a secularized society. It argued for the protection of human rights while sustaining biomedical development. Whereas the report is very pragmatic and liberal with regard to reproductive technology, it also argues for the regulation of medical experiments and further ethical discussion concerning genetic technologies. However, the report was characterized by a technocratic attitude that seeks to leave ethics out of law (Achen, 1997).

A central concern was to regulate human medical experimentation. Therefore, a commission was established to draft appropriate law and to provide the legal foundations for its successor, the Danish Council of Ethics. The commission had difficulties defining ethics, but concluded that ethics regards protecting human rights and respecting individual autonomy (Achen, 1997, p. 93). The commission touched upon the concepts of integrity and dignity and formulated very strict demands to the scientific research ethics committees that evaluate research on human beings, formulating special rules for the protection of vulnerable populations. It concluded that research projects involving subjects who cannot give informed consent, especially if there is significant risk to the subject's health, should only be permitted if there is a very good reason to presume that the result will meaningfully benefit the individual.

The commission was characterized by a Kantian approach that was very critical of utilitarian reasoning. Ethics is defined as the search for the good life, a collective vision of which is to some degree expressed in international human rights declarations (*Betænkning nr. 1185*, 1989, pp. 23ff.). This was the beginning of the presence of ethics in the preparation of appropriate laws, which became very visible in general public debate. Marxist, Christian, and utilitarian positions are present as well as theological visions for the protection of nature. With the creation of various ethical commissions, however, ethics slowly became an integrated part of the legislative process as "negotiated norms" (Achen, 1997, p. 103).

A criticism of the research ethics system, however, is that it focuses on legitimate research rather than on regulating the moral conduct of medicine. It is argued that physicians managed to frame research ethics as a legal issue in a way that allows them to maintain control over the health care system. Moreover, those who hold this point of view argue that the whole research ethics committee system fails to contribute to the adequate protection of individuals. The fact that the system does not work on problems related to hospital ethics committees is a good example of this situation. Physicians defined "ethics" as "research ethics" and, therefore, kept hospital ethics committees out of the health care system. Ethics became restricted to certain well-defined areas of invention and research, avoiding the establishment of ethical standards for clinical practice. The irony of this development is that the medical establishment is very proud of the research ethics committees, which it promotes as an example of the high ethical standards at Danish hospitals.

This view that clinical ethics is under-developed contrasts with the extended moralization of Danish law. Laws on organ transplantation, human medical experimentation, and reproductive technology, suggest the existence of significant ethical discussion. Each refers to the basic ethical principles of autonomy, dignity, integrity, and vulnerability, although they do not have direct constitutional content. Also, the Danish Center for Human Rights has contributed to this development of respect for the principles in relation the human person in Danish society, and there is no a change of attitude towards basic legal questions. The Danish Center for Human Rights actively promotes human rights and informed consent in health care institutions.

With regard to the regulation of reproductive technologies, *The Price of Progress* (1984) argued for very liberal propositions given the pluralism of family forms and the desire of the infertile to conceive and bear biologically related children. But after the Danish Council of Ethics was established the debate became more principlist. Members of the Council were critical towards the potential for reification of the woman's body, commercialization, anonymity, and changes to traditional family relationships brought about by such new reproductive technology (*Kunstig befrugtning. En redegørelse*, 1996). In 1994, IVF was accepted as a medical treatment. In 1997, a law on reproductive technologies was enacted according to which artificial insemination is only permissible with egg and sperm cells that have not been genetically modified (*Lov om kunstig befrugtning i forbindelse med lægelig behandling*, 1997). Surrogacy in connection with artificial insemination is not permitted. Also, the woman must not be older than 45 years of age. The development of the fertilized egg must not happen outside the womb of the mother and eggs taken from fetuses or dead women cannot be used. Furthermore, it is not permissible to sell fertilized or non-fertilized eggs. Donation of eggs must only occur as a part of the *in vitro* fertilization treatment of the donating woman, such that only eggs left over from the treatment of one woman can be donated to another. Donor anonymity is a presupposition of artificial insemination. Eggs may be stored at most for two years, and thereafter they must be destroyed. Artificial insemination proceeds only on the basis of written informed consent and can only be given to women, who are married or living as part of a stable heterosexual couple. Fertilization of lesbian or single women is forbidden.

Denmark does not have a general law regulating the field of genetics. In the 1992 law regulating medical experiments, every experiment aiming at cloning, creation of hybrids, and chimeras is forbidden. According to the 1997 law on reproductive technologies, genetic investigations of fertilized ova may only occur where there is a risk that the child will have a genetic disease. Again, sperm and egg cells must not be genetically modified. This has been the general attitude, since *The Price of Progress* (1984) introduced the distinction between eugenics and therapeutic use of gene technology. Gene therapy on body cells is still at the experimental stage, but germ line therapy is not permitted. The Danish Council of Ethics promoted body cell gene therapy after a hearing on the subject was held (*Genterapi, en debatdag*, 1995). The Council has also discussed dignity and integrity regarding the Human Genome Project (Bo Andreassen Rix m fl., 1991).[4] Some members were worried about the influence of the Human Genome Project on personal privacy. While DNA testing is used in legal practice, the use of genetic testing for life insurance and in the labor market, without special medical reasons, is not permitted. Great efforts have been made to secure the protection of genetic information under the law. However, it has been argued that existing legislation does not give the individual sufficient legal protection (Etisk Råd, 1991). More legislation on protection of personal integrity from the use of information about health is necessary (Nathan, 1990).

The attitude toward embryo experimentation of *The Price of Progress* (1984) was very liberal. When abortion is permitted, there can hardly be weighty arguments against embryo experimentation. Further, the embryos in question were destined to die and, therefore, are not considered future human beings. However, the report argued that embryo experiments should be restricted to the context of fertility treatment and therapeutic research to prevent disease (*The Price of Progress*, 1984, pp. 57ff.). In contrast, many argue for issuing gradual protection of the fetus (Rehof, 1989, pp. 62ff.). *The Price of Progress* also refers to the dignity of the embryo and the autonomy of the mother. Given current regulations, however, there exists no legal prohibition of the creation of embryos for research.

There has also been much discussion of the problem of prenatal diagnosis. The debate has centered on the role of suffering in human life and the implied change of our concept of normality through the extended use of prenatal diagnostics. In this context, respect for human dignity stands in opposition to utilitarian considerations of costs and benefits, which earlier had been predominant (*Redegørelse om fosterdiagnostik*, 1990, pp. 39ff.). The need of a just humanistic vision of human beings was emphasized (1990, pp. 39ff.). Recently, the efficiency of prenatal diagnostics has been seriously questioned, because many healthy children are aborted. However, prenatal diagnostics is permitted for women over 35 years and for women with a risk of hereditary diseases.

There was significant disagreement about organ transplantation in Denmark before the 1990 law on the inspection of the dead body, autopsy, and transplantation. In the beginning, the debate on transplantation was closely linked to the discussion of medical prioritization. In addition, many were critical of utilizing brain death criteria for harvesting organs for transplantation. The result was legislation that, in addition to affirming brain death as the foundation of organ procurement, establishes brain death as the functioning concept of death. The law states that a person's death can be defined as (1) the irreversible cessation of respiration or functioning of the heart or (2) the ceasing of every brain function (*Lov om ligsyn, obduktion og transplantationer*, 1990). The Danish debate on organ transplantation was marked by a high degree of symbolism because of an argument made for the close connection between the ordinary conception of death and the criteria for organ procurement. This was partly due to skepticism toward brain death in the early days of the Danish Council of Ethics. The technical definition of brain death was conceived as a change of the ordinary social conception of death. In Denmark, defining death criteria was a question about how to understand death, and there was no wish to change the problem into a mere question of how most easily to procure organs for transplantation. In 1998, the Danish Council of Ethics issued a statement confirming the existing "opt in" structure of organ donation and the centrality of informed consent to donate.

In Denmark, euthanasia is not permitted, since it is not considered to be the job of medical science to kill people. The organization of medical doctors is against the formalization of euthanasia as a medical practice, even though Danish standard of practice includes extended pain relief treatment of terminal diseases. There are many arguments for keeping an absolute distinction between active and passive euthanasia. It is possible to refuse certain treatments as well as to execute a living will, in which one refuses curative care under certain conditions. The right to refuse treatment was made concrete in the law for professional doctors in 1992. Danish physicians want, to a large degree, to respect patient autonomy in connection with life-prolonging treatment. Lately, there has been intense public debate on the question of euthanasia. The Danish Council of Ethics established a working group that, after various hearings, came forward with a proposal on euthanasia that refused to legalize euthanasia (*Appleton-retningslinierne om ophør med behandling*, 1989; *Etisk råds redegørelser om eutanasi*, 1995; and *Eutanasi? – en redegørelse*, 1996). Many argued that euthanasia on request would be a violation of human dignity (*Aktiv dødshjælp*, 1996, pp. 13ff.) because it would imply death without care. Moreover, it would further challenge the symbolic and real prohibition of killing in penal law (*Aktiv dødshjælp*, 1996, pp. 15ff.).

Extended interest in the moral treatment of animals, nature, and the living world has recently emerged. In 1986, the law on gene technology and the environment established some utilitarian values of sustainable development. This law was more pragmatic than moral (Achen, 1997). The Council of Ethics for Animals was created in 1987. This Council is also working within the framework of utilitarian ethics to establish ideals of animal welfare as fundamental for legislation. The Council of Ethics for Animals has had great success in making considerations of animal welfare important in industry and agriculture. The public debate reflects this concern for the protection of animals and nature. Perhaps public pressure is one of reasons for the establishment in November, 1997 of the so-called "BIOTIK" group of the Ministry for Trade and Economics, which establishes ethical guidelines for the treatment of the environment and animals in food production and, to some extent, the application of genetic technology to humans. The group agreed on ethical ideas for the regulation of gene technology and issued a report entitled, *The Gene Technological Choice* (*Det genteknologiske valg*) in 1999. The Center for Ethics and Law, represented in the commission by Professor Peter Kemp, had a significant impact on the work of the commission. The report, aroused much attention in the media, proposed a set of ethical principles for the regulation of genetic technology. Central among the proposed guidelines are the four basic ethical principles: autonomy, dignity, integrity, and vulnerability. Using this report as a central reference, the Danish government presented these principles to the Parliament, whose members were quite in favor of utilizing the principles to establish regulations on the use of genetic technology on animals and the environment.

IV. The Role of the Danish Council of Ethics

As the Danish Council of Ethics is a major source of the emergence of bioethics in Denmark, I now turn to the bioethical debates in this Council (Koch & Zahle, 1997). Because of the lack of hospital ethics committees, the importance of the Danish Council of Ethics has increased. The Danish Council of Ethics has influenced the increasing interest in ethics among physicians, nurses, and other health care professionals. These professional groups have set up ethics groups and tried to introduce ethics into their educational curricula.[5] In so doing, they regularly rely on contributions from the Danish Council of Ethics.

In its debates, many different moral points of views are represented. Many have argued for a somewhat utilitarian view of ethics, which would facilitate scientific progress and the treatment of patients in hospitals. Others have presented a deontological position, criticizing new technologies and emphasizing the importance of human dignity and integrity. In addition, a phenomenological understanding of ethics, based on a communicative view of treatment in close connection with an ethics of care, can also be found in the work of the National Council of Ethics. However, the work of the Danish Council of Ethics has mostly been casuistic and case-oriented, based on the analysis of different particular bioethical problems to develop proposals for action, rules and legislation. In such case studies, there are no definite ethical views. Instead, the analyses reveal many different perspectives on clinical ethics (Rendtorff & Kemp, 2000, pp. 161-170). The mandate of the Council is rather broad, but one of its main tasks is to help and advise Parliament formulate laws on research ethics committees and reproductive technologies. Thus, the Council has the double function of providing Parliament with advice while also contributing to national debates on ethical issues in medicine related to new technologies (Koch & Zahle, 1997, pp. 334-335).

The constitution and membership of the Council of Ethics reflect a concern for the democratization of moral decision-making as a dialogue between scientists and lay people. Of the seventeen members of the Council, the Minister of Health appoints eight members, while nine members are appointed by Parliament. Of these seventeen members, there should be representation from the medical–scientific community as well as from other scientific fields, law, philosophy, psychology, and so forth. As mentioned, a substantial number of the members of the Council should be lay people who have manifested a public interest in issues of ethical importance (Koch & Zahle, 1997, p. 337).

Over the years, many views on ethics have been presented in the debates of the Council. It has been argued that the task of the Council is to find already-existing consensus in Danish society about ethical matters. But the work of the Council has in practice been to construct, form, and create a new consensus on and awareness about bioethical issues. Before the emergence of the Council, there was little public interest in such matters. Moreover, it has been proposed that the function of the Council is to avoid a slippery slope towards the abuse of medical technology. It is true that the Council has helped bring about greater awareness of ethical questions. But many critics still think that it is a very difficult responsibly to regulate technological development. Some even argue that the establishment of the Danish Council of Ethics has helped to set parliamentary members free from party politics when it comes to ethical issues. This is good, since they can now vote independently according to personal consciences; but, it also manifests the danger of isolating ethics from traditional national party-oriented discussions.

The double function of giving parliamentary advice and participating in national debates has influenced the environment of clinical ethics in Denmark in a number of ways. Ethics is seen as a new kind of medical regulation. The process has resulted in an awareness of the many different stakeholders in debates on clinical ethics. It involves both users/clients/patients of hospitals and health care systems, workers and professionals, and a number of lay people, who are concerned with the development of medical technology. The national hearings organized by the Council of Ethics are good illustrations of how the debates involve many different stakeholders. Most of the major conflicts and possibilities of consensus among the stakeholders have been revealed in these meetings (Koch & Zahle, 1997, p. 340ff.).

The view taken by the Council of Ethics has typically concentrated on defining some of the most common understandings of ethics in the Danish debates. In the report on reproductive technologies (*Redegørelse for kunstig befrugtning*, 1995), the Danish Council of Ethics lists the following positions on reproductive technologies in Denmark: (1) an autonomy-based view, arguing for personal self-determination as the major value; (2) an humanistic "samaritan" position, appreciating the need to care for the vulnerable and weak as the most important concern; (3) an individualistic, consequentialist position, based on a utilitarian positive attitude towards medical science and technology; (4) a community-based communitarian vision of the relation between human beings in society; and (5) a Christian and conservative position, arguing for the protection and respect of the dignity of human life (1995, p. 64). With these positions in mind, the Danish Council of Ethics has addressed many different fields of clinical ethics.

Very early in its history, the Danish Council of Ethics contributed to the future structure of the Danish system of research ethics committees. This was some time after the special parliamentary commission was set up to formulate the law on the issue of research ethics committees.[5] The work of the Danish Council of Ethics helped to improve the basis and practical realization of the law. It was found significant for the Danish system of committees that a separate legal structure be established. As indicated, a strict separation between research ethics and hospital ethics was established and research ethics committees were not linked directly to particular hospitals but were established on a regional basis.

Another important development from the beginning of the Council was an elaboration of organ transplantation systems, thus the Council has also worked on the concept of brain death. It contributed to a polarization of the debate, because many of its members were very skeptical of the brain death criterion. In this debate, there was significant disagreement between Parliament and the Danish Council of Ethics, with the Council presenting a very critical opinion of medical technology.

Moreover, the Council has contributed to a very principlist debate on issues related to human procreation. The debate in the Danish Council of Ethics was so profound that it opened up for many new themes, making the Danish approach less legalistic and pragmatic. It included discussions of eugenics, reproductive freedom, genetic manipulation, and so forth (Etisk Råd, 1995). In relation to prenatal diagnostics, the Council of Ethics was very skeptical of a utilitarian, cost-benefit analysis. It argued that the risks and benefits of the technology were basically equal.

With regard to euthanasia, inspired by Dutch developments, the Council of Ethics initiated the discussion on euthanasia in Denmark. A great number of hearings, reports and proposals for resolutions were produced (Etisk Råd, 1996).[6] Many of the most influential physicians wanted to have more open legislation on euthanasia. The result was, however, a rather skeptical attitude towards the Dutch solution. Even though there was great pressure from certain elements of society, the Danish population did not want to change existing legislation. It seems that the Danish people want to keep the ambiguity of the "gray zone" between active killing and passive pain treatment grounded in the principle of double effect.

These different understandings of ethics are related to making decisions in concrete cases, which is a matter of reflective judgment (Rendtorff & Kemp, 2000, p. 56 ff.). In this context, different dimensions of medical treatment are evaluated in the light of the basic ethical positions. Reflective judgment considers clinical realities in order to formulate a clear connection between diagnosis, therapy, prognosis, and treatment. It considers the tension between patient as person and patient as object in order to formulate the right connection between ethics and medical treatment. This need for reflective judgment is stressed by the lack of ethics committees in the hospitals. In this situation, physicians have greater personal responsibility for making correct decisions.

Given the lack of ethics committees in hospitals and the major role of the Council of Ethics in the Danish discourse on clinical ethics, many critical voices have arisen. Indeed, the lack of hospital ethics committees has been highly criticized. Consequently, only legal instruments are used to enforce the protection of patients in clinical settings. In addition, many critics have stressed problems of communication between physicians and patients. For example, Lone Scocozza's (1994) book argues that communication between research subjects and physicians for informed consent is a failure and does not really exist. Alleged arrogance on the part of the medical profession is blamed for contributing to the distance between medical professionals and other health care workers. The need for ethical education at both the individual and organizational level is mentioned by many as a way of improving the role of clinical ethics in hospital decision-making.

In 2001, the Danish Council of Ethics, together with the Central Scientific Ethical Committee, made a statement on xenotransplantations. It was said that transplantation of animal tissue and organs to human beings had to be carefully scrutinized with regard to risk and ethical problems before it could be an acceptable treatment (*Det Etiske Råd*, 2001, pp. 15-16). Together, the Council for Animal Ethics and the Danish Council of Ethics also debated the problem of cloning of animals and human beings. The two Councils issued a joint report investigating problems of therapeutic and reproductive cloning, including stem cell research. The two Councils agreed to oppose reproductive cloning of any form, but they disagreed about therapeutic cloning and stem cell research. While the majority was in favor of such research, a minority was opposed because of their conception of the status of the human embryo (*Det Etiske Råd*, 2001, pp. 11-12).

V. Organizational Ethics and Professionalism in Danish Hospitals

The Danish Council of Ethics and the system of research ethics committees are examples of external systems influencing the formation of clinical ethics in Danish hospitals. Such formalized systems do not exist internally as a part of the organizational structure of hospitals. Ethical discourse has, however, had an impact on the organization of Danish hospitals. An increased emphasis on professionalism has been seen among Danish health care personnel due to legislation on patients' rights and patient autonomy. A striking feature of this change is the increased significance of professional and organizational learning in Danish hospitals. Danish professional caregivers are becoming aware of the need to integrate moral education into the curricula for health personnel. Nurses, physicians and other members of the care-giving team are receiving ethics training in their basic education and in the education offered to increase their professional competence once they are working in hospitals.

A. Professional and Organizational Learning

Bioethical education is integrated into theoretical and practical teaching as well as into the development of competencies of action and judgment of health care professionals, nurses, and therapists (Hounsgaard & Eriksen, 2000). But there is also an understanding of the need to educate and teach patients, clients, and hospital users. It is very important to recognize competence in ethics as a matter of organizational learning. Here, not only health care professionals but all members of the organization take part in the organization's learning to improve practices and functions.

In Denmark, conceiving of the hospital as a learning organization has been done against the background of a number of different theories of learning. The necessity of teamwork in a very technically sophisticated environment makes organizational learning a matter of increased reflection. Theories of knowledge management emphasize the social character of knowledge. The emergence of ethics in this context is a part of the social construction of knowledge within the organization. The creation of practical knowledge happens with the interaction among individuals and organizations (Nonaka, 1994). A hospital is a knowledge intensive organization and ethics can be understood as an important kind of practical knowledge that should be generated in organizational interactions.

From the perspective of theories of knowledge management, the informal ethics of protective responsibility and respect for patient dignity are understood as unspoken, tacit knowledge related to particular individuals within organizations. It can be argued that it is the aim of organizational learning and knowledge creation to make such tacit ethical knowledge explicit in order to use it in the treatment and care of patients. The discussions of ethical learning aim at institutionalizing ethical reflection as a part of organizational behavior.[7]

Ethical competencies in clinical hospital settings are, therefore, not only functions of theoretical knowledge but are also consequences of practice. These involve the capacity to react to very different social situations. It has been debated whether there might be a conflict between theoretical presuppositions and practical knowledge. Reflection and the exercise of good judgment requires the capacity to develop professional knowledge. In this way, ethics is an integral part of health care workers' professional capacities.

B. Values-Driven Management in Hospitals

Concern for clinical ethics has led to further changes in the management of Danish hospitals. Values-driven management has been proposed for improving the ethical culture of hospital (Hildebrandt & Schultz, 1997, pp. 345ff.). It is possible to situate concerns for ethics at the level of quality management and values-driven management in the health care sector. Health professionals at many different levels of Danish hospital organizations are taking part in the management of the hospital. This is important because it stimulates professional and moral activities at all organizational levels. Many ethical issues are discussed at the management level of health care organizations. In many cases, such discussion takes place in an interdisciplinary framework, but it is also the case that different groups of professionals (e.g., nurses, physicians, and so forth) are formulating their own particular guidelines for management activities.

In the case of values-driven management or total quality management, we can emphasize the communicative dimensions of decision-making. Many different stakeholders should be involved in this process (e.g., patients, physicians, nurses, and other health care workers, and social groups, who have an interest in the health care sector). In each case, management can be considered a relational ability of managers' capacities for coping and relating to the organization environment. This stakeholder theory of values-driven management need not be based on individual interest; stakeholder theories can be seen from the perspective of the common good. Stakeholder management appreciates values and individuals in relation to common organizational standards as well as in relation to social conceptions of the good (Argandona, 1998). Health care management requires a particular ability to communicate with all stakeholders of the organization. It involves a strategic process that has an impact on organizational culture in order to increase the standard of excellence in the organization.

Total quality management is a program used in some Danish hospitals for improving the quality of organizational culture (Fly & Hounsgaard, 2000, pp. 125ff.). It is based on an increased efficiency and excellence of all the dimensions of the organization. This quality improvement program does not manifest a radical change of the history, tradition, and culture of the organization. Rather, it aims at improving existing standards within the organization. For example, applied to a Danish hospital, the program established the following prioritization: (1) patient satisfaction, (2) employee satisfaction, (3) efficient use of resources, and (4) competition with other hospitals. This program was designed to include the whole organization and construct a common language of quality, with the quality of patient care as a primary focus of concern.

Values-driven management can be seen in the perspective of theories of organizational culture. At issue is the improvement of organizational culture in formulating new values for the organization. Values-driven management can be related to organizational learning and changing organizational behavior. To work with values is a major way to change and improve the ethical values of the organization. It is a way of constituting communities of professional organizational reflection in a very similar way to hospital ethics committees (Fly & Hounsgaard, 2000, p. 180). To improve the level of profession and quality, values-driven management in hospital organizations involves: (1) a vision of human well-being, (2) a vision of organizational well-being, (3) open communication about daily practices, (4) continuous dialogue, learning and conversation about the organization, (5) the process of formulating long-term visions of the future of the organization (Fly & Hounsgaard, 2000, p. 183).

The particular model of values-driven management that has been used in Danish hospitals is called DIALOGOS.[7] This model considers dialogue essential to hospital management. Management is a communicative process where all stakeholders are heard. DIALOGOS is closely related to organizational learning. It identifies basic values aimed at organizational improvement. Finally, learned experiences are measured in a process of reporting. This consists of a written final report.

On this basis, the following steps determine the process of the dialogue. (1) Identification of values: At this stage, basic values of the organization are identified. This includes determining and questioning basic values from different stakeholders. The prejudices of different professional groups are especially discussed. (2) Analysis: On the basis of the preliminary identification, the possible scenarios of collaboration are identified. In addition, possible scenarios of conflict are identified. (3) Dialogue with stakeholders: On the basis of the analysis, meetings with all stakeholders are conducted. Basic interpretations of interests are described. Furthermore, possible solutions to conflicts and different problems are proposed. (4) Coordination: Finally, representatives of different stakeholders are included in a process of coordination to define the best possible outcome of the process. Experiences from the process are collected. On this basis, proposals for organizational change are put forward to the executive board of the organization in order to improve the organization.

Values-driven management based on dialogue with all stakeholders is systematized organizational intervention aimed at learning and developing flexibility by accounting for all stakeholders, which creates the foundations for organizational improvement (Meyer, 1997, p. 358). It is an important aspect of this model of dialogue that it includes all stakeholders of the organization. This opens the organization to a wider understanding of problems and possibilities. Therefore, values-driven management is an important way of improving clinical ethics in the hospital.

VI. Conclusions

In conclusion, the Danish bioethical situation can be interpreted as "weakly normative" (Achen, 1997), in that a predominately pragmatic, bureaucratic legal system has slowly become more open to ethical issues. There has been a great deal of legislation in particular fields of bioethics, but no overlapping use of ethical principles. There is still a 'strong utilitarian trend among decision-makers, but there is a move toward stronger concern for basic argumentation. The establishment of the Danish Council of Ethics has made the debate more principlist and profound. This means that the basic principles of autonomy, dignity, integrity, and vulnerability are becoming a more integrated part of bioethics and biolaw[9] due to their very extensive debate in the public. In addition, there is an emerging interest in professionalism, organizational learning and values-driven management in Danish hospital organizations. This concern does not exclude concern for basic ethical principles as an integrated part of organizational ethics.

Notes

1. These reports included: The Price of Progress, *Fremskridtets pris, etiske problemer ved gensplejsning, kunstig befrugtning og fosterdiagnostik*, Ministry of the Interior, 1984.

2. See *Lov nr. 350 af 13 juni 1973*.
3. Among others a publication of the Lawyer Linda Nielsen about genetic integrity comparing the situation in Denmark and Italy.
4. Ulla Hybel (1998): *Forsøgspersoner, Om den retlige beskyttelse af mennesker,der deltager i biomedicinsk forskning*, (Research Subjects, About the Legal Protection of Human Beings, who participate in Biomedical Research) København. This book is a major discussion of the development Danish system of ethics committees for protection of research subjects.
5. The comission came up with the following report: *Betænkning nr. 1185, Forskning på mennesket, Etik/Jura*, (1989) Sundhedsministeriet, København. English translation: *Research involving Human Subjects, Ethics/Law* (1989), Ministry of Health, Copenhagen.
6. Etisk Råd (Danish Council of Ethics): *Eutanasi? En redegørelse* (1996), (Euthanasia, a Report), København.
7. Torbjørn Meyer from Copenhagen Business School developed DIALOGOS. He has used this model at two Danish hospitals as research examples in a Ph.D dissertation in 1996. He has done pioneer research on such an installation of ethics in hospitals. See Torbjørn Meyer: "Værdibaseret ledelse på hospitalet" ("Value-based Management in the Hospital") (1997) in Steen Hildebrandt & Majken Schultz: (1997) *Fokus på sygehusledelse* (Focus on Hospital Management), Copenhagen, p. 345 ff.

Bibliography

Achen, T. 1997. Den bioetiske udfordring. Et retspolitisk studie af forholdet mellem etik, politik og ret i det lovforberedende arbejde vedrørende bio- og genteknologi i Danmark, Norge og Sverige. [The bioethical challenge. A legal policy study of the relationship between ethics, politics and law in the preparatory work regarding bio- and gene technology in Denmark, Norway and Sweden]. Linköping.

Appleton. 1996. retningslinierne om ophør med behandling [Guidelines for stopping treatment] (ugeskrift for læger – 11 december 1989 – videnskab og praksis) and Etisk råds redegørelser om eutanasi: *Aktiv dødshjælp – er der behov for nye regler*, [Active euthanasia, Is there a need for new regulation] Det etisk råd 1995 and *Eutanasi? – en redegørelse*, (Euthansia, A Report) Det etiske råd, 1996.

Argandona, A. 1998. The stakeholder theory of the common good. *Journal of Business Ethics* 17.

Basic Ethical Principles in Bioethics and Biolaw Research Group (2000). *Basic ethical principles in European bioethics and biolaw*. Copenhagen and Barcelona: European Commission.

Bo Andreassen Rix m fl. 1991. *Kortlægningen af det menneskelige genom* [The mapping of the human genome]. København: Det Etisk Råd.

Det Etisk Råd. 1990. Redegørelse om fosterdiagnostik [Report on embryo diagnostics]. København: Det Etisk Råd.

Det Etisk Råd. 1991. *Redegørelse om følsomme personoplysninger* [Statement about sensitive personnel information], p. 5ff. København: Det Etisk Råd.

Det Etisk Råd. 1991. *Redegørelse om beskyttelse af følsomme personoplysninger*. København: Det Etisk Råd.

Det Etisk Råd. 1994. A dynamic theory of organizational knowledge creation. *Organizational Science* 5(1): 16.

Det Etisk Råd. 1995. Genterapi, en debatdag. [Gene therapy, a hearing]. *Proceedings*. København.

Det Etisk Råd. 1995. *Redegørelse for kunstig befrugtning* [Report on artificial insemination]. København: Det Etisk Råd.

Det Etisk Råd. 1996. *Aktiv dødshjælp. En redegørelse* (p. 13ff.). København: Det Etisk Råd.

Det Etisk Råd. 1996. *Eutanasi? En redegørelse* [Euthanasia, a Report]. København: Det Etisk Råd.

Det Etisk Råd. 1996. Kunstig befrugtning. En redegørelse [Artificial insemination, a report]. København.

Det Etisk Råd. 1999. Betænkning nr. 1185. Forskning på mennesket, Etik/Jura. [Research on human beings, law/ethics, Sundhedsministeriet]. Copenhagen.

Det Etisk Råd. 2001. *Årsberetning.* [Yearly report] (pp. 15-16). København: Det Etisk Råd.

Dübeck, I. 1997. Personers rettigheder. København: Jurist – og Økonomforbundes Forlag.

Fly, M. & Hounsgaard, L. 2000. *Faglig ledelse i sundhedsvæsenet* (p. 125ff.). København: Gyldendal Uddannelse.

Hildebrandt, S. & Schultz, M. 1997. *Fokus på sygehusledelse* [Focus on hospital management]. Copenhagen: Munksgaard.

Hounsgaard, L. & Eriksen, J.J. (eds) 2000. *Læring i Sundhedsvæsenet* [Learning in Health Care]. København: Gyldendal Uddannelse.

Jensen, L.B. 1991. På patientens præmisser. København: Det Etisk Råd.

Kemp, P. 1992. *Det uerstattelige [The Irreplaceable]*. København: Spektrum.

Kemp, L. & Rendtorff, J. 1997. *Den bioetiske vending* [The Bioethical Turn]. København: Spektrum.

Koch, L. & Zahle, H. 1997. *Et Etisk Råd af sagkyndige og lægfolk* [An ethical council of experts and lay people]. Juristen.

Lov om kunstig befrugtning i forbindelse med lægelig behandling, diagnostik og forskning mv. af 10 juni 1997: i Lovtidende A 1997, Hæfte 84.

Lov om ligsyn, obduktion og transplantationer m.v. af 13 juni 1990: Kapitel 1: Dødens konstatering.

Meyer, T. 1997. *Værdibaseret ledelse på hospitalet* [Value-based management in the hospital]. In: S. Hildebrandt & M. Schultz (eds). *Fokus på sygehusledelse* [Focus on hospital management] (p. 345 ff.). Copenhagen: Munksgaard.

Ministry of the Interior. 1984. *Fremskridtets pris, etiske problemer ved gensplejsning, kunstig befrugtning og fosterdiagnostik* [The reports (The Price of Progress)].

Nathan, M. 1990. *Retlig regulering af arvelige sygdomme* [Legal regulation of hereditary disease]. København: Det Etisk Råd.

Nonaka, I. 1994. A dynamic theory of organizational knowledge creation. *Organizational Science* 5(1): 21ff.

Rehof, L.A. 1989. *Behandling og forsøg med fostre* [Treatment and research on embryos]. København: Det Etiske Råd.

Rendtorff, J.D. 1999. *Bioetik og Ret, Kroppen mellem person og ting* [Bioethics and law, the body between person and thing]. København.

Rendtorff, J.D. & Kemp, P. 2000. *Basic ethical principles in European bioethics and biolaw. Autonomy, dignity, integrity and vulnerability*, Volume 1. Copenhagen and Barcelona: European Commission.

Ross, A. 1979. *Livets Hellighed contra individets autonomi. Ugeskrift for læger.* København.

Ulla, H. 1998. *Forsøgspersoner, Om den retlige beskyttelse af mennesker, der deltager i biomedicinsk forskning.* København.

Warnock Committee. 1984. *Warnock Report*, United Kingdom.

Part IV: Asia

Part IV Data

13 Turkish Perspectives in Bioethics

Sahin Aksoy

I. Introduction

Medicine has always existed in human society, since illness and disease have always been among humanity's greatest concerns. In the ancient world, those who were believed to have the power to cure illnesses were feared and respected (Coleman, 1985). Thus their professional behavior and personal morals was as important as their healing capabilities. The earliest known regulation of the responsibilities and duties of medical practice can be found in the Code of Hammurabi, written some 5000 years ago, which details certain of the social and legal rules a healer should follow in his medical practice (Porter, 1997, pp. 45-46). Still, Hippocrates is known as the father of medicine in the West especially given his influence on the social and moral aspects of the healing arts. During the 10th and 11th centuries, while scientific medicine was still developing, the social and ethical side of medicine was practiced in accordance with Ibn-i Sina's interpretation of Hippocrates. After a long period in which the church exerted significant pressure in every sector of life, medicine began to be practiced in a liberated and modern way from the 17th-18th centuries onwards (Conrad, et al., 1995, pp. 371-476).

However at the end of the 18th century, the physician's image in society was that of a "jealous, backbiter, money-lover and butcher-like machos" (Shyrock, 1966, pp. 151, 176). So, physicians were unloved but needed people. Obviously, this image was not ideal for a profession such as medicine. Concern with this situation led some to argue for the regaining of the traditional good image of physicians as well as for the regulation of the practice of medicine. In 1803, Dr. Thomas Percival, a Manchester physician, published *Medical Ethics: or, a Code of Institutes and Precepts, Adapted to the Professional Conduct of Physicians and Surgeons* (Percival, 1803). This is known as the first usage of the concept of "medical ethics" in the literature. After Percival, "medical ethics" became a frequent and ubiquitous concept.

Medical and technological developments of the 20th century, such as the discovery of DNA and its structure (Watson & Crick, 1953), renal transplantation (Merrill, et al., 1956), oral contraceptives (Vaughn, 1970), heart transplantation, description of brain death (Report, 1968), safe abortion (Callahan, 1970) and *in vitro* fertilization (Edwards & Steptoe, 1980), pushed the boundaries of medicine, leaving doctors almost helpless to tackle the social and ethical implications of such advanced biomedical technologies. Efforts to overcome and address such concerns resulted in the establishment of a discipline by the name of "bioethics" (Jonsen, 1998). While the concept of "bioethics" was first used by Dr. Van Rensselaer Potter (1971) in the context of the survival of the biosphere, the field has developed with the contributions of scholars from various fields such as medicine, philosophy, law and theology. Although the birth of bioethics occurred in the United States, its development and perfection carries on in many countries around the world.

II. Medical Education

Medical ethics education has been in the curriculum of medical schools in Turkey since the 1960s (Pelin & Ors, 1995). With courses entitled "Medical Deontology", first year medical students are taught moral sensitization and the development of ethical awareness regarding the moral problems which arise in various areas of medical activity (Arda & Pelin, 1995). Initially, such courses were taught together with the history of medicine classes; however, from the 1990's onward, the trend has changed, and the courses have been placed in the 1st and 4th (or 5th) years of medical school. The curriculum includes bioethical concerns as well as issues in clinical ethics. Although teaching methods may vary from one school to another, it is usual to mix lectures with time spent on case studies and small group discussions.

Turkey is a large country with a population of 70 million people from different ethnic backgrounds. The percentages of men and women are almost equal. It has a young population, with approximately 60% under the age of 20 (Republic of Turkey, 1990). The major religion in Turkey is Islam, which accounts for some 95% of the population; although there are Jews, Christians, and other faith traditions. While Turkey has a secular governmental system, since such a great majority of citizens are Muslims, religion plays a significant role in ethical reasoning in the public mind, though not necessarily in the minds of professional bioethicists.

There are sixty medical schools in Turkey, public and private. Although there are courses on medical ethics and bioethics in each institution, only ten are taught by a staff member with a postgraduate degree in medical ethics; the remainder are taught by "experienced" and "wise" physicians.

In Turkey, only persons with an undergraduate education in one of the health sciences, such as medicine, dentistry, pharmacy, nursing, and so forth, can pursue a postgraduate education in medical ethics. In this regard, the bioethics trends in Turkey are different than in Western Europe and the United States, wherein most of the field's "grandfathers" and practitioners are social scientists, philosophers, and theologians, rather than medical scientists (Jonsen, 1998). Drawing solely on medical professionals profoundly affects, in a negative way, the level and the depth of bioethical discussions in Turkey. Therefore, an important goal for Turkish bioethicists is to encourage social scientists, philosophers, theologians and others to contribute to the field and thereby to enrich the discussions.

Scholars who work in the field of bioethics organized and established the Turkish Bioethics Society in Ankara on September 28, 1994. The major aims of the Society were to contribute to the progress and development of bioethics and its education, and to develop its relations with health professions and other disciplines. The Society has provided an atmosphere of communication and discussion both in Turkey and internationally as well as the development of courses for undergraduate and postgraduate education. It organizes conferences, symposiums, seminars, and congresses, provides relevant and timely publications, encourages and supports the dissemination of bioethical research, and introduces the subject to the public, consistent with these aims. It also aims to provide closer cooperation among the membership in order to notify the appropriate parties when faced with unacceptable medical behavior, or faults due to disrespectful attitudes, as well as to inform the general public about bioethical updates when required. The Society has organized five national congresses with the participation of international scholars.

In addition to the Turkish Bioethics Society, other non-governmental organizations include the Turkish Philosophical Association, which established a bioethics section in 1990, and the Turkish Medical Association, which is interested in medical ethics issues and founded an ethics committee in 1993 (Arda & Pelin, 1995). Despite all such educational and organizational efforts, significant evidence of the negligence and misuse of moral principles implies that more effort should be paid to biomedical ethics.

A central concern of bioethics is to make appropriate choices that we can live with, for improving individual lives and seeking the public good (Macer, 1994). This philosophy has been followed as Turkey has established rules and regulations to govern particular ethical and legal issues in the fields of medicine and biotechnology.

III. Abortion

Although it takes longer to change understandings of the morality of abortion in the public conscience, the legality of it may change overnight (Aksoy, 1997a). In the early years of the Turkish Republic, after the War of Independence, population growth was desired and abortion was banned. However, with changing socio-economic and socio-cultural circumstances, abortion has since been legalized (Arda & Pelin, 1995). When the law on population planning was declared in 1983, Turkey became one of the most liberal countries in terms of abortion. According to this law, abortion is allowed up to the 10th week of pregnancy, if it does not harm the pregnant woman's health. After this time, it is possible to terminate pregnancy with the approval of two physicians if the mother's life is in danger, if there is a possible danger in the period following the pregnancy, or if the fetus has a serious disorder. If the woman is married, the written consent of the husband is sought in every case (*Official Bulletin*, 1983). After passage of this rather liberal law, the number of abortions exploded in the country. Studies indicate that one in every six pregnancies is terminated with induced abortion (Kocoglu, 2001). This is very interesting, given that Turkey is a relatively traditional society and such a choice is not entirely compatible with the prevailing ethical and religious norms. Possible reasons for this shift include the ways in which poverty may encourage people into disregarding their religious beliefs, or perhaps modern lifestyles have induced them into falling away from their traditional ethical and religious values.

IV. Euthanasia

In the beginning, there were very few people who supported euthanasia in Turkey (Oguz, 1996). However, research conducted in different locations in Turkey indicates that health care professionals, especially nurses, support assisted-suicide and euthanasia (Bahcecik, et al., 1998; Ersoy & Altun, 2001; Akcil, et al., 1998). Despite such findings, both passive and active euthanasia remains unlawful in Turkish Criminal Law. While passive euthanasia is considered to be unintentional killing (Turkish Criminal Law, Article 455), active euthanasia is punishable as intentional killing (Turkish Criminal Law, Article 448) (Artuk, 2001). Moreover, euthanasia is absolutely forbidden according to Islamic teaching (Rispler-Chaim, 1993, pp. 94-99). Although this is the case, the trend among health care professionals and an ever larger percentage of educated people to support euthanasia can only be interpreted as the falling away of traditional moral and religious values (Aksoy, 2000). The growing trend toward non-traditional morality has been observed in every sector of life within the last one or two decades in Turkey.

V. End of Life Decision-Making

In Turkey, there has not been much research conducted on end of life decision-making, but the general attitudes of professionals and the educated are quite similar to their views regarding euthanasia. Traditional beliefs and values play an important role in this process. A recent study (Aksoy, et al., unpublished) conducted among 200 volunteers (half of whom were health care professionals) indicated that Turkish people typically want to make their own individual decisions regarding the end of life, and that they do not want their families to be told. However, they do not allow relatives to make their own decisions and prefer to speak on behalf of them. In such cases, they neglect personal autonomy in the name of being more protective. Significantly, our research indicated that the majority of health care professionals (89%) wish to know if they are diagnosed with cancer, but that they would prefer not to inform their close relatives of a cancer diagnosis since they believe that "their relatives cannot tolerate this bad news". Among the general public, while 61% wish to know their own diagnosis, only 29% would allow their relatives to know of their own cancer diagnosis for similar reasons.

Hospice care does not exist in Turkey, except in some newly established hospice look-alike nursing homes. Our survey also indicated that 47% of the general public would not wish to send their relatives to hospices, even if they did exist, since they see this as an indication of disrespect toward their parents. This attitude may be due to traditional beliefs derived from Islam, which are central to Turkish culture, that it is very important to look after one's parents when they are ill or elderly. Nowadays, despite so much degeneration in the cultural framework, it is good for the social health of the society to see that respect for parents remains unchanged.

The findings suggested that everyone must have the right to die in his "own bed" in peace. However, health care professionals are more reluctant, compared to the general public, to stay in the hospital during their final hours. The figures are 33% and 54% respectively. As stated in the previous section, there is a kind of acceptance of euthanasia, especially the passive sort, among the Turkish community. Approximately 20% of those surveyed think the extra effort to extend the life of a terminal or hopelessly ill patient is useless and wasteful.

VI. Organ Transplantation

Discussions about the legal and ethical aspects of organ transplantation started in the 1960s after the first successful organ transplant. In many cases of chronic renal or liver failure and chronic heart disease, organ transplantation represents the only viable treatment. The demand for organs needed for transplantation is increasing rapidly, but organ donation has always fallen far short of the needed amount. The situation in Turkey is no better than in other countries, and is perhaps worse. The president of the Turkish Organ Transplantation Association told *The Times* that, while approximately 30,000 patients are waiting for transplantation, more than 80,000 patients are being treated for chronic renal diseases (Ozsaglam, 1999). Every government in the world has encouraged its citizens to donate organs and has passed laws to regulate organ transplantations (WHO, 1991).

The Turkish Parliament passed "the law on the procurement, preservation, grafting and transplantation of organs and tissues" in 1979 (*Official Gazette*, 1979). This law sets out the necessary conditions for organ procurement from living persons and cadavers. Significantly influenced by similar laws in European countries, it prohibits both commerce in human organs as well as advertising for donors. Under the law, donors must be over 18 years old and competent. Informed consent is an essential component of the donation process, thus the law requires that a mentally incompetent person's organ donation be declined. If the donor is married, the spouse's consent is required. With regard to cadaver donation, following much international law, brain death is equated with real death. The confirmation of death is made by a team consisting of one radiologist, one neurologist, one neurosurgeon and one anesthesiologist. Doctors who certify the death of the donor may not be involved in the transplantation team.

The concept of brain death was "invented" after the first transplantations of the 1960s (Ad Hoc Committee of the Harvard Medical School, 1984). While legal regulations and religious rulings are rather liberal and permissive in Turkey, some Turkish scholars argue that brain death cannot be equated with real death (Aksoy, 2001). Moreover, research conducted in Turkey has indicated that it is very questionable to assume that donors are strictly altruistic volunteers (Erek & Apaydin, 1999). The researchers rightly argue that living donors are under significant social pressure to donate their organ to relatives when needed. Thus, the consent they give is not necessarily fully voluntary and altruistically motivated. From a traditional religious point of view, Turkish people have no theoretical problem donating and accepting organs for transplantation, since the Presidency of Religious Affairs of Turkey issued a public release in 1980 that it is allowed by Islam (Religious Affairs High Council, 1980). But for some reason, such as suspicion of a fair distribution of organs or of doctors' possible negligence in their final minutes of life, and so forth, the number of donations are far less than the pressing need.

VII. Genetic Engineering, Cloning and Stem Cell Research

Genetic engineering and cloning are the current issues keeping scientists and moralists busy in discussion. Apparently it is more meaningful to get into such discussions when the technology is available in the respective country. Cloning and stem cell research are not usual practices in Turkey. Therefore, there does not exist direct legal regulation on such matters. But, in agreement with the general trend across the world, the Turkish Government and Presidency of Religious Affairs has declared that human cloning is morally unacceptable in principle, while animal cloning is welcomed. However, there are different views among Turkish bioethicists, some of whom argue that the entities involved do not possess sufficient moral standing for one to be against either human cloning (Aksoy, 1997b) or stem cell research (Aksoy, 2002).

VIII. Ethics Committees

Next, I turn to consideration of institutions and organizations that were established to improve the quality of bioethical discourse in the country, as well as to develop the excellence of the health care service.

Ethics committees and review boards play an important role in protecting the rights of both experimental subjects in scientific research and patients in health care institutions. Ethics committees and review boards began to flourish in Europe and the United States in the 1960s and 1970s (Solbakk, 1991). In Turkey, there was no legal regulation of research on human beings until 1993. In that year, the amendment relating to drug research was issued. The main objectives of the regulation were to establish a central ethics committee as well as local ethics committees, and to provide administrative control over research on human subjects (Arda, 2000a).

Up to that point, there had been no compulsory clinical ethics lectures in the medical curriculum, so it was also proposed that research ethics committees play an educational role, making physicians aware of moral problems and contributing to the training of research teams. However, on January 29, 1993, the Ministry of Health issued legislation, "Research on Human Beings by using Drugs and Chemical Substances", which raised some problems regarding research ethics committees. For example, the Central Ethics Committee has no medical ethicist as a member, and there is no ethical concept other than "consent" in their operational procedures (Arda, 2000b). But over the years, ethics committees have become inseparable parts of clinical and research activities. Almost every medical school has an institutional ethics review board that deals with research applications.

IX. Publications and Conferences

Publications are important for a field not only for recognition in the scientific community but also to share knowledge among scholars. General medical journals have accepted papers on medical ethics, but the first Turkish journal devoted solely to the field was the *Turkiye Klinikleri Journal of Medical Ethics* (or the *Turkish Journal of Medical Ethics*). It was published three times a year from 1993 to 1998, and biannually from 1999 until 2001. In 2002 the journal changed its name to *Turkiye Klinikleri Journal of Medical Ethics, Law and History* and is now published quarterly. The journal has broadened its scope so as to attract a larger audience. The journal is bilingual, with Turkish and English abstracts. Its international advisory board enables the journal to publish very high quality articles.

In terms of conferences and scientific meetings, the Turkish bioethics community was well organized from early on. National bioethics conferences have continued under the organization of the Turkish Bioethics Association since 1994. The meetings are held every two years with the participation of scholars from all around the country. These meetings contribute significantly to the general discussion and to the development of bioethics in Turkey.

X. Conclusion

Bioethics is becoming more and more popular in the international community. Since the world has become a global village, it is no longer possible to live in an isolated moral world. Most major projects are conducted with the cooperation of different countries, under the purview of various legal systems and moral traditions. Moreover, almost every country has a population comprised of people from various cultural and religious traditions. Therefore, it is crucial to be aware of the perspectives of diverse cultures and nations.

In this article, I have presented a Turkish perspective on bioethics. This may help the international bioethics community, not only because there are millions of Turkish people living in Western Europe and the United States, but also because Turkey is a unique country which is at the junction point of the East and the West, Europe and Asia, geographically as well as culturally. It is interesting to observe a nation that had been the leader of the Islamic world for ten centuries, but which in the last eight decades has committed itself to becoming westernized. This fact reflects a change of attitude on legal texts as well as the general public consensus.

Bibliography

Ad Hoc Committee of the Harvard Medical School. 1984. A definition of irreversible coma. *Journal of the American Medical Association* 252: 677-680.

Akcil, M., Bilgili, N., Turkan, S.K., Yardim, M. & Yildiz, A.N. 1998. Universite Son Sinif Ogrencilerinin Otanazi Konusundaki Gorusleri [Views of final year university students on euthanasia]. *Proceedings of the Third National Bioethics Symposium*: 149-158 (in Turkish).

Aksoy, S. 1997a. Abortion: the destruction of life. *Eubios Journal of Asian and International Bioethics* 7(2): 52-54.

Aksoy, S. 1997b. "Dolly the sheep" ve Getirdikleri ["Dolly the sheep" and beyond]. Presented at the *Third Turkish Medical Ethics Symposium*, Ankara, Turkey, 23-25 October (in Turkish).

Aksoy, S. 2000. Can euthanasia be part of "good-doctoring"? *Eubios Journal of Asian and International Bioethics* 10(5): 152-154.

Aksoy, S. 2001. A critical approach to the current understanding of Islamic scholars on using cadaver organs without prior permission. *Bioethics* 15(5/6): 461-472.

Aksoy, S., Cevik, E. & Edisan, Z. The attitudes of Turkish people on end of life decision making. Unpublished research prepared for publication.

Aksoy, S. 2002. Ethics of stem cell experimentation. Presented at the *Third International Conference of Bioethics*, 23-30 June, Chungli, Taiwan.

Arda, B. & Pelin, S. 1995. Bioethics in Turkey. *Eubios Journal of Asian and International Bioethics* 5: 64-65.

Arda, B. 2000a. Evaluation of research ethics committees in Turkey. *Journal of Medical Ethics* 26(6): 459-461.

Arda, B. 2000b. The experience of the research ethics committees in Turkey. *Medical Law* 19(3): 493-500.

Artuk, M.E. 2001. Hukukcu Gozuyle Otanazi [Euthanasia from a lawyer's perspective]. In H. Hatemi & H. Dogan (eds), *Medikal Etik* (pp. 42-60). Istanbul: Yuce Publication.

Bahcecik, N., Alpar, S.E., Yildirim, Y., Temiz, G., Ozen, C. & Keles, S. 1998. Hemsirelerin Otanazi Konusundaki Gorusleri [Nurses' views on euthanasia]. *Proceedings of the Third National Bioethics Symposium*: 339-348 (in Turkish).

Callahan, D. 1970. *Abortion: law, choice and morality*. New York: Macmillan Company.

Coleman, V. 1985. *The story of medicine*. London: Jill Norman Books.

Conrad, I.C., Neve, M., Nutton, V., Porter, R. & Wear, A. 1995. *The western medical tradition*. Cambridge: Cambridge University Press.

Edwards, R. & Steptoe, P. 1980. *A matter of life: the story of a medical breakthrough*. London: Morrow Ltd.

Erek, E. & Apaydin, S. 1999. Organ Transplantasyonu ve Tibbi Etik [Organ transplantation and medical ethics]. In H. Hatemi & H. Dogan (eds), *Medikal Etik* (pp. 17-28). Istanbul: Yuce Publication.

Ersoy, N. & Altun, I. 2001. Hemsirelerin Yardimli Intihar Hakkinda Gorusleri ile Ilgili Bir Calisma [A study of nurses' views on assisted suicide]. *Turkiye Klinikleri Journal of Medical Ethics* 9: 49-55 (in Turkish).

Jonsen, A.R. 1998. *The birth of bioethics*. New York: Oxford University Press.

Kocoglu, G.O. 2001. Dusukler [Abortions]. *Hacettepe Public Health Bulletin* 22(3-4): 5-9.

Macer, D.R.J. 1994. *Bioethics for the people by the people*. Christchurch: Eubios Ethics Institute.

Merrill, J.P., Murray, J.E., Harrison, J.H. & Guild, W.R. 1956. Successful homotransplantation of the human kidney between identical twins. *Journal of the American Medical Association* 160: 277-282.

Official Gazette No. 16655 (1979). The law on the procurement, preservation, grafting and transplantation of organs and tissues. Law No. 2238 (03.06.1979).

Official Gazette No. 18057 (1983). Law for population planning. Law No. 2827 (24.5.1983).

Oguz, Y. 1996. Euthanasia in Turkey: cultural and religious perspectives. *Eubios Journal of Asian and International Bioethics* 6: 170-171.

Ozsaglam, D. 1999. *The Times*, 25 January.

Pelin, S.S. & Ors, Y. 1995. Medical esthetics from a historical and ethical point of view. *Eubios Journal of Asian and International Bioethics* 5: 35-36.

Percival, T. 1803. *Medical ethics: or, a code of institutes and precepts, adapted to the professional conduct of physicians and surgeons*. London, S. Russell. New Edition: C. Leake (ed.) 1927. *Percival's medical ethics*. Baltimore: Williams & Wilkins.

Porter, R. 1997. *The greatest benefit to mankind*. London: HarperCollins.

Potter, V.R. 1971. *Bioethics: bridge to the future*. Englewood Cliffs: Prentice-Hall.

Religious Affairs High Council Decision No. 13 (1980), Ankara.

Report of the Ad Hoc Committee at Harvard Medical School to Examine the Definition of Brain Death 1968. A definition of irreversible coma. *Journal of the American Medical Association* 205: 337-340.

Republic of Turkey, Prime Ministry State Institute of Statistics. 1990. [On-line] Available: <http://www.die.gov.tr/english/ISTATIS/ESG2/f.htm>.

Rispler-Chaim, V. 1993. *Islamic medical ethics in the twentieth century*. Leiden: E.J. Brill.

Shryock, R.H. 1966. *Medicine in America*. Baltimore: John Hopkins Press.

Solbakk, J.H. 1991. Ethics review committees in medical research in nordic countries: history, organization and assignments. *Healthcare Ethics Committee Forum* 3(4): 215-220.

Vaughn, P. 1970. *The pill on trial*. London: Weidenfield and Nicholson.

Watson, J. & Crick, F. 1953. The molecular structure of nucleic acids. *Nature* 4356 (25 April): 737.

World Health Organization. 1991. *Human organ transplantation*. Geneva: World Health Organization.

14 Bioethics in Bangladesh

Hasna Begum

I. Introduction: Education in Bangladesh

While many public universities include Peter Singer's *Practical Ethics* as one of the required texts for philosophy courses (Singer, 1979), bioethics as an academic discipline did not develop in Bangladesh until the 1990s. Bioethics in Bangladesh is associated with a kind of utilitarianism, closely related to Singer's theory, and other views dominated by the idea of "quality of life".[1] In Bangladesh, the curriculum of tertiary education lacks the multidisciplinary approach seen in other countries. This may be due to a misunderstanding of the importance of such an approach in educating students, who will become the policy makers and educators for future generations. It is a narrowly focused educational approach that fails to provide a holistic view of the problems of life, which is necessary to find the solutions to such problems, could not be recognized by the formulators of the curricula of the various disciplines and areas of study.

So one finds in Bangladesh that theories of aesthetics are not being taught to the students of fine arts and architecture during their undergraduate studies, and theories of medical ethics are not being taught to undergraduate medical students. Medical students are only informed about the oaths prescribed for medical professionals. Students of the humanities are quite ignorant of basic theories of science, and students of the sciences are similarly ignorant of the humanities, including philosophy, literature, basic economic theory, and other social sciences. Consequently, the majority of students possess a limited base of learning, which hinders the in-depth understanding of even their own subject. The lack of interdisciplinary studies thus makes their knowledge flimsy and shallow.

During the early 1990s, a realization among some academicians emerged which resulted in taking the first step in formulating curricula to introduce an interdisciplinary system into the educational curriculum. Many academicians were returning to Bangladesh after being trained in various modern Western European, Australian, and Asian universities with new ideas. They became confident enough to try the interdisciplinary approach in Bangladesh's academic world, realizing that this method may be necessary for understanding the complexities of contemporary curricula of life. These academicians proposed the introduction of related disciplines into the curricula of their respective fields of study.

As a result, we find a slightly changed approach, though not radically new, in the fields of philosophy, sociology, economics and various science subjects. But, unfortunately, many academicians still have the tendency to shy away from anything new which is not thoroughly familiar to them. They continued to resist any change to the curricula or to the educational system. The conflict resulted in introducing only a slight inclination towards an interdisciplinary approach to the curricula of different disciplines.

We find the same scenario with regard to bioethics in Bangladesh. Bioethics is a form of ethics developed from the application of both normative and meta-ethical theories to the problems of life. It is a study that also evaluates the consequences of the implementation of various old and new science-based technologies in the fields of natural and biological sciences from an ethical point of view. In Bangladesh, bioethical problems have been discussed since the mid-1980s by a few scholars who became acquainted with the subject during their stays overseas. The main focus had been related to the problems discussed in Singer's book, *Practical Ethics*, on topics, such as abortion, euthanasia, animal rights, and so forth. Later, the author of this article published several papers on the control of new human reproductive technologies in Bangladesh, evaluating them from various ethical perspectives, including, for example, informed consent, coercion, and so forth. Papers by others were also published during that period on abortion, environmental issues, animal rights, and so forth. But these papers are more of a reflection of what is already being discussed in the West without any contextual analyses or regional interpretations.

II. Bioethics in Bangladesh

Interest in bioethics is absent for various reasons. The foremost reason for this deficient amount of interest, as discussed above, is the lack of an interdisciplinary approach among the country's professionals. Bioethics as a discipline is a multidisciplinary study in which professionals and academicians of many disciplines (e.g., philosophy and theology, medicine and law) usually take part. In this country, physicians do not normally consider it their obligation to look into whether a particular health insurance company has a policy of balancing the profit of the company with the benefit of the clients. Anthropologists in Bangladesh do not consider the ways in which the implementation of technology destroys certain cultural traits of a particular society to be of interest. Legal experts feel no obligation to safeguard the interest of their clients against bio-technical interventions. Ethicists might not feel obliged to criticize laws believed to be unethical, since they would think that their obligation is only to do their particular job. This typical apathy is, perhaps, due to the political and economical condition within the country itself: everyone is busy with his or her own self-interest, since the conditions of the country are not congenial to easy survival.

It is difficult to envisage the scope of the development of bioethics in the near future in Bangladesh. The reasons are many; here are just a few:

(1) In 1999, a draft of the National Education Policy was presented by a government committee, the members of which were prominent educators. As of this writing, that policy has not been accepted by the Cabinet, which has an inherent reactionary lenience towards religious education. So this country is yet to have its own National Education Policy.

(2) Only on November 8, 2000, did a committee of health professionals present the first draft of the National Health Policy to the Prime Minister of the country. It was then sent to the Cabinet for discussion and final acceptance.

(3) Bangladesh has no national bioethics association. The author attempted to form one, but no more than two ethicists or other professionals were interested.

(4) Due to the lack of interest in bioethics (even among ethicists), there is not even a government proposal in place for the formation of a national bioethics commission.

Such factors are detrimental to the development of bioethics as a discipline, since bioethical discussions need a multidisciplinary approach in the educational system. A declared national health policy is also needed to provide general guidelines for an approach to the population's health. This would further aid those who are interested in the study of bioethics in this country.

A few other astounding facts should be mentioned here to clarify how backward this country is in the appreciation of bioethics. First, no hospital in the country has an ethics committee, which implies that the hospitals deem them unnecessary.[2] There is an ethics committee for the International Centre for Diarrhoeal Diseases Research, Bangladesh (ICDDRB), which is internationally funded, mostly by the World Health Organization. But it is interesting to note that no ethicist is on this ethics committee, which makes the name of the committee a misnomer.

Second, there are a few serious national and international organizations (e.g. ICDDRB, BIRDEM, Bangladesh Medical Research Council [BMRC]), which are conducting research on medical and biomedical issues. But no organization is thus far interested in researching the ethics of medical and biomedical research.

III. Conclusion

In spite of such a dearth of interest in bioethics and of so many hindrances to the development of bioethical studies, the scope of such studies in this country is widely available. From an ethical point of view, there are ample candidates for critical evaluation: family planning programs within the country, water pollution from arsenic and other harmful industrial wastes, environmental air pollution by vehicle emissions, unethical practices by health professionals in relation to patients and other subordinates (e.g., doctors' behavior with nurses), biomedical research involving humans by national and international research organizations and/or individuals, and implementation of technology in the agricultural sector, and so forth.

It can be safely stated that Bangladesh is an untrodden, rich ground for a bioethicist to do research on many important biomedical topics present within the country. For the purpose of creating interest among national and international researchers on bioethics, a national association of bioethics must be established soon. The country's government should also form a national bioethics commission, whose main agenda should be promoting bioethical research, as well as guarding the interest of the population against any harm done to them by national or international aggression through old and new technological interventions.[3]

Notes

1. "News", Bangladesh Television, 8 November 2000.
2. This is confirmed after discussion with Professor Liaquat Ali, Coordinator, Biomedical Research Group, BIRDEM, Dhaka, on 6 December 2000.
3. For more information, see also Begum, 1993, 1994, 1996, 1997, 1998, 2001; Begum and Hemberg, 1998.

Bibliography

Begum, H. 1993. Family planning and social position of women. *Bioethics* 7(2&3): 218-223.
Begum, H. 1994. Vaccine contraceptives: wisdom, optimism, and combatting the potential for abuse. *Reproductive Health Matters,* 4, November.
Begum, H. 1996. Violence in Islamic texts and its relevance to practice. *Women Heritage and Violence.* Calcutta: Jadavpur University.
Begum, H. 1997. Issues related to implementation of reproduction technology in Islamic society. *Bioethics* 11(4): 341-347.
Begum, H. & Hemberg, H. 1998. Health care, ethics and nursing in Bangladesh: a personal perspective. *Nursing Ethics* 5(6): 535-542.
Begum, H. 1998. Relevance of genetic information in a developing country. *IAB News*, Issue 8, Autumn.
Begum, H. 2001. Poverty and health ethics in developing countries. *Bioethics* 15(1): 50-56.
Singer, P. 1979. *Practical ethics*. Cambridge: Cambridge University Press.

15 Bioethics in China

Ya-li Cong

I. Introduction: Characteristics of China's Bioethics

A. *The Definition of Bioethics in China*

It is first necessary to define "bioethics" and "medical ethics" in China. According to an American definition of "bioethics":

> The term "bioethics," as it was first used by the biologist Van Rensselaer Potter, referred to a new field devoted to human survival and an improved quality of life, not necessarily or particularly medical in character. The term soon was used differently, however, particularly to distinguish it from the much older field of medical ethics. The traditional domain of medical ethics would be included within this array, accompanied now by many other topics and problems (Callahan, 1995, p. 250).

Most scholars in China, on the contrary, place bioethics within the domain of medical ethics. They regard medical ethics as a broader category, where bioethics is a branch of medical ethics. For example, the first book with "bioethics" in the title was published in 1987, and the author, Ren-zong Qiu, wrote that "bioethics" is an extension of medical ethics (Qiu, 1987, p. 6). Zhi-zheng Du thought that bioethics and medical ethics should not be taken as two unrelated branches of learning; bioethics is not only the inheritance but also the development of medical ethics (Du, 2000, p. 155). Until now, most Chinese scholars did not isolate bioethics from medical ethics. When mentioning "bioethics", they usually mean that the content is related to biomedical technology and dilemmas such as euthanasia, test tube babies, cloning, and organ transplantation. Bioethics, as a new period of medical ethics, emerged in the late 1980s, with evidence of several cases of euthanasia and artificial insemination by donor. Currently, many issues of bioethics are not very urgent for most clinicians and the field of medicine generally in China, but bioethics will become more important over time (Du, 2000, p. 147).

B. *The Characteristics of Medical Ethics in China*

Just like the status of Hippocrates in Western medical ethics, Si-miao Sun (581-682 A.D.) is the symbol of traditional medical ethics in China. His *On the Absolute Sincerity of the*

Great Physician was the first full-length explicit statement on medical morality. Unlike Hippocrates, who emphasized rules of behavior (e.g., do not perform abortions for women, respect the privacy of patients, and so forth), Si-miao Sun emphasized relationships: treat patients just as if they were members of one's own family, without regard for personal financial interests. This reflects certain characteristics of medical ethics in China: for example, attending to patients' emotional side and not simply to their rational side; maintaining a harmonious relationship with patients not by signing contracts, but through the physician's love for the patient and by the patient's gratitude to the physician; and, although the relationship between different people is not equal, the physician treats each person equally. Generally speaking, if we take American bioethics as an example of Western style bioethics, scholars of both the East and the West tend to use such comparisons as: individualism versus communitarianism, autonomous versus familial decision-making, individual development and perfection versus commitments to family and filial piety, or contract versus trust (Nie, 2000, p. 246). But this does not adequately represent the characteristics of Chinese bioethics, so we must deepen the analysis by understanding the cultural background of China.

1. *Emphasis on a harmonious doctor–patient relationship.* In China, the doctor–patient relationship refers not only to the relationship between physician and patient, but also to the relationship between the physician and the patient's family members. Physicians interact with the family as a whole rather than with the patient as an isolated individual, and this directly characterizes many special aspects of medical ethics in China. Traditionally, physicians pursued a good relationship with their patients, treating patients as family members; in other words, maintaining a good relationship depends on inner love instead of external restraints.

Equality is not the character of the doctor–patient relationship in China. Obedience to the physician is a psychological habit of the common people; however, even more important is the physician's focus on the interests of his patients. The traditional paternalistic model was strengthened by the system of protectiveness following the establishment of the People's Republic of China (PRC), which still has deep roots in the current psyche of physicians, patients, and their family members. The protective system (which was clearly emphasized in article three of the law: "The norms of medical ethics and measures for their implementation for health care personnel", issued by the Ministry of Health in 1988) is not only favored by physicians but also by many patients. If family members do not tell the patient the diagnosis, few patients claim that it is their right to know the information. Some enjoy being cared for and are content with everything being decided and done by family members; furthermore, they may feel abandoned if they must decide everything for themselves. Family members tend to believe physicians and hope that physicians will help them to make appropriate decisions. So, the paternalistic model of the doctor–patient relationship still plays a dominant role in clinical practice, but the present situation in China is not optimal.

2. *Family autonomy and informed consent.* Unlike modern Western societies, where the patient is autonomous and gives his own informed consent, in China, the family is autonomous and usually gives the informed consent on behalf of the patient. For example, physicians first disclose the diagnosis or the results of an examination to a family member instead of to the patient. The patient and his family are always regarded as a unit. In the physician's eyes, the patient's family fully represents the patient's interests. When

the physician needs informed consent, he will discuss the medical situation with the family members, one of whom will make the decision. Deeply affected by the paternalistic model, family members even tend simply to accept the physician's treatment suggestions. The typical example of this is that a family member (who is usually the leader of the family) signs the consent form for surgery, while the patient does not even know the details of the procedure before the surgery, let alone consent on his own behalf.

A recent development regarding human rights in China should be mentioned. Within the last decade, more and more people are demanding respect for basic human rights, especially patients' rights. Only since September 1, 2002, when the Ministry of Health and the State of Drug Administration co-issued a new notice about how to write a standard medical record, has it become permissible for a patient himself to sign the forms authorizing surgery and certain other risky procedures. This development is only a trial, however.

3. *Medical ethics as the closest combination of general ethics and medicine.* In ancient China, medical books were mostly written in the classic Chinese literary style, which was rather abstruse and difficult for people to understand. It was commonly recognized that in order to become a medical doctor, one must read a vast range of books, particularly the Four Books and Five Classics (Peng, 2000, S. 23). These books themselves are full of moral statements (many books in ancient China were about moral behavior and personal cultivation), and so naturally they were deeply influential. "Confucian physician" was another name for the physician, which showed the close combination of general ethics and medicine.

Benevolence is the core of general ethics, and self-cultivation is key; so it is also in medical ethics. The purpose of medicine is to save people by love, which was also the goal of Confucianism, so the intrinsic goals of medicine and Confucianism are the same. Benevolence became the theoretical foundation of medical ethics during that time. Bu Lin, a famous physician of the Song Dynasty, once said: "if there is no permanent morality, there is no medical practice"; this saying is still very familiar to many physicians. In the Song and Ming dynasties, many Confucians rushed into the field of medicine, creating a unique circumstance of Confucian medicine. Shi-gong Chen (1555-1636 A.D., Ming Dynasty) noted in his "Five Commandments and Ten Requirements for Physicians": the first requirement is to understand Confucianism, the second is to understand medicine (Ben-fu Li et al., 1996, p. 14). Interestingly, this article is the only standard Chinese work collected in the appendix of Volume 5 of the *Encyclopedia of Bioethics* (first edition). Similarly, Ting-xian Gong, a physician in the Ming Dynasty, also expressed the same idea in his "Ten Requirements of Physicians": the first requirement is to have a benevolent heart, the second is to understand Confucianism, the third is to master the knowledge of the pulse, the fourth is to know the causes of disease, and the tenth is to never attempt to make money (Li, 1996, p. 14).

China's ethics differs from the ethics of other cultures, especially in its emphasis on self-cultivation. Many doctors of different historical periods held the view that the doctor's self-cultivation was of great importance. As one physician noted, a doctor should rectify himself first, then he should know the principles of medicine (Zhang, 2000, p. 158). These ideas could help physicians refrain from doing wrong actions.

Being connected closely with politics is another important characteristic of Chinese general ethics (Tai-heng Liu, 2000), and this is true also for medical ethics. We can understand Chinese medical ethics as a feudal and socialist style of medical ethics, and this affects some current issues of medical ethics in China, especially those that stem from health care policies.

4. *The lack of strict organizational professional codes.* Medical education and practice in China were characterized by individuals and the family, with medical associations or organizations lagging behind. There was no need to formulate universally accepted professional codes (Zhang, 2000, S. 10), since the core of benevolence was shared by all.

II. The History of Chinese Medical Ethics and its Development

It is commonly accepted that the history of medical ethics in China can be divided into four phases: feudal Confucianism's medical morality, intermediate period medical ethics, socialist medical ethics, and contemporary medical ethics. Bioethics is a new chapter in contemporary medical ethics.

A. Feudal Confucianism's Medical Morality[1]

1. *Ethics, once established, had a strong connection to politics.* China's culture is mainly a kind of ethical culture, and China's philosophy is an ethical philosophy. During the 2000 years of the feudal system,[2] the division of labor was not developed, and society stressed the importance of human science, not natural science; agriculture, not industry and business. Every family was an independent productive unit, and the patriarchal clan system was the foundation for family regulation.

Since its establishment as the dominant school of ethics, Confucianism was combined closely with politics. Its creator, Confucius (551-479 B.C.), based most of his ideas on the patriarchal clan system; he dreamt of establishing a benevolent society and advocated his ethical, political, and educational thoughts towards this goal. Benevolence was the core of Confucianism, and the benevolent government was esteemed. The way to rule a country was by morality, not by law. He and Mencius (Mengzi, another great scholar of Confucianism) thought that people had an innate nature of kindness: all men have a sense of compassion, a sense of shame, a sense of respect, and a sense of discriminating right and wrong. These good virtues existed at first as seeds in the mind of everyone, so that every man, no matter whether he is the emperor or a common person, has the capacity to become a sage. It is necessary, however, to cultivate and temper oneself in one's social life. As a result, these virtues were also regarded as the foundations of medical virtues. Emphasis on the doctors' moral cultivation forms a major component of Chinese medical morality.

Zhong-shu Dong (179-104 B.C.), a great scholar, propagandized Confucianism and persuaded an emperor of the Han Dynasty to believe in the efficacy of Confucianism for consolidating his rule in 134 B.C.; since then, all emperors have held only Confucianism in great esteem, rejecting all other schools of ethics. Zhong-shu Dong developed the Confucian school, establishing a well-organized ideological system, the core of which are the "three cardinal guides" and the "five standards". The "three cardinal guides" suggests that the ruler guides the subject, the father guides the son, and the husband guides the wife. In all three, the latter must be absolutely loyal to the former. The "five standards" are: *ren, yi, li, zhi,* and *xin. Ren* (benevolence) means to love other people, not ourselves; *yi* represents justice, righteous, and rectifying ourselves, not others; *li* means difference, obedience, and people being in different hierarchies according to different standards; *zhi* means not only knowledge, but also an ability to identify what is morally right or wrong;

xin means honesty, promise-keeping, and doing what one says one will do. In Chinese, the word "ethics" is represented by two words *lun* and *li*; the former means different hierarchies, and the latter means that people in different hierarchies should obey different rules. The greatest success of Zhong-shu Dong was that he combined the school of *yin*, *yang*, and five phases[3] with the ethical idea of the three cardinal guides and the five standards. Zhong-shu Dong used the natural law to show the reasons for ethical standards, and the common people were instilled with the idea that they must obey these standards that represent morality; otherwise, they would be immoral and be punished by "heaven" (the natural God). In the *Miraculous Pivot*, one of the two bibles of ancient Chinese medical literature, it was noted that a man who mastered medicine could keep the ordinary people as well as himself in good health, so that a harmonious society could be formed and maintained (Zhang, 2000, S. 9). It is clear that general ethics was the foundation of political government: it connected morality, health, and society naturally and closely. Zhong-yan Fan, a famous scholar and statesman, once said: if you cannot become a good prime minister, then become a good physician.

The well-being of the total human person consists of being a cultivated person, having good human relationships, and living in a well-ordered society. This was demonstrated clearly in "the great learning" through eight steps: investigation of things, extension of knowledge, sincerity of the will, rectification of the mind, cultivation of personal life, regulation of the family, national order, and world peace (Soo, 1987, p. 698). It is insufficient if we think of personal cultivation only on the level of behavior and moral standards. The reason why self-cultivation is the most important step in Chinese moral practice is that it is the essential link of the eight steps: the former four are the foundation of cultivation, and the latter three are the effect of cultivation (Jiao, 1997, p. 383). Mengzi once said: if we can take care of our own parents and extend this care to other people's parents, and love our own children and extend this love to other people's children, then the world is under our control. So, politics is not only connected to the ethical ideas of the people but also to their behavior. This can be shown by a well-known Chinese antithetical couplet: the sound of wind, the sound of rain, the sound of reading, all we can hear; the affair of family, the affair of country, the affair of the world, everything for which we should care.

Continuing on the eight steps listed above, the next step after self-cultivation is to serve the family well, for only after that can you serve the country and the world well. Confucianism instructed people to tell right from wrong by self-examination, rather than by proposing external standards or codes of conduct to restrict general behavior, which is one reason why China lacks a professional code of medical morality.

2. Filial piety and the doctor–patient relationship. Following the three cardinal guides, Confucianism took the relationship between father and son as the foundation for all other relationships. As a human being, the most important responsibility is to repay one's parents. *Filial Canon*, an ancient book on filial piety, noted that filial piety starts with loyalty to parents, then loyalty to the emperor, and ends at self-cultivation (Chen, Y.,1985, p. 229). The idea behind filial piety is that if the people are loyal, it is impossible for them to rebel, and society will be stable. Loyalty to one's parents means respecting and obeying them, not disgracing them, supporting them, and remembering them after they die. Among the three most "unfilial" things, having no children is the worst. In the Tang Dynasty, not being loyal to one's parents was one of the ten crimes.

Young children should be obedient to their parents, but parents in their old age should be obedient to their adult children, especially when they are sick. This is an important reason why doctors need only to receive informed consent from family members, instead of from the patient himself. Another interesting historical fact is that an important motive to learn and practice medicine was to care for one's parents in case they became ill.

To generalize from loyalty to parents to loyalty to the emperor is a common way of thinking in China. When the interest of the family conflicts with that of the country, then sacrificing the happiness of the family is advocated; this is regarded as "great filial piety". The extreme case is when a person dies for a just cause, while a less extreme case is when a person sacrifices his own happiness for the happiness of his whole family. So, Chinese traditional morality emphasizes not the rights of the individual, but one's responsibility to the community. Similarly, the rights of the physician are not central, but rather the responsibility of the physician to his patients; as a result, physicians usually make decisions according to their own judgment in the interest of their patients, without getting the patient's (or a family member's) informed consent. Currently, many Chinese have begun to pay significant attention to "individual rights", but we still cannot say that the principle of autonomy is first among moral principles.

3. *The effect of Taoism and Buddhism on medical ethics.* Generally speaking, the traditional culture of China was the result of the co-existence of three religions. Although less obvious, the philosophy of Taoism and Buddhism exerted a strong influence on Chinese society. Confucianism was the dominant school and always forms the mainstream of thought in society (Cai, 1996, p. 55); the ideas of other religions that conflicted with Confucianism were typically rejected.

In contrast to Confucianism, the philosophy of Taoism is that one should do nothing but live a natural life and not be involved in social trouble; then one will not lose anything, and in this way can people reach the state of immortality. Buddhism, to some extent, is similar to Taoism. Influenced by the spirits of *karma* or "preordained fate", many Buddhists practiced good deeds by practicing medicine. Si-miao Sun wrote in his *On the Absolute Sincerity of the Great Physician*: being a great physician, one should relieve tension and calm the mind, and not have any desires or needs. This should be the realm of Buddhism. Moreover, from the title of his article, "Five Commandments and Ten Requirements for Physicians", we can see that Shi-gong Chen was also affected by the five commandments of Buddhism.

After absorbing the essence of Taoism and Buddhism, Neo-Confucianism was developed systematically in the Song and Ming Dynasties (Chen, S.-F., 1996, p. 286). Compared with the other four standards, *ren* (benevolence) was highlighted as the only core, and it is explained as being the only one from "heaven's law" and not from human nature. Similar to religious doctrines of the Western Middle Ages, the natural desires of people were strictly constrained, which formed the main reason why China has a strong tradition of restraining one's desires and of not emphasizing individual rights and autonomy, but rather duties and the priority of the family's and country's interests.

Another factor which needs to be mentioned is the methodology of the golden mean. The advantage of the golden mean is that it builds harmonious relationships: it can reconcile everything and even absorb the useful ideas of Taoism and Buddhism. One of its problems, however, is that it cannot make opposing sides argue and discuss and, as a result, it is sometimes difficult to progress. To summarize, it is not surprising that, because of the rigid feudal system, the period of feudal medical morality lasted for more than 2000 years. What the scholars in a different dynasty did was to explain the words of the schol-ars of a previous dynasty. The 2000 years of the feudal system was just a closed cycle of intellectual repetition. What changed was only the *name* of the dynasty, not the *content* of the dynasty. The same was true for Chinese feudal medical morality.

B. The Intermediate Period of Medical Ethics

The Opium War (1840) forced China to open its doors to the rest of the world. The cycle of the feudal system could no longer continue. The medicine of the West came into China, bringing its values along with it.

After the final dynasty, the Qing, was abolished by Zhong-shan Sun (Sun Yatsen) in 1911, and the Republic of China was set up, the rule of Confucianism lost its political roots and bases. Zhong-shan Sun was deeply influenced by Western culture, so he accepted the ideas of humanitarianism and held the ethical ideal of combining the cultures of the East and West (Chen, S.-F., 1997, p. 106). Some young intellectuals, such as Du-xiu Chen, Da-zhao Li, and others, were influenced by Western thought and were involved in the revolutionary activities. Marxism, as a political ideology, was almost totally new and different from both Confucianism and Western democracy. However, once con-verted, Du-xiu Chen became one of its most forceful promoters. Chen criticized Confucianism sharply in the Movement of May 4, 1919, arguing that traditional Chinese morality made son auxiliary to father, wife auxiliary to husband, and people auxiliary to emperor, and all of these relationships resulted in a slave morality and killed human nature and individual personality (Chen, S.-F., 1997, p. 149). So, Chen thought, only if people eradicated the old ideas could they establish a new communist party. All of this paved the way for the Chinese socialist style of medical ethics.

The Chinese Medical Association was established in 1915 and, just like the condition of medicine, medical ethics was in an intermediate state between West and East. For the first time in the 1910s, Feng-bin Yu translated the newest edition of the "Ethical Standards of the American Medical Association" as a reference for Chinese colleagues (Xu, 1998, p. 122). In 1932, Guo-bin Song wrote *The Ethics of the Medical Profession*, the first systematic book of medical ethics, and it still regarded *ren* and *yi* as the two basic components of ethics. He emphasized the physician's personality and three kinds of basic relationships: between physician and patient, physician and physician, and physician and society (He, 1988, pp. 226-227).

C. Socialist Medical Ethics

Marxism is a kind of political ideology and, being the absolutely dominant school in China, it affected the formulation of socialist medical ethics, which is also a continuation of the tradition of ethics closely connected with politics. Chairman Mao wrote for the Chinese Medical University in May 1941: "rescue the dying, heal the wounded, and serve the people wholeheartedly". This penetrated into all medical professionals and because the forerunner of the socialist principle of medical ethics. During the War of Resistance against Japan (1937-1945), Chairman Mao published "In Memory of Dr. Norman Bethune" and "Serve the People": he called on people to learn from Dr. Bethune, who came from Canada and dedicated himself to the care of Chinese soldiers. Chairman Mao argued: if one died for the people, it was a worthy death and it weighed more than Mount Tai; otherwise, it was lighter than a feather. The essay on Bethune was viewed as an incomparable formulation of medical ethics during the Maoist era (Qiu, 1995, p. 1486).

After the People's Republic of China was established in 1949, socialist communism was the basic principle in the field of general ethics and can be expressed as: "I for everybody and everybody for me" – but the former was emphasized. Under its guidance, a very new style of DPR was formed. Almost everyone could enjoy equal medical care and the relationship between different people was equal, too. Physicians treated patients for the country and patients accepted the treatment also for the country; there was no conflict of interest, so naturally the DPR was very good.

In the 1950s, China followed the Soviet protectiveness model of medicine. This ideology argued that the psychological relationship of the patient to his or her disease was so significant that patients should be protected from all unpleasant stimuli, which might retard the healing process. It is the duty of health care professionals to mobilize all the strengths of the patient against his or her disease and to develop this attitude of strength in the patient (Pang, 1999, p. 249). Also, the tradition of family was still central, so the patient's right of informed consent was usually ignored.

D. Contemporary Medical Ethics

Contemporary Chinese medical ethics can be dated from 1979, when a medical dialectic conference was held in Guangzhou. This conference was sponsored by the Chinese Society for Dialectics of Nature and the China Association of Science and Technology.[4]

The most important year in the history of medical ethics in China is 1981, because the first national medical ethics meeting was held in Shanghai that year. Participants came from 21 provinces and autonomous regions. This meeting became the cornerstone of contemporary medical ethics in China. Some basic issues (e.g., the content of the subject, its principles, and so forth) and some special issues (e.g., euthanasia, organ transplantation, medical experimentation, and so forth) were discussed. The most important result was the determination of "the principle of socialist medical morality"[5]: Rescue the dying, heal the wounded, prevent illness, cure disease, implement revolutionary humanism, and maintain the health of the people wholeheartedly. Also, the summary of the meeting and a proposal to offer a medical ethics course in medical schools were both passed by the first meeting, which were reported by the Xinhua Agency. The Ministry of Health and the Chinese Science Society also reported the news.

The second national medical ethics meeting was held in 1982 in Dalian, where more participants attended; the third meeting, in 1984, was in Fuzhou; the fourth, in 1986, in Nanning; the eighth, in 1995; the ninth, in 1997; the tenth, in 1999; and the eleventh, in 2001.

On December 15, 1988, the Ministry of Health formulated a code of conduct for health care personnel. The name of the code is "The Norms of Medical Ethics and Implementation Measures for Health Care Personnel" and is composed of 11 articles. In article three, seven clauses were written about the moral standards in detail: relieve the pain of patients as much as possible, respect the patients and treat them equally, maintain confidentiality, implement protective treatment, respect other colleagues, and keep improving. This is the first time the concept of patients' rights is mentioned.

Medical students swear an oath after enrollment, but it is not the Hippocratic Oath, but the one promulgated by the Ministry of Education of China in 1991. The oath for medical students in China is:

A patient's health relates to us, a patient's life relies on us.
I solemnly swear upon arriving at this sacred medical school:
I will pledge myself to consecrate my life to the medical profession;
I will love my country, be loyal to my people, and I will abide by medical morality;
I will give to my teachers the respect and gratitude which is their due;
I will practice my profession with conscience and dignity;
I will advance medical science continuously and diligently;
I will relieve a patient's suffering by all means, maintain the honor and noble traditions
    of the medical profession.
Rescue the dying, heal the wounded, face hardship, and devote myself to the develop-
    ment of the medical profession and the health of human kind (Zhang, 2000, p. 411).

The revolution of 1911 and the movement of May 4 brought about the collapse of the traditional Chinese social structure, but the traditional Chinese values never completely disappeared. Even after the Great Cultural Revolution in late the 1960s and 1970s, when
many traditions were criticized, some ideas from Confucianism are still alive in social life.
Also, people's attitudes have gradually changed from sanctity of life to quality of life and
from fear of death to facing death and hospice realistically. At the same time, because of
these changes, many ethical issues have emerged.

III. Specific Topics

A. Bioethics in General

1. *Important institutions of medical ethics in China.* The Medical Ethics Association, a
branch of the Chinese Medical Association, was established in October 1988. The chairman of the first class was Zhi-zheng Du, director of the journal *Medicine and Philosophy*.
Now, Professor Ben-fu Li, director of the department of medical ethics at the Beijing
University Health Science Center, is the chair of the second class. There are four special
committees in the Medical Ethics Association: education, law and regulation, learning
exchange, and academics. Below the Medical Ethics Association, there is the level of the
Association found in most of China's 30 provinces. The Medical Ethics Association has
not practiced a system of membership.

Until now, the Medical Ethics Association has drawn up and passed at least five ethical papers: "Hospitals Should do a Morality Examination and Establish Medical Morality Files" (draft 1990); "Organizational Regulations of Medical Ethics Committee" (1995),
"On the Measurement and Ethical Requests Towards the Final Phase of Chronic Diseases",
"The Ethical Principles of Organ Transplantation", and "The Rights and Responsibilities
of Patients" (1998).

Since the early 1990s, medical schools, institutions, and scholars have communicated
and collaborated with scholars from other countries. In 1992, China became a member of
the International Association of Bioethics (IAB). In November 1995, the East Asian
Conference on Bioethics was held in Beijing and at that conference the constitution for the

East Asian Association of Bioethics was established. In addition, China became a member of the Asian Bioethics Association (ABA) in November 1998 in Tokyo.

The Chinese Nursing Association, established in 1909, does not have a branch of nursing ethics yet, and there is no specialized journal of nursing ethics. An important conference on the drafting of the 21st century ethical norms for Chinese nurses was held in April 2000. The draft is composed of 21 clauses and divided into five parts: general rules, respect for life and raising the quality of life, respect for the rights and personalities of people, clearly knowing the demands of society and working as a team for the people's health, and continuously improving and ensuring high quality of nursing care (Pang, M.-C.S. 2000, p. 518).

2. *Important personalities in bioethics.* Zhi-zheng Du, Ren-zong Qiu, Zhao-xiong He, Hong-zhu Zhang, Ben-fu Li, and Da-pu Shi are famous scholars in the field of medical ethics. Zhi-zheng Du's *Outline of Medical Ethics*, published in 1985, was the first systematic textbook of medical ethics after the cultural revolution of the 1960s and 1970s. Ren-zong Qiu's *Bioethics*, published in 1987, was the first bioethics book in China and it contains many fresh ideas and cases from the West, digging the virgin land of this new field, and developing it with the help of many scholars from foreign countries. Zhao-xiong He's *History of Chinese Medical Morality*, published in 1988, provided abundant materials on medical ethics from ancient to current China. Hong-zhu Zhang's *Survey of Chinese and Foreign Medical Moral Standards*, published in 2000, contains a full and accurate treatment of moral codes. Ben-fu Li's *Textbook of Medical Ethics*, published in 1996, is a useful textbook for medical students.

China does not have a journal specifically called "bioethics" or "nursing ethics" in the mainland, but two journals have much influence in this field: *Medicine and Philosophy* and *Chinese Medical Ethics*, whose initial issues were published in 1980 and 1988, respectively. Other journals that also publish articles in medical ethics are: *Medicine and Society, Morality and Civilization, Research of Natural Dialectics, Philosophy Trend, Chinese Journal of Hospital Management, Medical Education, Chinese Journal of Nursing*, and the social sciences editions of the academic journals of some leading medical schools. Also, there are some newsletters, e.g., the newsletter of the Chinese Medical Ethics Association, the Chinese Bioethics Newsletter (Hong Kong), and newsletters from each province where medical ethics branches are established. Also, the first dictionary of Chinese medical ethics was published in 2002.

3. *The dominant bioethical theory of China.* Objectively speaking, China does not have dominant bioethical theories by the names of "deontology" and "utilitarianism", but in fact we utilize the ideas of both. The difference is that China traditionally weighs deontology over utilitarianism. If we say (albeit reluctantly) that the dominant theory in China is a virtue theory that is rooted in Confucianism, then Chinese medical ethics is also a virtue theory. "That ethics highlights a spirit of self-sacrifice and self-cultivation, a high sense of responsibility, modesty, self-control, devotion, and other virtues" (Nie, 2000, p. 240). Its ideas include sanctity of life and a duty-based ethics of medicine, and it still emphasizes that public benefits should be given priority over individual benefits, when they conflict (Wu, 1994, p. 370).

The four principles of Western bioethics (autonomy, beneficence, non-maleficience, and justice) were introduced into China in 1988 by Ren-zong Qiu's series of papers in the *Chinese Journal of Nursing* (Qiu, 1988, pp. 59-60, 115-117, 177-179). These four principles were commonly accepted among the medical ethics scholars, especially in the academic field, and they were taught to medical students. But the former socialist principles are more familiar among clinicians. The understanding of the four principles among scholars is also interpreted in a Chinese way: "In the field of medical care, both Chinese and Americans would accept the principle of respect for autonomy and the principle of beneficence as ethically relevant. ...Americans would give more weight to this principle of respect for autonomy, whereas Chinese would give more weight to the principle of beneficence" (Fan, 1997, pp. 196-197).

Two basic arguments have always existed throughout the history of China: one concerns the nature of humankind (whether it is good or evil), the other concerns the conflict between *yi* and *li* (which is more important, justice or self-interest?), which is something like the conflict between deontology and utilitarianism. Because of the dominant status of Confucianism, people tend to think the nature of humankind is good and prefer *yi* to *li*. Zhong-shu Dong's words, quoted by almost every Confucianism scholar, are: "no matter what you do, you should only care if it is just, you should not care [about] the benefit and effect" (Chen, Y., 1985, p. 268). So, the dominant ethical theory in China is almost deontological. This does not mean there is no notion of utilitarianism, but it could not become more important nor become mainstream. During the last two decades, some scholars have discussed the idea that China should set up an ethical theory that combines humanitarianism and utilitarianism in order to resolve many bioethical dilemmas. In fact, more and more people in Chinese society hold some utilitarian values, especially after the market economy began in the early 1980s, but we still cannot say that it has become the dominant theory yet.

B. Professionalism: The Patient-Health Care Professional Relationship

1. *The current condition of the doctor–patient relationship in China.* Currently, China is undergoing the darkest period of the doctor–patient relationship in its history: more and more patients sue hospitals and doctors, and many cases of medical disputes have been shown on television, which further aggravates the condition of the doctor–patient relationship. It is reported that in Beijing in 2001 there were 500 occasions when a patient hit a physician. The most serious case was when a patient killed his physician because the physician could not cure his leukemia after the patient had run out of money.

Generally speaking, a crisis of trust exists between patients and physicians: physicians do not open their hearts to patients, but only think of how to protect themselves from being sued. Previously, physicians held the belief that even if they are only one percent certain about a procedure, they will try their 100 percent best. But now they will do surgery only when they are 100 percent certain that it will succeed.

2. *The complicated reasons behind poor doctor–patient relationships: from the perspective of the doctor.* When inquiring into the causes of poor doctor–patient relationships, different questionnaires draw different conclusions, but most show that the main reason is the bad attitude and quality of service of doctors. After that, a common complaint is that doctors do not have a high sense of respect for patients. Some departments are too busy, where a physician regularly must treat 60 outpatients per day; they cannot bear the pressure of so much work and cannot deal with so many relationships. Afraid of being sued, many physicians do not do their best to treat patients, so the quality of

service cannot be guaranteed. Moreover, some physicians ask patients to have unnecessary examinations and prescribe expensive drugs for financial reasons, which are important reasons for conflict. Finally, doctors doubt that patients are able to face the risks
and unforeseen reactions of drugs and surgery, so they are reluctant to perform these
procedures.

3. *From the perspective of the patient.* The sense of individuals' and patients' rights has
increased in China very rapidly, but the doctors' attitudes have not changed at the same
rate. Patients have different demands: many patients think medical service is too expensive to afford, some are not satisfied with the environment of the hospital, and it is difficult for physicians to meet every patient. Some patients have the misunderstanding that
modern medicine can cure most diseases.

4. *From the perspective of government policy and hospital management.* The insurance system in China has not developed well: the government does not provide enough
funding for the hospitals and, as a result, the hospital lays the economic task on doctors.
Small hospitals cannot survive and large hospitals are too crowded. Hospitals usually
charge more than patients should pay and the way of appraising a medical accident or
medical malpractice incident is unfair, since the appraising institute usually just makes
excuses for the hospital and physician. Patients are not even allowed to see their own
medical records and even the courts are sometimes prohibited by hospitals from copying
the medical records of a patient who is suing a physician. Access to medical records
should become easier after April 1, 2002, when the law on "Regulation of Medical
Accidents" was issued. The law allows medical records to be copied by patients, and the
system of appraising medical accidents and malpractice is also reformed and has become
more transparent.

C. Reproduction: Birth Control
1. *The background of birth control.* After the People's Republic of China was founded,
the population rose rapidly, the main reasons of which (besides the traditional idea of
"more children, more happiness") were the need for a stable society, the good health care
insurance system, and the preventative health policy. Plus, because of Chairman Mao's
closed-door policy and his slogan "more people, more strength" (to fight against imperi-
alism), from only 1962 to 1972 the Chinese population increased by 300 million. At the
end of the 1970s, Xiao-ping Deng saw clearly the relationship between the population
and the economy, so the Chinese government decided to control the size of the population
by making this an explicit requirement in the "Constitution of the People's Republic of
China" in 1982. By February 15 1995, China's population had reached 1.2 billion (see
"Chinese White Paper of 1995 on Family Planning", http://www.xinhuanet.com/zhengfu/
jingtai/zf_bps199501.htm).

2. *Different attitudes towards family planning.* The "Chinese White Paper on Population and Development in the 21st Century" stated that the traditional idea of "marry earlier, bear earlier", "more children, more happiness", and "bear children for the aged" had
changed gradually to "marry later, bear later", "bear less, bear healthier", and "boy and
girl are the same". (http://www.xinhuanet.com/zhengfu/jingtai/zf_bps200005.htm).

Economic factors play an important role in controlling the population, and it is common sense that people do not want too many children, but there remains a disagreement

about whether the one child policy is totally accepted. A questionnaire and interview done on the spot by Xinxiang Medical College of Henan province shows that more than 50% of those interviewed want two children, 30% want one child, but more than 50% prefer one boy, especially in the undeveloped regions (more than 70%). People want to have a boy to succeed the family line and to care for them when they become old (Liu, 2000, pp. 38-39). So the conflict between people and the policy lies in "one boy" to a great extent. "Handing down the family name from generation to generation" is a very strong tradition, and only a boy can continue the family name. This conclusion is similar to that of a report of Jing-neng Li:

> According to the National Statistic Bureau in 1989, among married women in Liaoning province and Beijing, correspondingly 79.7% and 86.4% want two or two more children; moreover, in Guangdong, Gansu and Guizhou provinces, more than 90% want two or two more children. Most of them prefer boys. Another 850 women of 20 villages in 20 counties, 50.55% couples hope to have two children, 45.41% hope to have three or more children; meanwhile, they show the preference of boys (Li, 2000).

But another survey showed a different result: "A survey by the Chinese Society of Sociology found that a majority of peasants in the villages near cities want two or more children, whereas the majority of respondents in cities are satisfied with one child" (Qiu, 1995, p. 1487). The "Chinese White Paper of 1995 on Family Planning" stated:

> Though we had succeeded in family planning, it is not balanced in different regions. Some regions still have a high ratio of birth, and the working method and service level need improvement in most countryside and some undeveloped regions. Also, some new problems emerge: sex ratio, the population to age, etc. (http://www.xinhuanet.com/zhengfu/jingtai/zf_bps199501.htm).

3. *The ethical issues of family planning.* Together with economic change, some traditional biases in Chinese society seem alive and well. Several Chinese population studies have shown that the male-to-female sex ratio increases sharply for second and subsequent births. Connected to this is that more female babies than male babies die in infancy. A "Study on the Abnormal Phenomena of Sex Differentials in Infant and Child Mortality in China" revealed that the gap in mortality between female and male infants was highest in regions where women have relatively low social status and the economic conditions and medical care are relatively poor (Han, 1999, p. 11).

Besides the sex ratio, the most controversial issue is informed consent about contraception, which does not stem from cultural tradition but from the low quality of family planning workers. A case happened in a village of the Heilongjiang province where the fact that the wife could not become pregnant almost made the couple divorce. Only when a county physician came to the village with an ultrasonic machine did the wife discover that an IUD had been placed inside her without her consent after she had an abortion three years prior. The case is now being heard (2001b). In fact, this kind of case is not unique, especially in the countryside, and the government has become aware of its danger. In the "Chinese White Paper on Population and Development in the 21st Century", in the section on the aims of population and development, the first goal is to practice the service of reproductive health and to develop the informed selection of the methods of contraception. (http://www.xinhuanet.com/zhengfu/jingtai/zf_bps200005.htm)

D. Reproduction: Abortion

The reality of abortion in China is that most people do not regard it as an ethical issue. This is related not only to the policy of family planning but also to the traditional idea that a human being begins at birth. Also, if an issue is already legislated, it is common sense in China that most people will not re-think it from the angle of ethics. But physicians face a serious ethical problem when a fetus, especially older than seven months, is born alive after a failed abortion; this situation was at its worst during in the 1980s.

Presently, many young women face premarital abortions and their potential dangers – the main reason for infertility is abortion (and a greater number of abortions increases the risk). Even if a post-abortive women can become pregnant, the child will likely have a low birth weight. Although RU-486 (a legal prescription drug widely used for early-term abortions) may not be sold in drug shops, it is clear from media reports that it can be easily purchased. So, the non-prescription use of the drug may lead to complications stemming from the lack of a physician's examination and supervision.

E. Reproduction: Artificial Insemination and In Vitro Fertilization

1. *Cases related to reproduction technology.* The first child of artificial insemination by donor (AID) was born in the Hunan province in 1982, and the first test tube baby was born on March 10, 1988 in Beijing. Through 1997, 90 test tube babies were born in China (Ni, 2000, p. 174). In 1988, the first conference on social, ethical, and legal issues in reproductive technology was held, just after the first legal case concerning AID, which happened in Shanghai in 1987. The couple could not have a child because of the husband's infertility and, after an agreement between the husband and wife, they finally had a child through AID. But the husband's older brother said the whole family could not accept such a child and they even drove the wife away. Then the wife sued the husband and they divorced. Another interesting case began on August 8, 2001, when a woman named Xue-li Zheng wanted to have a child through AID for her husband, who had been sentenced to the death penalty because of murder. The Middle Court of Zhoushan city of Zhejiang province did not allow it and the wife appealed the decision to the high court (2001c). With the execution of Zheng's husband in January 2002, her hope has vanished.

2. *The management of reproduction technology.* Based on the infertility rate (7-10%), a huge number of families need the help of reproductive technology, but many problems have emerged because of poor management of the clinics (e.g., using famous individuals' sperm donations to set up sperm banks for profit, the high price for a test tube baby, the widespread use of *in vitro* fertilization for profit, and the low utilization ratio of regular sperm banks).

Two laws, "Management Measure of Artificial Reproduction Technology" and "Management Measures of Sperm Banks", were put into effect on August 1, 2001. The law required strict standards on technological equipment and quality of medical professionals; it also requires a medical ethics committee at each clinic. Surrogate motherhood was also temporarily forbidden. Before this law was published, an older sister became pregnant for her younger sister; they both agreed that the mother of the child was the younger sister but, according to hospital policy, only the woman who gives birth to the baby is the mother on the birth certificate, so the hospital could not change the name of the mother.

Concerning human cloning, the Ministry of Health (1997) published a statement of "do not approve, support, allow, or accept" it on March 19, 1997.

F. Death and Dying: Euthanasia and Physician-Assisted Suicide
1. *The brief history of euthanasia in China.*[6] The first court case regarding euthanasia happened in the Hanzhong region of the Shanxi province in 1986; it did not end until 1992, when the physician was declared innocent. On December 24, 1987, several institutions (the Chinese Academy of Social Science, the Chinese Association for Dialectics of Nature, Beijing Hospital, and so forth) held a conference on euthanasia, and a month later it was broadcast on the radio by China Center People's Broadcast Station, which had a great effect on the population. Several hundred listeners wrote letters to the broadcast station, one of whom was Ying-chao Deng, wife of first Premier En-lai Zhou. She wrote that accepting euthanasia is a Marxist materialist attitude, that she will accept it if she is in the final phase of life, and that she will not want to use artificial instruments to prolong her life.

In July 1988, the first conference on euthanasia was held in Shanghai, and participants included physicians, ethicists, and lawyers. In 1991, a computer scientist named Ting-ying Zhou of the Chinese Academy of Science attempted euthanasia several times and finally died through euthanasia with the agreement of her husband, children, the leader of her work unit, and the hospital. It was a typical positive example of euthanasia, and no legal issues were raised in court. On September 8, 1994, a peasant, Xiu-yun Wu, in the final phase of liver cancer asked to be euthanasized because of the pain, and her husband finally gave her a bottle of pesticide, and she died. The local court sentenced her husband to three years in prison.

In October 1994, the second conference on euthanasia was held in Shanghai. On August 7, 1996, the whole edition of the *Health News* (the largest newspaper in the field of health) was dedicated to euthanasia (1996). It mentioned that some hospitals secretly perform euthanasia. On November 1, 1999, a patient in Guizhou province who was suffering from final phase liver cancer asked for help for euthanasia through the media, which drew attention to euthanasia once more in China (Zhou, 1999, pp. 51-52). A 67-year-old-son (in Shanghai) of a 92-year-old-mother was sentenced to five years in prison for euthanasizing his mother (who could only move a finger and a toe after leaving the hospital, and the doctor said any improvement was impossible). The court judged that such behavior violated criminal law; however, in considering that he exhibited filial piety to his mother when she was hospitalized, he was given a lenient penalty of five years in prison (*Health News*, 2001e).

2. *Current opinions toward euthanasia.* Taboo and fear are a common psychological fact toward death. Filial piety requires that people care for their parents and prolong their lives, which is in conflict with modern medical technology and the new value of pursuing quality of life. On the one hand, under such a social environment, adult children think they should prolong life by all means – no matter what the quality of life is; on the other

hand, it lengthens the suffering and dying process of patients. But the condition is complicated in China, since sometimes economic factors contribute to reasons for euthanasia.

Almost every questionnaire about euthanasia shows that most people support it, especially medical professionals; but doctors dare not do it because of the lack of protection from the law. In 1992, 1994, and 1995, about 30 representatives of the National People's Congress put forth a proposal about euthanasia, but it was rejected. An interesting fact, though, is that people who support euthanasia are usually against it when the patient is a family member. Sometimes, although the patients are in much pain, their family members will deny the patient's request for euthanasia. The reason behind this is their responsibility to prolong the patient's life; otherwise, their conscience will not be clear and, moreover, some people are afraid of society condemning them for being impious to their parents. So some people argue that what family members think is usually for their own interests, rather than for the interest of the patient, so they suggest that it be regulated by law, to help those whose decision cannot be respected by family members (2001a).

Also, financial and other practical factors affect people's attempts to make a just judgment. As one physician wrote: in China, the condition they usually encounter is that many patients in the final phase of a disease ask to stop treatment or to be euthanasized, not because they cannot bear the pain, but because they are afraid it costs too much and do not want family members involved in debt, or it is too hard for family members to take care of them day and night (Dong, 1999, p. 60).

3. *Issues of brain death*. The ethical issues of brain death have been discussed for several years, and, though China does not have a law on brain death, many people are accepting it gradually. On March 1, 2001, the Long March Hospital of the Shanghai Second Army Medical University announced that half a year before they had done the first organ transplant surgery where the organ was obtained from a brain-dead young man (his kidneys saved two uremia patients). When this news spread, it did not raise much ethical debate. Legislative work on brain death is being done.

G. Death and Dying: Hospice Care and Care of the Dying

Hospice began in China in the mid-1980s, being mainly concentrated in large cities, such as Beijing, Tianjin, and Shanghai. The tradition of the first-aid medical model is commonly used to save terminally ill patients. The reason for this is that Chinese people still regard the first-aid model as according with the demands of filial piety, although to some extent it only relieves some psychological pressure for the family members, rather than for the patient.

One ethical issue of hospice is the low quality of service because of the lack of formal and systematic training. Most hospices are something like an old guardhouse, where only food and drink can be provided, and little effort is spent promoting a good quality of life and good ethical practices. The support from government policies, the medical welfare system, and the insurance system is not developed yet, and the government cannot cover these costs currently, so it seems that mainly the private hospices will occupy the market. The first hospice facility in Shanxi province was set up in September 1998; it is a joint-stock cooperation facility and serves mainly terminally ill patients, provides psychological and spiritual support for family members, and also provides funeral services (1998). This shows that hospices are being set up in most provinces and not only in large cities. Hospice has a bright future, because China is becoming an aged society.

H. Ethics of Pain Management

Not much ethical discussion can be heard regarding pain management in contemporary China. It is estimated that China will have 16 million new cancer patients every year: 30% of whom cannot bear the pain, and 80% of pain cannot been controlled effectively (2001d). Morphine and other similar medicines can now be used relatively freely, whereas several years ago they were under strict control. On the one hand, physicians are afraid of the serious side effects of such medicine, and most patients and their family members agree; on the other hand, physicians usually do not trust their patients very much, so they probably do not provide enough medicine to relieve pain.

The government encourages scientists to combine traditional medicine and therapy with Western medicine. Traditional Chinese therapy sometimes controls pain well.

I. Access to Health Care

1. *The current condition and the ethical problem of the health care system of China.* China has made significant progress on raising its population's level of health, which is mainly due to the socialist health care system: "consistent policy of prevention first, fully extended primary care services, ... good coverage of medical care" (Peng, 2000, S. 23). The greatest progress is that the life-expectancy has risen from 35 years before the People's Republic of China to 68.55 in 1990, to 70 in 1997 (http://www.moh.gov.cn/digest99/ TF2-141.html), and to 71.8 in 2000 (http://www.xinhuanet.com/zhengfu/jingtai/ zf_bps200101.htm).

Since 1949, when the People's Republic of China was founded, China developed three kinds of health care systems: labor protection (for workers of factories), public medical service (for government employees), and rural cooperative medical service (for peasants) (Cong, 1998, p. 594). Before 1980, the health care system covered almost all people, although it could only provide a low level of health services. After the open-door policy, when China began free market economics, the government fixed the position of the hospital at "public welfare enterprise". But the government does not provide a sufficient budget for hospitals, which can be shown from the percentage of total national financial expenditure on health care: 1998, 2.62%; 1990-1995, 2.37%; 1985-1990, 2.53%; 1980-1985, 3.10% (http://www.moh.gov.cn/digest99/T11-127.html). On the one hand, the economic support for hospitals declined; on the other hand, the price of drugs and examinations is becoming increasingly expensive, so that common people can hardly afford it. From the statistics of 1999 published by the Ministry of Health, we can see that 59.49% of hospital profit was from drugs for outpatients and 47.17% from inpatients (http://www.moh.gov.cn/digest99/T2-47.html).

The table below (Table 1) shows the various kinds of health care systems and the percent of people using them. Previously, only three kinds of care existed and covered almost all people; now, however, the percent of self-paid patients forms the majority. From this, we can see that most people shoulder nearly all the burden of their health care expenses. Medical insurance is just starting in some cities for employees of the government or of foreign companies. "Whole medical plan" is similar to medical insurance, but it is mainly for workers: participants pay a sum of money, then they usually receive 80 percent of the hospitalization costs. Outpatient clinic costs, however, usually cannot be refunded.

One important ethical issue stemming from the health care system is the "greater inequity in health care access, as underlined in the recent *World Health Report 2000* in

Table 1. The constitution of the health care system (in percent of population).

Item	Total of City and Village	City	Village
Free public service	4.91	16.01	1.16
Labor protection service	6.16	22.91	0.51
Half labor protection service	1.60	5.78	0.19
Medical insurance	1.87	3.27	1.39
Whole medical plan	0.39	1.42	0.04
Cooperation service	5.61	2.74	6.57
Self-paid	76.40	44.13	87.32
Others	3.04	3.73	2.81

(Source: http://www.moh.gov.cn/digest99/T2-59.htm)

which China ranked 177 out of 191 countries in terms of the equity of access to health care" (U.S. Embassy Beijing, 2000b). The inequity can also be shown from the distribution of medical resources: 80% of resources went to cities and 80% of that went to large hospitals (Wang, 1999, p. 124).

2. *China has not formed an idea of a "right" to health care.* Trying to fix the problems resulting from the health care system, the government has been reforming the system in the past decade. The government started the "basic medical insurance system for workers in cities and towns" in 1999, where workers and companies, paying 2% and 6% of the worker's salary, respectively, co-pay a basic insurance fee. In the "China white paper of the development of Human Right of 2000", it is noted that, by the end of 2000, 43 million workers had enrolled in this basic health care insurance (http://www.xinhuanet.com/zhengfu/jingtai/zf_bps200101.htm).

Article 45 of the "Constitution of People's Republic of China" notes that citizens have a right to receive help from the country when they are old, ill, or lose the capacity to work; article 98 of the "General Rule of Civil Law of People's Republic of China" notes that citizens have a right to life and health; however, it is not a common idea that citizens have a right to health care. They tend to think that health care is mainly a kind of special consumer good, which may be primarily due to the idea of the market economy prominent during last two decades. There is not much discussion about the two-tiered system in China, and most scholars do not know it well. Considering the diversity of people and of the values they hold, as well as their different abilities to afford health care, the government will probably provide different levels of health care for citizens.

J. Ethics Consultation and Committees: Medical Ethics Committees and Their Role in Hospitals and Clinics

The committee of law and regulation, which is a specialized committee of the Medical Ethics Association, drafted the regulations of medical ethics committees in 1989, and the formal file was passed by the Medical Ethics Association in 1995. Different from the American style, the Chinese medical ethics committee is not totally independent in clinical practice, but is "under the leading of the party and administration of hospital", according to a clause of one of the regulations (Medical Ethics Association, 1997, p. 15). So, although some medical ethics committees were established in certain large hospitals in the early 1990s, they were not true ethics committees, because they were primarily led administratively rather than ethically.

The Ministry of Health Medical Ethics Expert Committee was established in March 2000. The Ministry of Health emphasized the importance of this committee, the aims of which are to regulate the behavior of physicians and medical researchers, to protect the interests of human subjects, and to provide ethical advice for the Ministry itself. One regular function of this committee is to review the ethics of international projects or projects sponsored by the Ministry that are related to human experimentation.

The Good Clinical Practice Act was passed by the State Drug Administration in 1999. Chapter 3 of this act requires the establishment of a medical ethics committee in each institute of clinical pharmacology. This means that ethics consultation and committees have started to play a role in some clinical practice; the next step is to provide training for the members of ethics committees.

K. Other Issues

1. *AIDS will be an urgent issue in near future.* It is officially reported that 11,170 cases of HIV infection exist in China, including 338 cases of AIDS. But some experts estimate that the total number of HIV and AIDS is 300,000-400,000 (Wang, 2000, p. 48). Common people would like to connect AIDS with immoral sexual behavior first, although in fact the primary way (about 70 percent) it is transmitted is by drug use (which is also regarded as immoral). So the most serious issue that faces HIV-positive and AIDS patients is that they are rejected by society. The extreme solution that several organizations propose is setting up an "AIDS patient concentration camp" to try to stop the rapid spread of the disease in the area. Thirty-one deputies of the National People's Congress proposed an amendment to China's Criminal Law that would make it a crime intentionally to spread HIV (U.S. Embassy Beijing, 2000a). Some scholars argue that China should adopt a strategy of clinical tolerance to resolve the ethical dilemmas created by HIV infection and AIDS (Wang, 2000, p. 57).

2. *Research ethics has a bright future in China.* An increasing number of biomedical research collaborations are done between China and other countries, and a system of informed consent has been gradually established. On October 6, 1998, the Ministry of Science and Technology and the MOH co-published "Interim Measures for the Administration of Human Genetic Resources" (1998) to regulate the behavior of researchers. In October, 2001, the Sino-U.S. conference on protection of human subjects was held in the Yunnan province; Chinese and American experts discussed many ethical issues, which will become a solid base for the near future of research ethics in China. Because of varying cultures, there will be different understandings and implementations of informed consent between China and collaborative countries, which is also an important ethical issue within the research itself.

IV. Conclusions

In the narrow sense, the discussion of bioethics is still mainly found in the medical colleges and the academy, and it is still a common phenomenon that clinicians do not think that bioethics concerns them. Even in the broad sense of medical ethics, only a very small percentage of clinicians really participate in the activities of medical ethics and few show their medical students the ethical aspects of their clinical practice. So, the most serious problem facing the future of bioethics in China lies not in the barrier from traditional culture, but in the divorce of medical ethics and the clinical practice.

Effective methods to resolve the above problem are as follows:

(1) What medical students do, represents the future of medical ethics and, to prevent passing on the current state of poor doctor–patient relationships to medical students, we must continue medical ethics education to those medical teachers who lead medical students in clinical practice. We should make use of the tradition that holds that students easily follow their teachers.
(2) Establishing a medical ethics committee in every hospital is an effective way to link medical ethics theory to clinical practice and, as a result, it can raise the ethical sense of medical professionals.
(3) Encourage multidisciplinary scholars to participate in the activities of bioethics and to spread the knowledge of bioethics to common people.
(4) The basic way to resolve many of these issues is to develop the economic conditions of China, which is the primary cause of inequality in the health care system. Of course, unjust health policies also constitute an important factor.
(5) It is fundamental that a systematic theory and set of principles of bioethics with a Chinese character be established. It must fit the special conditions of the Chinese, because many moral problems, such as euthanasia, artificial insemination by donor, and so forth, have an important relation to China's unique cultural situation. We should not simply borrow a Western theory; we must stand on the land of China – after all, it is the fountainhead of bioethics in the future.

Notes

1. Here I use "medical morality" and not "medical ethics" mainly because many Chinese scholars think "medical ethics" during this period had not developed as a discipline yet; while there were many moral standards, they lacked systematic theories and principles.
2. To understand the background, here is the brief chronology of Chinese history: Xia, 2100-1600 B.C.; Shang, 1600-1066 B.C.; Zhou, 1066-256 B.C.; Spring–Autumn, 770-476 B.C.; Warring States, 475-221 B.C.; Qin, 221-206 B.C.; Han, 206 B.C.-220 A.D.; Three Kingdoms, 220-265 A.D.; two Jin, 265-420 A.D.; South and North Dynasties, 420-479 A.D.; ... Sui, 581-618 A.D.; Tang, 618-907 A.D.; ... Song, 960-1279 A.D.; ... Yuan, 1271-1368 A.D.; Ming, 1368-1644 A.D.; Qing, 1644-1911 A.D.; Republic of China, 1912-1949; People's Republic of China, 1949-present.
3. This school, which was well accepted by common people, meant that everything has two opposite aspects – yin and yang, which are antagonistic to each other. Five phases represents five materials – gold, wood, water, fire and earth – which are the elements of the world. By mutual promotion and restraint, they form the natural law of the world. In regard to medicine, it means that people will remain healthy as long as they are able to live in accordance with the underlying law of yin, yang, and the five phases.
4. In China, we do not have a special major in medical ethics. Some experts today majored in natural dialectics, now called "the philosophy of science and technology".

5. We call this "the principle of socialist medical morality" to distinguish it from Western-style principles: nonmaleficence, beneficence, autonomy, and justice. Even today, many Chinese physicians might not know these Western principles, but they are familiar with the socialist principle.
6. When mentioning euthanasia, we mean active euthanasia. Passive euthanasia is commonly done in Chinese medical practice.

Bibliography

_____. 2001a. *Beijing Youth Newspaper*, 7th edition, December 2.

_____. 2001b. *Guangming Daily*, January 6.

_____. 1996. *Health News*, August 7.

_____. 1998. *Health News*, September 17.

_____. 2001c. *Health News*, October 23.

_____. 2001d. [On-line]. Available: <http://www.999.com.cn/professional/medicine/special/anlesi/200104/8107120010412.htm>.

_____. 2001e. [On-line]. Available: <http://www.999.com.cn/professional/rule/200110/10630320011011.htm>.

Cai, Y.-P. 1996. *History of chinese ethics*. Beijing: Dongfang Press.

Callahan, D. 1995. Bioethics. In W.T. Reich (ed.), *Encyclopedia of bioethics (2nd ed.)* (pp. 249-252). New York: Macmillan.

Chen, S.-F. 1996. *History of chinese ethics*, Volume 1. Beijing: Beijing University Press.

Chen, S.-F. 1997. *History of chinese ethics*, Volume 2. Beijing: Beijing University Press.

Chen, Y. et al. 1985. *History of chinese ethics thoughts*. Guizhou: Guizhou Peoples Press.

Cong, Y. 1998. Ethical challenges in clinical care medicine: A Chinese perspective. *Journal of Medicine and Philosophy* 23(6): 581-600.

Dong, Q.-Y. 1999. Some issues of euthanasia against morality. *Chinese Medical Ethics* 3: 60-63.

Du, Z.-Z. 1985. *Outline of medical ethics*. Nanchang: Jiangxi People's Press.

Du, Z.-Z. 2000. *New research of medical ethics*. Henan: Henan Medical University Press.

Fan, R.-P. 1997. Three levels of problems in cross-cultural exploration of bioethics. In K. Hoshino (ed.), *Japanese and western bioethics*. Dordrecht: Kluwer Academic Publishers.

Han, S.-H. et al., 1999. A study on the abnormal phenomena of sex differentials in infant and child mortality in china. *Chinese Journal of Health Statistics* 16(1): 11-13.

He, Z.-X. 1988. *History of Chinese medical morality*. Shanghai: Shanghai Medical University Press.

Jiao, G.-C. 1997. *General introduction of Chinese ethics*. Taiyuan: Shanxi Education Press.

Li, B.-F. et al., 1996. *Medical ethics*. Beijing: Beijing Medical University Press.

Li, J.-N. 2001. [On-line]. Available: <http://www.999.com.cn/public/sex/special/people/200106/9291420010626.htm>.

Liu, J.-R. 2000. The basic trend of Chinese culture of reproduction. *The Journal of Medicine and Society* 13(6): 37-39.

Liu, T.-H. 2000. The contemporary value of Chinese traditional morality. *Morality and Civilization* 1: 41-45.

Medical Ethics Association. 1990. Hospitals should do a morality examination and establish medical morality files (draft).

Medical Ethics Association. 1995. Organizational regulations of medical ethics committee.

Medical Ethics Association. 1997. The regulation of medical ethics committees. *Journal of Chinese Medical Ethics* 5: 15.

Medical Ethics Association. 1998. On the measurement and ethical requests towards the final phase of chronic diseases.

Medical Ethics Association. 1998. The ethical principles of organ transplantation.

Medical Ethics Association. 1998. The rights and responsibilities of patients.

Ministry of Health. 1997. Statement on Human Cloning. March 19.

Ministry of Science and Technology & Ministry of Health. 1998. Interim measures for the administration of human genetic resources [On-line]. Available: <http://www.usembassy-china.org.cn/english/sandt/generesourcesreg10-98.html>.

Ni, H.-F. et al. 2000. *Bioethical dilemmas in the 21st century*. Beijing: High Education Press.

Nie, J.-B. 2000. The plurality of Chinese and American medical moralities: toward an interpretive cross-cultural bioethics. *Kennedy Institute of Ethics Journal* 10(3): 239-260.

Pang, M.-C.S. 1999. Protective truthfulness: The Chinese way of safeguarding patients in informed treatment decisions. *Journal of Medical Ethics* 25: 247-253.

Pang, M.-C.S. et al. 2000. Use the way of Delphi to write Chinese nursing ethical rules of new century. *Chinese Journal of Nursing* 35(9): 517-518.

Peng, R.-C. 2000. How professional values are developed and applied in medical practice in China. *Hastings Center Report, Special Supplement* 30(4): S.23-26.

Qiu, R.-Z. 1987. *Bioethics*. Shanghai: Shanghai People's Press.

Qiu, R.-Z. 1995. Medical ethics, history of contemporary China. In W.T. Reich (ed.), *Encyclopedia of bioethics, (2nd ed.)*. New York: Macmillan.

Qiu, R.-Z. 1999. Medical ethics. *Chinese Journal of Nursing* 23(1): 57-60; 23(2): 115-117; 23(3): 177-179.

Soo, F. 1987. Contemporary Chinese philosophy. In B. Carr et al. (eds), *Companion encyclopedia of asian philosophy*. London: Routledge.

U.S. Embassy Beijing. 2000a. [On-line]. Available: <http://www.usembassy-china.org.cn/sandt/sandtbak-hp.html#AIDS>.

U.S. Embassy Beijing. 2000b. Human research subject protection in China: Implications for U.S. collaborators [On-line]. Available: <http://www.usembassy-china.org.cn/english/sandt/humanresearchsubjectprotection.htm>.

Xu, T.-M. et al. (eds). 1998. *A Comparative study on Chinese-Western medical ethics*. Beijing: Beijing Medical University Press.

Wang, H. 1999. The management of hospitals in China: problems and solutions. *Chinese & International Philosophy of Medicine* 2(1):121-138.

Wang, Y.G. 2000. A strategy of clinical tolerance for the tolerance of the prevention of HIV and AIDS in China. *Journal of Medicine and Philosophy* 25(1): 48-61.

Wu, Z.H. 1994. Conflicts between Chinese tradition ethics and bioethics. *Cambridge Quarterly of Health Ethics* 3: 367-371.

Zhang, D. & Cheng, Z. 2000. Medicine is a human art: The basic principles of professional ethics in Chinese medicine. *Hastings Center Report, Special Supplement* 30(4): S. 8-12.

Zhang, H.Z. et al. 2000. *A survey of Chinese foreign medical moral standard*. Tianjin: Tianjin Ancient Books Press.

Zhou, Q.H. 1999. Important events of euthanasia in China. *Chinese Medical Ethics* 1: 51-52.

16 Bioethics with Chinese Characteristics: The Development of Bioethics in Hong Kong

Gerhold K. Becker

By Chinese standards, Hong Kong is a rather small place; it is, however, truly unique and intensely bustling. While the total population had fallen by 1 million to about 600,000 in 1945 due to the Japanese occupation of Hong Kong, and the ensuing flight of large numbers of people back to China, the 1950s saw it rise again and reach 2.5 million. Since then, the population has steadily increased to its current level of 6.7 million people, who are crammed into three main areas: Hong Kong Island, the Kowloon peninsula, and the so-called New Territories. Hong Kong Island, originally 78 sq km, with ragged terrain that includes steep slopes as well as beautiful beaches, has over the years been significantly expanded with stretches of land reclaimed from the sea. The same is true for the Kowloon peninsula, the smallest of the three areas (46.8 sq km), which nonetheless houses 30% of Hong Kong's total population. The average population density here is 44,210 per sq km. In districts such as Mong Kok it topped 140,000 per sq km at 1986 figures, making Kowloon one of the most densely populated areas in the world.

Nearly all (95%) of Hong Kong's population is ethnic Chinese, with the major non-Chinese ethnic groups comprised mainly of Filipinos and Indonesians (representing the work force of about 240,000 domestic helpers), as well as British nationals. The dominant language is Cantonese (*Gwongdunghua*), yet one third of the population claims to be able to speak Mandarin (*Putonghua*) as well. Hong Kong has one of the highest living standards in Asia: the median monthly income of its working population has increased by 93% over the past ten years to about HK$10,000. (Domestic household incomes increased by 88% over the same period to about HK$18,700.)

I. Hong Kong Bioethics in Its Socio-Cultural Context

Hong Kong's complexity derives from its remarkable history as a prosperous and extremely successful British colony whose average per capita income has by now surpassed that of its former British masters. As a result of the Opium War (1840-42), Hong Kong was ceded to Britain and occupied by British troops on 26 January 1841. A contemporary article in *The Bombay Gentlemen's Gazette* estimated the total population to stand at about 7800, comprised of "smugglers, stone cutters and vagabonds" (Dyson, 1986, p. 1). In the jaundiced view of an early Treasurer, Robert Martin, Hong Kong was a "small, barren, unhealthy, valueless island, the expenditure on which outstripped revenue by a ratio of some 10 to one" (Dyson, 1986, p. 1). The 99-year lease from China of the New Territories on 9 June 1898 sealed Hong Kong's fate, when the Sino-British Joint Declaration in 1984 stipulated the colony's return to the motherland on 1 July 1997. Hong Kong's status as a Special Administrative Region of the People's Republic of China with a high degree of autonomy and its own legal and economic system has been defined in its Basic Law.

A. Dual Identity

The "kaleidoscope of cultural images" (Siu, 1996, p. 177) that is characteristic of the Hong Kong way of life may occasionally suggest that the people of Hong Kong lack a specific cultural identity. While it is true that "Hong Kong as an historical space encompasses vastly different cultural affiliations" (Siu, 1996, p. 193), it is equally true that a distinct cultural identity has been fashioned by the dual forces of traditional Chinese culture and Western economic liberalism, which has significant implications for the contemporary bioethical discourse in Hong Kong. The stunning economic success of Hong Kong is reflected in a prevailing materialistic attitude, which seems to be a "deep-seated value entrenched in the minds of Hong Kong people" (Ho & Leung, 1997, p. 335). This attitude has been attributed to the two main forces of value transmission and socialization, i.e., the education system and the family. While a large proportion of the population is almost exclusively concerned with economic issues and tends to focus on economic stability and growth, the so-called post-materialist values, particularly those which foster an awareness of individual liberties and rights, remain largely underdeveloped (Ho & Leung, 1997, p. 354).

In the past, governance in Hong Kong was exercised by the authoritarianism of benign and enlightened rule which perpetuated the state-dominated social order of traditional Chinese society (Postiglione, 1992, p. 29). Its moral sensitivities derived from a precarious balance between the needs of political stability and the questionable legitimacy of the colonial authority in Hong Kong. As Siu-kai Lau and Hsin-chi Kuan have pointed out:

> The establishment of colonial rule in Hong Kong was based until several decades ago on military force. In the long span of colonial rule, subtle versions of the doctrine of the economic prowess and cultural superiority of the white people, and the civilizing mission of the colonizer, had occasionally emerged to justify colonial dominance. Still, there has not been an elaborate, systematic theory, explicitly articulated, to buttress the legitimacy of authority in Hong Kong (Lau & Kuan, 1988, p. 19).

This uncertainty is reflected in the general provision of public education, which represents – alongside the family – the most significant moral resource in a Chinese society. For many years, access to education was extremely limited on the grounds, as stated in a government report in 1950, that "free education is right and proper for territories where the population is stable and the cost of providing it falls equally on all classes" (Sweeting, 1990, p. 88). It was not until 1978 that the provision of nine years of free and compulsory education was achieved. Even so, the scarcity of post-secondary schools allowed only 8% of students access to local universities and thus forced large numbers to further their studies overseas. In the early 1990s, it was estimated that one in fifteen of those with higher education had obtained their qualifications outside Hong Kong (Wong & Ng, 1997, p. 235).

This situation is particularly characteristic of Hong Kong physicians, almost all of whom studied abroad or at least spent a significant amount of time during their medical training at overseas institutions, most notably in the United Kingdom, the United States of America, and Australia. This fact may also explain the remarkable degree of similarity between approaches to bioethics in Hong Kong and in Western countries. In 1979, during one of the first bioethical fact-finding missions to China and Hong Kong by a group of foreign bioethicists after the end of the infamous Cultural Revolution, Tom Beauchamp noted, somewhat surprised: "The Hong Kong Chinese have virtually the same approach to medicine and the same bioethical problems to which we are accustomed in the United States." In particular he mentioned issues of informed consent, the allocation of health care resources and institutional ethics review board mechanisms for research. And he concluded his report on Hong Kong bioethics with the observation that the Chinese in Hong Kong are not only concerned with virtually the same set of problems as their Western counterparts, but "are at least as well on their way to resolving those problems as are we" (Beauchamp, 1979, pp. 49, 51).

While this statement is correct as far as it goes, it is obvious that Hong Kong has developed its own form of socio-cultural identity, which clearly has implications for bioethics. Regarding their verdict of a total absence of bioethics in mainland China (Engelhardt, 1980), the bioethicists from the Kennedy Institute of Ethics have been charged with an inadvertent ethnocentric view and with "cultural myopia". Since they were locked in "the social and cultural matrices of their ideas" (Fox & Swazey, 1984, p. 339; Nie, 2000), they were unable to discover anything other than that with which they were already familiar. In the case of mainland China, this led them to conclude that there was no medical ethics to speak of, and, in the case of Hong Kong, they failed to appreciate the influence Confucianism and the moral values of traditional Chinese society in general still exert on bioethical discourse in Hong Kong.

B. Health Care and Health Care Reform in Hong Kong

The co-existence of classical Chinese and modern Western moral traditions has clearly influenced the development of health care in Hong Kong and the government's role in the provision of public health services (Hong Kong Government, 1974, p. 1991). The government's health care policy stipulates that everybody in Hong Kong should be able to receive adequate medical treatment regardless of individual means. To this end, the government provides a range of services and facilities to complement those available in the private sector and to meet the needs of the general population, in particular the needs of the less affluent patients. As a result, patients pay only a nominal user fee for services at public clinics and in public hospitals, which are financed through general tax revenues. This "cornerstone" of government policy (Hong Kong Government, 1990, p. 156) has repeatedly been emphasized, from the first White Paper on the *Aims and Policy for Social Welfare in Hong Kong* in 1965 to the relevant statements of the current administration.

At the same time, Hong Kong subscribes to a *laissez faire* policy that keeps market interference at a minimum and allows the private sector both in business and in health care extensive opportunity to develop services that cater to the specific needs of those who can afford them. This is reflected in the discrepancy between the use of outpatient and inpatient care. While about 85% of outpatients consult private physicians and only 15% government-employed physicians, the picture is quite different in the case of inpatient care, with only 8% of the patients seeking admission to private hospitals and the other 92% relying on public hospitals (Hsiao, 1999; Fan, 1999b).

In 1990, the government established the Hong Kong Hospital Authority as a statutory body under the Hospital Authority Ordinance to manage all public hospitals in Hong Kong (44 public hospitals and 49 specialist outpatient centers). In December 2000, the number of hospital beds in Hong Kong was 33,102, representing 4.8 beds per 1000 inhabitants. Medical doctors in public clinics and hospitals are now employed by the Authority. The Hospital Authority's Community Based Nursing Service provides post-discharge rehabilitative nursing care and treatment to the sick, the elderly and the disabled through its 36 nursing centers and 12 psychiatric nursing offices. Nursing homes are run by missionary groups and large non-profit organizations like the Tung Wah Group of Hospitals and the Po Leung Kuk.

The overall health care expenditure of Hong Kong in1996 figures stands at 4.6%, almost equally divided between the government's public health expenditure (2.5%) and that of the private sector (2.1%). In comparison with Western countries, Hong Kong has spent much fewer resources to achieve "at least as good health outcomes (in terms of life expectancy for both men and women, infant mortality rate and maternal mortality rate) as the other countries" (Fan, 1999b, p. 556). The comprehensive range of health and social services and improvements in the standard of living have fostered a high level of general health, and Hong Kong's health indices remain among the best in the world. In 2000, the infant mortality rate was 2.9 per 1000 live births (down from 19.0 in 1970), the post-neonatal mortality rate stood at 1.2 and the average life expectancy at birth was 77.2 years for males and 82.4 years for females (according to figures provided by the Department of Health and the Hospital Authority).

One sector, however, that has been repeatedly criticized for lagging behind in the overall development of health care is that of psychiatric rehabilitation. It has been alleged (Yip, 1997) that the need for psychiatric rehabilitation was almost entirely ignored up to 1948 and acknowledged only in the 1950s and early 1960s. While for many years the government's commitment to psychiatric rehabilitation was seen as insufficient, greater public awareness of the need for treating psychiatric patients in recent years as well as the contribution to psychiatric care by NGO's have led to remarkable improvements.

Apart from receiving government support, hospitals are also funded by charitable organizations (e.g., the Community Chest), the Hong Kong Jockey Club, corporations and individuals. Missionary groups too play a significant role in providing hospital services: Protestant organizations operate seven hospitals with 3749 beds and 18 clinics, while Catholic organizations are in charge of six hospitals and 13 clinics.

In November 1997, the government's Health and Welfare Bureau commissioned a study on the overall health care provisions in Hong Kong, their problems and their future development. An interdisciplinary team from Harvard University's School of Public Health led by Professor William Hsiao was given the task to diagnose Hong Kong's health care system on the basis of the following two principles: "Every resident should have access to reasonable quality and affordable health care. The government assures this access through a system of shared responsibility between the government and residents, where those who can afford to pay for health care should pay" (Hsiao, 1999, p. 87).

In its report (published by the government for public consultation in 1999), the Harvard team concluded that, in terms of access and utilization, resource distribution and financing, Hong Kong has a relatively equitable system and has benefited from improvements in quality and efficiency as a result of the 1990 reform and the establishment of the Hospital Authority. Yet it also pinpointed "three interrelated weaknesses" with regard to the quality of care, the allocation of public funds and the sustainability of the current system of public health care provision. While care is seen as highly variable and doubts were expressed about the adequacy of the rankings of patient satisfaction about the health care services provided, the most important result of the study suggests that the current system of health care is unsustainable. The team concluded that there was a "need to seriously rethink and redevelop an overall coherent health care policy and health care financing/ delivery system that will meet the needs of the population of Hong Kong" (Hsiao, 1999, p. 82). As a solution, the report recommended the establishment of a comprehensive Health Security Plan (HSP) and a savings accounts scheme for long-term care. Each resident would be required to enroll in a health insurance plan (HSP), whose costs would be jointly born by themselves and their employers, and to contribute 1% of their salary to an individual savings account (MEDISAGE) for the exclusive use of purchasing individual long-term care policies upon retirement or disability.

The public consultation on the proposed health care reform provoked strong criticism from various quarters, including many bioethicists. From the perspective of a Confucian ethics of care, the Harvard team was charged with ignorance of the dominant values of Hong Kong and with a failure truly to understand Hong Kong society's basic moral vision by emphasizing equity as the overriding value for its health care system (Tao, 1999). Others suspected that the team's recommendations would result in a US-style managed care system, which in their view would be inconsistent with the local values of self-reliance and non-compulsion as the two primary values cherished by Hong Kong people (Au, 1999, p. 612). While the HSP was intended to increase patient choice, some suspect that it may in fact erode choice and constrain their freedom to seek the services they want and from whom they want them (Chan, Ho-mun, 1999).

In view of sustained critique and under the impact of the current economic downturn, the government put the implementation of the recommendations in the *Harvard Report* on hold. There are indications that it now favors a less radical and, for the average Hong Kong resident, less costly overhaul of the current health care system, which would also pay greater attention to cultural factors.

C. The Human Body in Chinese and Western Perspectives:
The Example of Organ Transplantation

The socio-cultural parameters of Hong Kong bioethics are particularly noticeable at the intersection of modern medical technology and traditional Chinese beliefs. One such example is transplantation medicine, which has challenged the traditional Chinese view of the human body.

In spite of significant differences, Confucianism and traditional Chinese medicine share some fundamental assumptions with regard to the human body and its relation to nature and society. "Confucianism has greatly influenced the Chinese medical perception of the body, and actually constitutes an organic part of the philosophy in which Chinese medicine evolved" (Nie, 1999, p. 202). Traditional Chinese philosophy accords to the human body a special dignity "and even sacredness" (Nie, 1999, p. 202) and severely restricts medical interventions and manipulations. These restrictions apply even to the dead body, which should be returned to the grave whole and intact.

Although transplantation of solid organs and bone marrow "are now well-established and successful procedures in Hong Kong" (Hawkins, 2000, p. 17), cultural factors have kept the rate of organ donation at considerably lower levels than in Western countries. Over the years, the organ donation rate has been steady at about 1-2 per million people (compared with a donation rate of 19 per million in Australia, 16-20 per million in USA, and 18 per million in most European countries with the exception of Spain, where the rate is even 22 per million). In 2000, over 3000 patients were on dialysis due to chronic renal failure. 1000 patients were on the waiting list for kidney transplants (Li, 2000, p. 8), while 100 waited for liver and 20 for heart-lung transplantation (Hospital Authority's Central Renal Registry). The first successful liver transplantation in Hong Kong was performed in 1991 (Queen Mary Hospital). From 1996-1999, a total of 168 kidney transplants have been carried out, where the median age of the recipients was 42. Kidney transplant patients had to face a median waiting time of 79.5 months (Chan & Wong, 2000, p. 14).

Surveys about public attitudes towards organ donation (Chan, et al., 1990; Li, 2000) have consistently confirmed that Hong Kong people usually want to preserve a "complete body" after death and believe that cadaveric organ donation will not only mutilate the body but also cause "pain" to the deceased. In addition, there is still great reluctance in the general public to accept brain stem death as a reliable criterion of the cessation of life. These cultural perceptions, which are deeply rooted in the Chinese philosophical and medical traditions, are not shared by the medical community, which has tried to alleviate the shortfall of transplant organs through public education campaigns and by relaxing the criteria for cadaver donor acceptability. Several organizations (including the Hong Kong Liver Foundation, the Hong Kong Kidney Foundation and the Hong Kong Society of Transplantation) have been established to educate the public about the benefits of organ transplantation and to promote a better understanding of organ harvesting. The Hong Kong Liver Foundation has launched public education programs (including health exhibitions, television programs and seminars) with particular emphasis on schools and the grassroots.

The shortfall on transplant organs has also been attributed to a lack of concerted efforts in organ donation and the lack of awareness amongst doctors. To circumvent this problem, the Hong Kong Medical Association has set up a computer-based central organ donation registry, which facilitates the process of donor identification and shares information with transplant centers. Hong Kong has several organ transplant centers, of which the most important are those at Queen Mary Hospital and Prince of Wales Hospital (for liver and kidney transplantation) and Grantham Hospital (for heart and lung transplantation).

The allocation of transplant organs is managed by the transplant centers, which assess potential donors and recipients. Due to the shortfall of transplant organs, transplant centers tend to accept also marginal donors irrespective of age, adverse in-hospital events or the use of inotropes (Lo, Chung-mau, 2001, p. 16). Living donor liver transplantation (first performed at Queen Mary Hospital in 1993) and split liver transplantation (first performed on two adult recipients in 2000) have further expanded the range of organ transplantation and somewhat alleviated the consequences of the insufficient supply of cadaveric donor organs.

Transplant coordinators are responsible for counseling potential organ donors and facilitating the harvest process. In view of the dramatic discrepancy between supply and demand of donor organs, Hong Kong transplant centers have tried to ensure the equity in the allocation of cadaveric organs through objective criteria. Before 1994, the allocation of graft kidneys was based solely on the results of tissue typing (human leucocyte antigen, HLA) between donor and recipient (Hawkins, 2000). Since this system disadvantaged patients with uncommon HLA and did not factor in the time spent on the waiting list and favored younger patients, it was in 1994 replaced by a point-score system according to the factors of the patient's age, the time spent on dialysis and the ranking of patients by tissue typing. The system was further revised in 1996 and greater weight given to the time spent on dialysis. Ten additional points were accorded to patients less than 15 years old. Yet priority is still given to patients with zero HLA mismatches. The point score system has been regarded as a fair and equitable basis for the allocation of cadaveric graft kidneys, since it seems to have achieved its goal of serving more patients on long-term dialysis without discriminating against others and without negative effects on graft survival (Chan & Wong, 2000, p. 14).

Organ transplantation in Hong Kong vividly exemplifies the dual cultural identities that also characterize Hong Kong bioethics. On the one hand, organ transplantation, representing one of the greatest achievements of the dominant paradigm of Western medicine, has been whole-heartedly endorsed by the medical establishment and expertly utilized with great success. On the other hand, its comprehensive application to patient care is severely constrained by cultural perceptions deeply rooted in the alternative Chinese medical paradigm. The unresolved tension between these two models of medicine is reflected in the development of bioethics in Hong Kong.

II. Approaches to Bioethics

Hong Kong bioethics resembles "a melange of disciplines" more than "a coherent body of principles and methods appropriate to the analysis of some particular subject matter" (Jonsen, 1998, pp. 342, 345). In this regard, it is not different from developments overseas and shares with them similar conceptual problems. At the same time and to a considerable degree, it reflects the dual identity of its citizens, which has been shaped by the values of the Chinese cultural tradition, on the one hand, and the parameters of modern secular and pluralistic societies without dominant moral institutions and without strong moral coherence, on the other.

Bioethics in Hong Kong is comprised of many voices, yet, when it comes to deciding on ethical matters pragmatic views generally prevail. These are usually tempered by a certain degree of caution, as one would expect of a society burdened with socio-political uncertainty and divided loyalties.

While a 1992 survey on research in bioethics proved largely inconclusive and the conceptualization of ethics sketchy, much has considerably changed in the meantime. Academics with a demonstrated commitment to bioethics both in their teaching and in specific research projects are now found at all universities. The following five research areas are most representative of this new development:

- moral issues of biotechnology, particularly issues of genomic research, human cloning and gene therapy;

- moral issues at the beginning of life, including reproductive technology, abortion, and the moral status of the embryo;
- moral issues at the end of life, including issues of care for the terminally ill and euthanasia;
- moral issues in public health care policy, resource allocation, and financing;
- conceptual and methodological issues of bioethics in general and of bioethics in a Chinese or Confucian context in particular.

A. The Rehabilitation of Traditional Values in Medicine

In spite of its status as a British colony, Hong Kong has always remained a Chinese society firmly rooted in traditional Chinese beliefs and values. During its colonial past, the government-sponsored institutions of medical education and health care were exclusively based on the Western medical paradigm, while the practice of traditional Chinese medicine was officially ignored. Yet in spite of the lack of formal recognition and funding, Chinese medicine remained highly popular and was practiced alongside its Western counterpart.

Against opposition from the medical establishment but in line with its own aspirations to strengthen traditional Chinese values, the post-colonial government introduced measures to rehabilitate Chinese medicine by recognizing it as a legitimate form of health care and regulating its practice. The establishment of the School of Chinese Medicine at Hong Kong Baptist University and the introduction of the first government-approved five-year, full-time undergraduate program in traditional Chinese medicine in 1998-99 confirms the government's reorientation towards traditional Chinese values. As in mainland China, modern biomedicine, traditional Chinese medicine, and a combination of both are firmly established and co-exist alongside each other in Hong Kong.

The rehabilitation of traditional Chinese medicine in Hong Kong is certainly one factor in a remarkable shift towards a more pronounced focus on the development of a specifically Chinese bioethics. The process began, however, much earlier. In the years leading up to 1997, the impending return of Hong Kong to China prompted increased reflection on issues of cultural identity and on the possibility to harvest traditional Chinese moral resources in response to the questions posed by the development of modern medicine and biotechnology. While it is difficult to claim exclusive ownership for Hong Kong bioethicists in the emergence of a specifically Chinese or even Confucian bioethics, quite a number of its advocates are either Hong Kong-based or Hong Kong-born who settled later elsewhere (e.g., in Taiwan and Canada).

B. The Emergence of a Confucian Bioethics

The single most important factor for value formation in Chinese society has certainly been Confucianism. While it is true that Confucianism has made an indelible mark on Chinese society (Tu, 1989), it has neither been a monolithic doctrine nor was its influence exclusive. "Confucianism" as a generic term has no counterpart in Chinese but is of Western origin. Thus Confucianism can stand for many things and has been referred to as "a world view, a social ethic, a political ideology, a scholarly tradition, and a way of life" (Tu, 1989, p. 1). In spite of claims about the demise of Confucianism and its loss of appeal to the contemporary Chinese both in mainland China and Hong Kong, Confucianism as a moral world view and value-laden perspective on life continues to be highly influential. Although it would be anachronistic to expect the reappearance of a "Confucian civilization" (Levenson, 1968) revolving around a state-sanctioned ideology of rigid hierarchic relationships, Confucianism has been invoked to buttress the claim of the existence of distinctively "Asian" values at the core of a comprehensive socio-political theory that could provide a full-fledged alternative to the Western human rights tradition (Bauer & Bell, 1999; Bell, 2000). Political analysts in Hong Kong have recently even argued that current government policies largely reflect this claim and can best be explained in terms of a deliberate reversion to the political values of a Confucian past which focused on authority, obedience and social stability rather than on liberal democratic yearnings (Shaw, 2000).

The Confucianism, however, that currently plays a particular role in the bioethical discourse seems less tangible and may be loosely described as a "tradition of philosophical thought" and "a cultural perspective" that is "generally endorsed by the Chinese and embodied in their way of life and practices" (Chan, Joseph, 1999, p. 213). As such, the "Confucian bioethics" (Fan, 1999a) that recently has been explored as a specifically Chinese response to ethical "cosmopolitanism" starts from the assumption that Confucian values are still at home in Hong Kong (as well as in Korea, Japan, Taiwan and mainland China). It is further presupposed that "particular Confucian metaphysical, cosmological, and moral convictions and assumptions" can be utilized in the construction of a "real bioethics" that has its place in the lives of Chinese individuals and their communities. This Confucian bioethics is supposed to stand out "as a significant communitarian bioethics that offers a coherent way of engaging the good life" (Fan, 1999a, pp. 2-3)

The phrase "Confucian bioethics" seems to suggest a uniform theory of bioethics. This is, however, misleading, since various versions of Confucian bioethics have been proposed. One of them is being explored by Hong Kong-born Confucian scholar Shui-chuen Lee, who now teaches in Taiwan. Lee seeks to develop his version of Confucian bioethics (Lee, 1999a) by utilizing Tsung-san Mou's Neo-Confucian ontology in the construction of an ethics that is able to integrate what Lee sees as "the two chief achievements of Western civilization", science and democracy (Lee, 1999b, p. 187). Taking the guiding principle of his version of Confucian bioethics from the *Doctrine of the Mean* and its teachings about the Tao that "works sincerely and thus produces things in an unfathomable way", Lee concludes that "Confucianism basically supports the employment of biotechnology in the relieving of human defects whether they are inborn or man-made". One of the consequences of this approach is that, from a Confucian perspective, "the use of IVF test-tube baby biotechnology for solving infertility" is morally as acceptable as human cloning (Lee, 1999b, p. 192).

It is an indication of the liveliness of the current debate about a Confucian bioethics that Ruiping Fan at the City University of Hong Kong arrives at exactly the opposite conclusion. Taking his point of departure from the moral significance of natural human relationships and constructing a Confucian notion of human dignity, Fan concludes that "any action or scientific innovation that jeopardizes the relation of parent and child violates human dignity. From the Confucian view, the cloning of humans destroys the relation of parent and child. Accordingly, it is morally unacceptable for Confucians to practice human cloning" (Fan, 1998, p. 196).

C. Confucian Ethics of Care

Another facet of the Confucian moral paradigm shaping the development of bioethics in Hong Kong is the strong emphasis some scholars have put on an ethics of care. In particular, Julia Tao (City University of Hong Kong) has argued that care and reciprocity rather than equality are the primary values that are most characteristic of Hong Kong and highly influential on governmental social policies:

> In Hong Kong, social policy has always been guided by the vision of a caring and compassionate society based on the central values of care and compassion. Hong Kong society's approach to social policy is a care-based approach which emphasizes the value of care more than equality (Tao, 1999, p. 572).

According to Tao, the ethics of care is firmly rooted in the core values of Chinese culture (Tao, 2000; 1998) and thus is of paramount importance for any attempt to understand more intimately the moral fabrics of Hong Kong society. It is also a particular Chinese contribution to the further development of bioethics in general.

The Confucian vision of the ideal community rejects the notion of mutually disinterested, independent and rational individuals. Instead, it starts from the assumption that individuals "are benevolently disposed to recognize and ... sympathetically care for others' well-being as if it were their own" (Tao, 1996, p. 22). Thus the ethics of care is based on the Confucian concept of human relatedness and relational agency. Care as disposition and practice is "a form of altruistic regard", since the "Confucian self is always a relational self, whose individuality is constituted by a web of unique role relations and by the way concrete responsibilities are performed by the self in each particular set of relationships" (Tao, 1999, pp. 576, 578). It follows that a Confucian ethics of care endorses neither universal moral claims nor a moral obligation of universal love. Instead it is based on "the twin principles of 'love by gradation' and 'care by extension'" (Tao, 1999, p. 581).

Opportunities for bioethical applications of a Confucian ethics of care abound in Hong Kong but are particularly relevant in the area of health care and reform of the health care system. It is therefore no surprise that the strongest critique of the *Harvard Report* and an assumed shift in government policy towards an exclusively market-driven system of health care was inspired by a Confucian ethics of care (Tao, 1999).

The other highly significant application concerns the care for the elderly. Filial piety (*xiao*) has always been regarded as the hallmark of a traditional Chinese ethics that is based on a conception of relational personhood. The paramount importance of filial piety in traditional Chinese family life is undisputed. *Xiao* has been described as "a respectful and obliging attitude towards the elders of the family, above all the parents" and as the cultivation of an attitude of care and obedience (Roetz, 1993, p. 53). Yet, in spite of the singular significance of filial piety in traditional China, contemporary Hong Kong society appears in need of additional inducements to observe the responsibilities owed to parents, particularly when they are getting older and need filial support and respect most. Nelson Chow has pointed out that despite all the rhetoric about filial piety in a Chinese society, the actual care for the elderly in the family today is weakening and being replaced by rather pragmatic considerations (Chow, 1992, p. 133).

Empirical investigations into the model of family care based on filial piety within an Asian context seem to corroborate Chow's conclusion. Yow-Hwey Hu's research into the suicide pattern of the elderly in Asian societies revealed that the elderly "are killing them-selves at rates up to five times higher than their own younger generations and eight times higher than their Western counterparts" (Hu, 1995, p. 202). Most vulnerable among the elderly are older women. In Hong Kong, their suicide rate per 100,000 population stands at 34.6 (in contrast, rates for Western women of a comparable age group range from only 2.6 to a high of 9.2). This suicide risk analysis apparently suggests that in practical life the traditional, Confucian-based ethics of care is being eroded and additional moral resources are needed to curb the rising incidents of abuse, neglect and ill treatment of the elderly.

D. Sino-Christian Bioethics

Another approach to bioethics is less concerned with constructing a specifically Confucian bioethics than with utilizing Confucian (and generally Chinese) and Christian moral resources in response to specific issues in medicine and health care. Its advocates expect it to enable them to identify deficiencies in the dominant Western bioethical dis-course and to offer remedies through a bioethics that is at the same time deeply Chinese and Christian.

One representative of this approach is Hong Kong-born Canadian bioethicist and the-ologian Edwin Hui, who has proposed a comprehensive and cross-cultural review of the foundations of modern bioethics and a re-examination of its key concepts that engages both Christian and Chinese alternative approaches. In view of its far-reaching implica-tions for modern bioethics, Hui has focused on the concept of personhood. Noting "a clear proclivity" in Western bioethics "to define human personhood in terms of higher-brain functions or some similar psychological criteria" (Hui, 2000, p. 95), he argues that such an approach is not only counter-intuitive and in conflict with basic human experi-ence but also unable to provide satisfactory answers to fundamental moral questions aris-ing at the beginning and the end of human life. He attributes these shortcomings in Western bioethics to the overwhelming influence of the Cartesian tradition on modern moral discourse and seeks to amend this conceptual bias through a re-evaluation of a Christian alternative: the relational ("perichoretic") conception of personhood as it was first developed in seventh-century Trinitarian theology. Hui claims that Christian Trini-tarian theology has laid the foundations for a relational understanding of creation upon which a conception of personhood can be constructed that does not share the shortcomings of the Cartesian tradition.

Interestingly, Hui finds in Confucianism a further reason for the rehabilitation of the Trinitarian concept of personhood and its application to contemporary bioethical dis-course. Against the backdrop of Christian onto-theology, the Confucian concept of *ren* (usually translated as *benevolence* or *humanity*) can be seen as "a serious attempt by the Chinese people to probe the relational dimension of human nature as an instance of the manifestation of the perichoretic nature of reality" (Hui, 2000, p. 104). As a relational term, *ren* constitutes personhood in a complex ontology of relationships that involves mutuality and commonality of the self and the other. Thus Confucian personhood is a continuous process of "person-making", which is grounded in "the relation that exists between the self and the other both of whom attain personhood in that matrix". Hui con-cludes that in this regard "the Confucian person bears resemblance to the Christian peri-choretic personhood in being an onto-relational concept" (Hui, 2000, pp. 109-110). He is confident that such relational understanding will modify the narrowly psychological and individualistic conceptualization of personhood and shed new light on issues that range from the use of reproductive technologies and fetal-maternal relationships to the treatment of comatose patients and euthanasia.

Similar attempts to tap both Christian and Chinese moral resources and engage them in the re-evaluation of modern bioethics have become rather popular in Hong Kong in recent years, particularly among Chinese Christians in academia. The most visible sign of this interest is the foundation in late 2001 of a new research center, the Center for Sino-Christian Studies, at Baptist University. According to its mission statement, the center reflects the acknowledgment within academia of the significance of the study of Christian thought as an integral component of Western culture for the renewal and modernization of Chinese society. The center aims at coalescing research in the field of Christian studies in the Chinese context and at exploring the cultural significance of Christianity for contemporary Chinese society. Its founding director, Ping-cheung Lo, has not only actively promoted the Chinese-Christian dialogue in Hong Kong and the Chinese mainland but also developed a strong research interest in bioethics. Although his main focus is on the development of a Christian bioethics that can offer guidance to Hong Kong society at large in its deliberation on difficult issues in modern medicine and health care, his profound understanding of the Chinese moral tradition has exerted an increasingly strong influence on the kind of Christian bioethics he envisages. This influence is particularly visible in more recent publications on a Confucian-based re-evaluation of issues at the end of life and of death with dignity (Lo, 1999b, 1999c, 1994, 1993). Lo has argued that much of the contemporary debate about physician-assisted suicide and voluntary euthanasia is marred by an underlying "impoverished vision of human life" that is absent in both Confucianism and "other major world religions". He suggests overcoming the "superficiality" of the "argument of 'death with dignity'" that has recently gained some currency in the bioethical debate by a more comprehensive vision of human life that is neither reduced to its biological dimension nor loses sight of the soul or spirit and what Confucianism calls the moral life (Lo, 1999a, pp. 326-327).

E. The Continuing Appeal of a Universal Bioethics

As one might expect, the project of a "Confucian bioethics" has found its most ardent supporters not among the Hong Kong medical establishment but among philosophers and ethicists in tertiary institutions. The call for the construction of a Confucian bioethics is, however, not unanimously supported by Hong Kong ethicists. Doubts have been raised whether a modern bioethics can be exclusively grounded on distinctly Confucian values and thus provide the answers to the moral issues of modern medicine and biotechnology. Although it has been claimed that "Confucian bioethics stands out as a significant communitarian bioethics that offers a coherent way of engaging the good life" (Fan, 1999a, p. 22), the very attempt to press Confucian bioethics into the matrix of a debate defined by liberalism or cosmopolitanism, on the one side, and communitarianism, on the other, seems to confirm the doubts about its ability to provide an original and resourceful alternative. Instead of bringing Confucianism into the rather narrow focus of this debate and taking sides, it seems that a true alternative conception of a Confucian bioethics would imply that it should transcend both versions of moral theory and, on the basis of its own unique moral tradition, be able to respond persuasively to the same set of moral issues the rival theories are supposed to resolve.

While it may be true that, from a Confucian point of view, modern medicine and biotechnology do not pose serious moral problems, the wholesale acceptance of modern science and its high-tech products has been attributed to conceptual shortcomings in such versions of Confucian bioethics. With regard to the Confucian understanding of personhood that has been frequently invoked to criticize the alleged individualism of "Western" ethics (Hui, 2000), Jiwei Ci at the University of Hong Kong has argued that Confucianism cannot offer the alternative its proponents suggest. He even claims that "Confucianism is vitiated by certain unattractive features that cannot be removed without reducing the Confucian relational concept of the person to an abstract and not very helpful notion of human relatedness". On his account, the concept is:

> either *over*determined, in the sense that it retains unattractive features of historical Confucianism [i.e., unquestioned social hierarchies] or it is *under*-determined, in the sense that the realization that persons and personhood are formed in the context of social relations does not determine the form that those social relations should take and therefore cannot by itself yield a distinctively Confucian concept of social relations (Ci, 1999, p. 325).

Jonathan Chan (Hong Kong Baptist University) has raised similar methodological questions from a Rawlsian perspective and asks how a Confucian bioethics might be able to give moral guidance other than to the few committed Confucians. Given that Hong Kong constitutes a pluralist "public sphere" of diverse moral communities where Protestants and Catholics, Muslims, Buddhists, and Taoists live alongside Confucians and where the overwhelming majority belongs to none of these but "keeps an open mind" about any traditional values of particular communities, Confucian bioethics is facing a dilemma:

> On the one hand, if the ethical rules and guidance in question are so heavily shaped by the comprehensive doctrines of the traditions of Chinese philosophy, then there is no reason to expect citizens who belong to other traditions to accept them. On the other hand, if the ethical rules and guidance in question have nothing, or too little, to do with the traditions of Chinese philosophy, then Chinese bioethics will lose its distinctiveness (Chan, Jonathan, 1998, p. 191).

Thus the picture of Hong Kong bioethics would be incomplete without reference to Hong Kong-based ethicists who continue to explore bioethical issues from the perspective of universal ethics that would nevertheless be sensitive to the moral intuitions of the Chinese tradition. Major issues that are being explored include the principle of human dignity and its relevance for contemporary bioethics (Au, 2000; Becker, 2002b, 2000a), conceptions of autonomy and liberty in the context of prenatal screening and diagnostics (Becker, 2002a, 1996a), informed consent (Pang, 1999, 1998a), the ethics of human cloning (Becker, 2000b, 1997; Chan, Jonathan, 2000, 1998), abortion (Li, Hon-lam, 1997, 1996), euthanasia (Chan, Ho-mun, 1997a), health care (Chan, Ho-mun, 1999, 1998), reproductive technology (Liu, 1991; Lo, 1996) and nursing (Pang, 1998, Pang & Shae, 1998).

The continued belief among Hong Kong bioethicists in the need for and the viability of a universal bioethics has also been confirmed by some highly visible and influential conferences, symposia and public forums. They include conferences organized by the Center for Applied Ethics at Hong Kong Baptist University (Biotechnology and Ethics, 1993; Reproductive Technology and Ethics, 1997; Bioethics and the Concept of Personhood, 1998), the Center for Comparative Public Management and Social Policy at the City University of Hong Kong (Individual, Community and Society: Bioethics in the Third Millennium, 1999; Ethics and Policy Choice in Health Care Financing, 1999; Quality Care Services for Elderly People, 1999, 2000; Values of Health Care and Fundamentals of Reform, 2000; Managing New Drugs: Ethical, Legal, Administrative, and Clinical, 2001) and by the Department of Philosophy at the Chinese University (International Conference on Applied Ethics, 1999).

III. Bioethics at Hong Kong Tertiary Institutions

Moral relationships in secular societies have been described as those of moral strangers, i.e.:

> persons who do not share sufficient moral premises or rules of evidence and inference to resolve moral controversies by sound rational argument, or who do not have a common commitment to individuals or institutions in authority to resolve moral controversies (Engelhardt, 1996, p. 7).

As far as Hong Kong bioethicists and their moral relationships are concerned, moral strangers seem to live side-by-side with moral friends, while the vast majority may simply fall into the category of moral acquaintances (Loewy, 1997, p. 3) whose diverse moral communities have still so much in common as to make the search for an overlapping consensus a meaningful enterprise.

In the 1995 opening issue of the *Chinese Bioethics Newsletter*, Si-Wai Man of the Chinese University of Hong Kong claimed to discover two main conceptual approaches in Hong Kong bioethics, which she characterizes as *static* versus *dynamic*. She associates the static approach as having emerged from the "long tradition of Christian concern for applied ethical issues", with variations existing "only as a result of divergence in interpretation of the Christian doctrines by different sects or denominations". In contrast to this, she notices a recent "more dynamic turn" in Hong Kong bioethics, signs of which she sees mainly in the fact that instead of academics, more "practitioners in their personal capacities" discuss ethical issues in the media without aiming at a systematic analysis and principled theory. Although this seems to take existing differences too far, it may be meaningful as an attempt to project the larger discussion about ethical "principlism", virtue ethics and communitarian approaches onto the unfolding canvass of Hong Kong bioethics.

A. *The Center for Applied Ethics*
One clear indicator of the emerging strength of bioethics research in Hong Kong was the establishment of the *Center for Applied Ethics* at Hong Kong Baptist University in 1992

(founding director: Gerhold K. Becker; director since 2000: King-tak Ip). The Center was (and still is) the first of its kind in Hong Kong and has been recognized as a leader in the whole region. Though deliberately not founded as a research center with an exclusive focus on bioethics, the Center has greatly facilitated bioethics research and the bioethical discourse in general through individual research projects, international conferences (see above), publications and its public lecture series. Major research projects and publications in bioethics include the following: Issues of doctor–patient communication (Smith, David, 1996); Chinese perspectives on suicides (Lo, 1999a, 1999c); age and gender as categories of analysis in decisions at the end of life (Weaver, 1998); prenatal screening (Becker, 2002a); human dignity and moral autonomy (Becker, 2002b); moral issues in the genetification of human life (Becker, 1998, 1996; Zimbelman, 1996a); the moral significance of personhood (Becker, 2000a); the ethics of scientifically assisted human reproduction policies in Hong Kong (Lo, 1996); the ethics of human cloning (Chan, 2000; Becker, 1997) and testing for HIV in Hong Kong (Zimbelman, 1996b).

Besides organizing various bioethics conferences and symposia, the *Center* launched an Occasional Papers Series as well as a newsletter entitled *Ethics and Society*. It is co-sponsor of the new Chinese-language *Journal of Chinese and International Philosophy of Medicine* (*Zhong Wai Yi Xue Zhe Xue*) and of the *Studies in Applied Ethics*, a special series of the Value Inquiry Book Series (VIBS), published by Rodopi (Amsterdam & New York).

B. Bioethics Teaching

Bioethics has arrived rather late at the educational scene of Hong Kong. Up to the early 1990s, ethics played only a marginal role in teaching and research. The two oldest universities distinguished themselves mainly by their different emphases on Western philosophy in the analytic tradition (University of Hong Kong) and on Chinese and Western comparative philosophy (Chinese University). While the universities together with the colleges in the liberal arts tradition included ethics in their curriculum (particularly within the context of general education), the focus of ethics teaching and research was largely on foundational issues and rarely widened to include topics of a more applied nature.

At present (2001), Hong Kong has seven publicly-funded universities under the government's University Grants Committee with about 70,000 full-time students in higher education. Only two of them, the University of Hong Kong and the Chinese University of Hong Kong, have full medical faculties or schools with several large teaching hospitals attached. This fact alone signals certain restrictions for bioethics teaching in institutions not involved in the training of medical students. While the medical research and practice at these two institutions is undoubtedly of the highest standard and has been internationally recognized for its excellence in a variety of disciplines, the development of ethics education within the medical curriculum has been relatively slow and piecemeal. As someone involved in ethics teaching at the Prince of Wales Hospital and Shatin Hospital said: "I believe that medical ethics is a relatively under-developed area in Hong Kong. This has a detrimental effect on patient care and the morale of doctors."

In general, medical ethics and bioethics are not offered as semester-long courses but integrated into the various components of the curriculum. Although students are faced with ethical issues throughout their five-year medical training, ethics teaching takes place predominantly in the context of patient care during ward rounds and bedside tutorials. Individual lectures on specific topics in medical ethics are offered at certain junctures in the medical curriculum and are usually taught by medical doctors with some specialization in ethics. Topics covered include a fair range of ethical issues, in particular organ donation and transplantation, consent to and refusal of treatment, confidentiality and patients' rights. Currently, a semester-long course in medical ethics proper as a required subject is only offered by the newly established School of Chinese Medicine at Hong Kong Baptist University. According to the course document, the objectives are to deepen ethical sensitivity in medical students, to provide them with the necessary conceptual and analytical skills for moral decision making in a clinical setting, to introduce the students to the moral values of the Chinese medical tradition together with those of the West, to stimulate their moral imagination through case studies and, finally, to clarify and reflect on the wider and foundational ethical issues of medicine.

An elective course at the University of Hong Kong, "Biomedical Ethics and Law", is not exclusively focused on medical ethics but covers also an introduction to the relevant laws of Hong Kong. In addition, a bioethics course (of 24 credit hours) has been offered over the last years as an elective by the Department of Zoology but is open to medical students too. This course explores the ethical implications in recent major advancements in biological and medical sciences and includes the areas of genetics, reproduction, disease diagnosis and therapy, transplantation, aging, dying, the environment, and the use of animals in research. According to the lecturer, this course has proven popular with students and received good feedback.

Courses in medical ethics are also offered in the various nursing programs at the two medical schools and the Polytechnic University of Hong Kong. The course "Ethical and Legal Aspects of Nursing" at the latter institution is a case in point. The course is an integral part of the Bachelor of Science in Nursing and introduces students to "biomedical principles and ethical theories" besides offering opportunities "for value clarification and self-understanding" of the students' moral stance. Selected models of ethical reasoning are being discussed "for their application in analyzing ethical issues in difficult care situations" (Course Document).

IV. Towards a Public Moral Discourse

Obviously, there is room for improvement regarding how Hong Kong medical schools integrate bioethics into their curriculum and prepare medical doctors for the many challenges ahead. The significance of adequate ethical education in medical schools and in professional life has been highlighted in recent controversies involving the monitoring role of the Hong Kong Medical Council. As the number of cases of alleged malpractice increased and the subsequent rulings of the Medical Council were seen as inadequate and lacking in transparency, a leading clinician and academic appealed to the public to "trust its professionals", because they had "received years of training, including in professional ethics" (Lam, 2001, p. 16). The comment sparked astonished reactions in the letter sections of local newspapers, and readers wondered whether such views were representative of the medical profession as a whole. In light of the strong public criticism of the Medical Council's handling of complaints against individual doctors, the Council instituted a comprehensive review of its complaints mechanism and accepted a government proposal to establish a central complaints office within the Department of Health. Similarly, the Academy of Medicine recommended to the Medical Council that continuing medical education units be linked to the annual registration of physicians.

The public attention that issues of professional ethics receive is just one indicator of a growing awareness in Hong Kong of the significance of medical ethics and of the need for public moral discourse. Reasons for this development may be found in a broad-based recognition of the extent to which advances in modern biology, medicine and biotechnology have begun to influence, and irreversibly so, the views people hold about fundamental aspects of life, health, disease and death. Although such heightened awareness of the ethical challenges in modern life is not exclusively confined to the fields of modern biology, medicine and health care, in Hong Kong it is characteristic of a developing public moral discourse that involves individuals from all walks of life and continues to exert influence on relevant government policies. It is typical of such public moral discourse that it is conducted simultaneously through the usual academic channels (journal essays, symposia, etc.), the news media (including editorials, comments and letters to the editor), as well as government-sponsored formal processes of public consultations.

The most impressive example of the existence of such moral discourse is the strong response by the public to the government's decision to regulate reproductive technology. The inherent complexity of this process, which raised numerous moral and legal issues, generated the most sustained bioethical debate Hong Kong has so far seen.

A. The Human Reproductive Technology Bill

In Hong Kong, artificial insemination has been available at least since the 1970s, although the first successful *in vitro* fertilization (IVF) did not take place until 1986 (Queen Mary Hospital). From 1986 to 1995, a total of 2578 treatment cycles in artificial reproduction were performed through a variety of techniques (GIFT: 192; PROST: 200; IVF: 1375), which resulted in 495 successful pregnancies.

In light of public unease about the new technology and its potential for abuse, the government concluded that the unfettered use of reproductive technology was morally controversial and socially undesirable. In November 1987, a regulatory framework for future legislation was set up and a Committee on Scientifically Assisted Human Reproduction (CSAHR) appointed, with representatives from the medical and legal professions, social work and psychology. Its terms of reference included the task to advise the government on the social, moral and legal issues arising from local developments in reproductive technology and to assess public reactions towards these issues.

After nineteen meetings, the Committee published in July 1989 an *Interim Report* on surrogacy and artificial insemination and conducted a public consultation both in English and Chinese, which produced 24 formal submissions. The Committee reviewed its earlier conclusions and presented in October 1992 its *Final Report* to the Executive Council with a total of 22 recommendations. Apart from the establishment of a statutory body and a licensing system for all reproductive service providers, the recommendations included provisions against the creation of embryos for research purposes and embryo research after the fourteenth day of fertilization as well as the prohibition of commercial surrogacy. Surrogacy should be generally allowed but subjected to a number of specific restrictions.

On the advice of the Executive Council, the Governor decided that the public should be consulted on these recommendations. The consultation period took place from April to September 1993, and a total of 30 written responses were received.

The reaction from the public to the government's approach towards reproductive technology was, however, not restricted to formal submissions to the Committee. A survey of local newspapers reveals a lively debate along moral lines of concern about these issues and thus confirms an emerging and sustained bioethical discourse in Hong Kong. While there was a broad consensus that the use of reproductive technology should be regulated by law and that embryos should not be created for research purposes, public response was more divided on the approach to surrogacy (Lo, 1996). Various commentators found the proposed ban of commercial surrogacy unnecessary and in conflict with the values of a liberal society that Hong Kong has been espousing for so long in the areas of business and trade. Yet, this view was strongly rejected by those who claimed to uphold specific Chinese values of family and social bonding. They argued not only for a ban of commercial surrogacy but of surrogacy itself and in all its forms, since it was considered to be in conflict with the traditional Chinese values of parenthood, a violation of filial relations and detrimental to the well-being of the children concerned; it was, above all, out of tune with the traditional Confucian concept of relational personhood (Tao & Chan, 1997). This perception was corroborated by a telephone opinion poll conducted in March 1999 by researchers from City University (Julia Tao, Ho-mun Chan, Anthony Fung) on public attitudes towards surrogacy and related issues (such as "male pregnancies"). A majority of respondents rejected both commercial and non-commercial surrogacy as "immoral" and "unnatural" and neither in the interest of the children born through such methods nor in accordance with human social (parental) relationships. A similar view was expressed by the Central Coordinating Committee on Obstetrics and Gynecology of the Hospital Authority, which proposed actively to discourage surrogacy and to make commercial surrogacy and its arrangement or advertising a criminal offence (Lee, 1997). It was, therefore, not surprising that the news of a couple paying HK$40,000 to a domestic helper to be the surrogate mother of their future child was met with public indignation and outrage (Smith, 1997).

In the light of the response from the public, the Executive Council endorsed in September 1994 the recommendations put forward by the CSAHR and decided that "a value-neutral attitude" should be adopted that neither prohibits nor promotes reproductive technologies. In accordance with the recommendations, a statutory body was established in December 1995 under the name Provisional Council on Reproductive Technology so as to draw up regulatory legislation and a licensing system for service providers. On 2 May 1996, the Provisional Council set up an Ethics Committee to examine the ethical and social dimensions of new developments in reproductive technology.

Recognizing the complexity as well as the daunting choices new developments in reproductive technology present to policy makers and individuals alike, the Provisional Council sought to adopt "a multi-disciplinary approach", which should ensure "the safe and informed practice of reproductive technology in a way that respects human life, the role of the family, the rights of service users and the welfare of children born through reproductive technology" (Mission Statement). In the same spirit, the Ethics Committee selected the following four moral principles as signposts for its deliberations:

(1) Human life in all its forms warrants respect and special moral consideration.
(2) The welfare of the child is of paramount importance.

(3) Personal autonomy and individual liberty must be duly safeguarded.
(4) Due recognition must be given to basic community values such as responsible parenthood, parental love, and the family.

The Provisional Council decided to carry out a two-month public consultation in 1996 (both in English and Chinese) to gauge the view of the public on three major issues arising from the currently drafted Human Reproductive Technology Bill:

- the licensing arrangements,
- sex selection achieved by means of reproductive technology, and
- the use of fetal (ovarian or testicular) tissue in infertility treatment and in research.

A total of 41 written submissions were received, most of which were from medical professionals and professional bodies, social service groups, religious bodies, academic institutions and organizations involved in the practice of reproductive technology. One submission represented the views of 183 individuals. 15 views were also collected from a call-in radio program, *Heart of the Matter*, and from articles/editorials published in newspapers.

With regard to sex selection, except for a few respondents who suggested that sex selection be prohibited completely, the majority view was that it should be allowed for medical reasons only, since it could avoid the birth of a child suffering from a serious sex-linked disease. This view was also supported by the Hong Kong Medical Association and the College of Obstetricians and Gynecologists. While a few respondents thought the prohibition of sex selection for social reasons would violate basic human rights, and the Gender Choice Center, which had offered relevant services in Hong Kong since November 1993, should be allowed to continue its operation, most respondents expressed great moral concern and feared the social consequences of sex selection. Particularly in a Chinese society, which has traditionally preferred male to female children, even to the extent that female infanticide is still not uncommon in some areas of contemporary rural China (Becker, Jasper, 2000, p. 237), respondents argued that sex selection on social grounds would ultimately erode the respect owed to each and every human person.

Incorporating these views into its recommendations, the Provisional Council decided to allow sex selection only for avoiding the birth of a child with a severe sex-linked genetic disease and stipulated that the need for sex selection must be certified by two registered medical practitioners and monitored by the future statutory Council. In spite of the acknowledged difficulty to define "severity of disease", the Provisional Council decided to draw up an open-ended list of sex-linked genetic diseases for guidance and reference purposes.

Although a few respondents considered that fetal ovarian/testicular tissue was a rich source of material for infertility treatment and its use would help infertile patients, most respondents did not regard such use as an appropriate solution for infertility treatment. With the exception of two respondents who indicated strong objection, all those who expressed views on these issues were in support of the use of ovarian/testicular tissue for research purposes as long as no embryo was formed.

In line with earlier recommendations by the CSAHR, which had been endorsed in the public consultation process, the Provisional Council supported the prohibitions of creating embryos for research purposes and of keeping or using an embryo after the appearance of the primitive streak. It strictly ruled against combining human and non-human gametes or embryos and against the cloning of embryos in all its forms. The Provisional Council considered research on so-called spare embryos morally and legally permissible, if such research was proven to be "essential" for the medical advancement and could not be achieved by any other means. For that purpose, it endorsed a two-tier system for approving embryo research projects comprised of institutional research ethics committees for internal vetting of research proposals and the future statutory Council as the authority for final approval. While the Provisional Council considered somatic genetic manipulation and therapy morally unproblematic, it banned germ-line genetic therapy, on the grounds that it poses unacceptable risks for individual patients and society alike.

To supplement the statutory requirements in the Human Reproductive Technology Ordinance and to regulate its practice, the Provisional Council drew up a draft *Code of Practice on Reproductive Technology and Embryo Research* and subjected it to a public consultation process in February 1999. The *Code* sets minimum standards, which aim to support the best clinical and scientific practice, to safeguard the health and interest of service users and to protect the welfare of children born through reproductive technology. The *Code* will assist the statutory Council to discharge its duties as the licensing authority for reproductive technology procedures and embryo research, and failure to comply with the *Code* may constitute grounds for refusal to grant or renew a license, or for suspension or cancellation of a license. The draft was sent to 180 reproductive technology service providers, medical and health related professional bodies, non-medical professional bodies, hospitals, tertiary institutions, academics and support groups for IVF and infertility services. While most respondents welcomed the draft Code as a meaningful regulatory tool, some criticized it as too conservative and paternalistic and, in particular, questioned the need to restrict reproductive technology services to legally married couples.

The Human Reproductive Technology Bill was finally approved by the Legislative Council on 23 June 2000. The new Bill incorporated all recommendations of the Provisional Council and in particular restricted reproductive technology services to legally married couples.

Taking into account the fundamental community values as they had been endorsed during the long process towards legislation, it seems fair to say that the stipulations in the Bill are based on the three fundamental principles of equal liberty, equal worth, and family integrity (Gould & Chan, 1995). Particularly the latter principle reflects the strong emphasis the Bill has placed on traditional Chinese family values and was the main reason for restricting the use of reproductive technology to legally married couples. As the Provisional Council stated in its *Report*, this provision is in accordance with the agreed community values of responsible parenthood, parental love and the family. Since marriage is considered by the community as having a unique personal and social value, the Provisional Council concluded it should be protected and strengthened by law and the restriction should be seen as a recognition of the value which the law and the community give to the institutions of marriage and family, particularly with regard to the welfare of the child. The principle that the welfare of the child is of paramount importance, which was adopted by the CSAHR and endorsed by the Provisional Council, has again been invoked. It argued that the complex legal, ethical, medical and social problems raised by reproductive technology, which affect not only individuals but also the common good, would be "seriously aggravated should reproductive technology services be not restricted to legally married couples and become generally available to all regardless of whether they are single or married or regardless of sexual orientation" (*Report*, 2000). The Provisional Council recognized, however, that exceptional circumstances could arise, which may arguably justify a departure from this norm. Such circumstances could concern previously married persons who were no longer parties to a marriage at the time of their application. In accordance with the recommendations of the Provisional Council, the Bill has empowered the newly established statutory Council on Reproductive Technology to circumscribe the exception by way of regulations.

V. Conclusion

Bioethics in Hong Kong has been as much shaped by the *genius loci* as by relevant developments overseas. Though it is too early to identify it in Hong Kong with a clearly defined discipline that can muster its own theoretical support, bioethics is much more visible as an ongoing public moral discourse about ethical decision-making within the context of modern medicine and health care. Thus bioethics as a securely established academic discipline has still some way to go to in finding its place in Hong Kong's tertiary institutions. A multi-disciplinary discourse with a particular focus on ethical issues in medicine, health care and the quality of life, however, is already firmly entrenched.

Bibliography

Au, D.K.S. 2000. Brain injury, brain degeneration, and loss of personhood. In G. Becker (ed.), *The Moral Status of Personhood: Perspectives on Bioethics* (pp. 209-217). Amsterdam/Atlanta: Rodopi.

Au, D.K.S. 1999. Constructing options for health care reform in Hong Kong. *Journal of Medicine & Philosophy* 24(6): 607-623.

Bauer, J.R. & Bell, D.A. (eds) 1999. *The East Asian challenge for human rights*. Cambridge: Cambridge University Press.

Beauchamp, T. 1979. Bioethics in Japan and Hong Kong. *The Kennedy Institute Quarterly*: 49-51.

Becker, G.K. 2002a. The ethics of prenatal screening and the search for global bioethics. In J. Tao (ed.), *Cross-cultural perspectives on the (im)possibility of a global bioethics* (pp. 105-130). Dordrecht: Kluwer Academic Publishers.

Becker, G.K. 2002b. In search of humanity: human dignity as a basic moral attitude. In M. Häyry & T. Takala (eds), *The future of value inquiry*. Atlanta/Amsterdam: Rodopi.

Becker, G.K. (ed.) 2000a. *The moral status of personhood: perspectives on bioethics*. Atlanta/ Amsterdam: Rodopi.

Becker, G.K. 2000b. Reproductive choice and moral responsibility: the challenge of human cloning. *Prajna Vihara Journal of Philosophy and Religion* 1(1): 1-31.

Becker, G.K. 1998. Ethical issues in medical genetics. In: S.T.S. Lam, M.H.Y. Tang, I.F.M. Lo & W.K. Chan (eds), (pp. 207-216). *Proceedings of the 1st Hong Kong Medical Genetics Conference*. Hong Kong: Publication of Hong Kong Society of Medical Genetics.

Becker, G.K. 1997. Cloning humans? The Chinese debate and why it matters. *Eubios Journal of Asian and International Bioethics* 7(6): 175-177.

Becker, G.K. (ed.) 1996a. *Changing nature's course: the ethical challenge of biotechnology*. Hong Kong: Hong Kong University Press.

Becker, G.K. (ed.) 1996b. *Ethics in business and society. Chinese and Western perspectives*. Berlin: Springer.

Becker, J. 2000. *The Chinese*. New York: The Free Press.

Bell, D.A. 2000. *East meets west: human rights and democracy in East Asia*. Princeton: Princeton University Press.

Chan, Ho-mun. 1999. Free choice, equity, and care: the moral foundations of health care. *Journal of Medicine and Philosophy* 24(6): 624-637.

Chan, Ho-mun. 1998. Social justice and the distribution of healthcare burdens and benefits. *Values & Society Series*, Vol. 2. Beijing: China Social Sciences Publishing House (in Chinese).

Chan, Ho-mun. 1997. The absurdity of euthanasia, patients right to self-determination, and the goals of medicine. *Values and Society Series*, Vol. 1 (pp. 74-101). Beijing: China Social Sciences Publishing House (in Chinese).

Chan Jonathan, K.L. 2000. Human cloning, harm and personal identity. In G. Becker (ed.), *The moral status of personhood: perspectives on bioethics* (pp. 195-207). Amsterdam/Atlanta: Rodopi.

Chan Jonathan, K.L. 1998. From Chinese bioethics to human cloning: a methodological reflection. *Chinese & International Philosophy of Medicine* 1(3): 49-71 (in Chinese; English abstract, 189-192).

Chan Joseph, K.L. 1999. A Confucian perspective on human rights for contemporary China. In J. Bauer & D. Bell (eds), (pp. 212-237). *The East Asian challenge for human rights*. Cambridge: Cambridge University Press.

Chan, A.Y. et al., 1990. Public attitudes toward kidney donation in Hong Kong. *Dialysis Transplant* 19: 242-257.

Chan, Y. H. & Wong, F.K.M. 2000. Highlights of the 5th annual scientific meeting of the Hong Kong society of transplantation. *The Hong Kong Medical Diary* 5(4): 11-15.

Chow, N.W.S. 1992. Family care of the elderly in Hong Kong. In J.I. Kosberg (ed.), *Family care of the elderly. Social and cultural changes* (pp. 123-138). Newbury Park: Sage Publications.

Ci, J. 1999. The Confucian relational concept of the person and its modern predicament. *Kennedy Institute of Ethics Journal* 9(4): 325-346.

Döring, O. (ed.) 1999. *Chinese scientist and responsibility: ethical issues of human genetics in Chinese and international contexts*, Vol. 34. Hamburg: Mitteilungen des Instituts für Asienkunde.

Dyson, A. 1986. Hong Kong in touch with the world. In B. Knight (ed.), *Hong Kong 1986* (pp. 1-13). Hong Kong: Government Information Services.

Engelhardt, Jr., H.T. 1980. Bioethics in the People's Republic of China. *Hastings Center Report* 10 (April), 7-10.

Engelhardt, Jr., H.T. 1996. *The foundations of bioethics*, (2nd ed.). Oxford: Oxford University Press.

Fan, R. 2000. Can we have a general conception of personhood in bioethics? In G. Becker (ed.), *The moral status of personhood: perspectives on bioethics* (pp. 15-27). Amsterdam/Atlanta: Rodopi.

Fan, R. (ed.) 1999a. *Confucian bioethics*. Dordrecht: Kluwer.

Fan, R. 1999b. Freedom, responsibility, and care: Hong Kong's health care reform, *Journal of Medicine and Philosophy* 24(6): 555-570.

Fan, R. 1998. Human cloning and human dignity: pluralist society and the Confucian moral community. *Chinese & International Philosophy of Medicine* 1(3): 73-93 (in Chinese; English abstract, 193-196).

Fox, R.C. & Swazey, J. 1984. Medical morality is not bioethics: medical ethics in China and the United States. *Perspectives in Biology and Medicine* 27(3): 336-360.

Gould, D.B. & Chan, H. 1995. Organs and embryos: ethical policymaking in a moral minefield. *Hong Kong Public Administration* 4(1): 95-109.

Hawkins, B.R. 2000. The role of tissue typing in transplantation. *The Hong Kong Medical Diary* 5(4): 17-18.

Ho, K. & Leung, S. 1997. Postmaterialism revisited. In: S. Lau et al. (eds). *Indicators of social development: Hong Kong 1995* (pp. 331-358). Hong Kong: Hong Kong Institute of Asia-Pacific Studies.

Hong Kong Government. 1974. *White paper on the further development of medical and health services in Hong Kong.* Hong Kong: Hong Kong Government Printer.

Hong Kong Government. 1991. *Social welfare into the 1990s and beyond.* Hong Kong: Hong Kong Government Printer.

Hu, Y. 1995. Elderly suicide risk in family contexts: a critique of the Asian family care model. *Journal of Cross-Cultural Gerontology* 10: 199-217.

Hui, E. 2000. Jen and perichoresis: the Confucian and Christian bases of the relational person. In: G. Becker (ed.), *The moral status of personhood: perspectives on bioethics* (pp. 95-117). Amsterdam/Atlanta: Rodopi.

Hsiao, W. et al. 1999. *Improving Hong Kong's health care system: why and for whom?* (Main report). Hong Kong: Hong Kong Government Printer.

Jonsen, A. 1998. *The birth of bioethics.* Oxford: Oxford University Press.

Lam, S. 2001. Phone row a loss to society. *South China Morning Post*, 2 May.

Lau, S. & Kuan, H. 1988. *The ethos of the Hong Kong Chinese.* Hong Kong: The Chinese University of Press.

Lee, Anita. 1997. Opposed to surrogacy. *South China Morning Post*, 13 May.

Lee, Shui-chuen. 1999a. *Confucian bioethics (rujia shenming lunlixue).* Taipei: Legion Press.

Lee, Shui-chuen. 1999b. A Confucian perspective on human genetics. In O. Döring (ed.). *Chinese scientist and responsibility: ethical issues of human genetics in Chinese and international contexts* (pp. 187-198) Vol. 34. Hamburg: Mitteilungen des Instituts für Asienkunde.

Levenson, J.R. 1968. *Confucian China and its modern fate: a trilogy.* Berkeley: University of California Press.

Li, P.K.T. 2000. Public attitudes towards organ donation in Hong Kong. *The Hong Kong Medical Diary* 5(4): 8-9.

Li, H. 1997. Abortion and degrees of personhood: understanding why the abortion problem (and the animal rights problem) are irresolvable. *Public Affairs Quarterly* 11(1): 1-19.

Li, H. 1996. Abortion and uncertainty. In G.K. Becker (ed.). *Ethics in business and society. Chinese and Western perspectives* (pp. 179-180). Berlin: Springer Verlag.

Liu, A. 1991. *Artificial reproduction and reproductive rights.* Aldershot: Dartmouth Publishing Company.

Lo, P. 1999a. Confucian ethic of death with dignity and its contemporary relevance. *Annual of the Society of Christian Ethics* 19: 313-333.

Lo, P. 1999b. Medical and philosophical issues in determining death. *Chinese & International Philosophy of Medicine* 2(3): 1-28.

Lo, P. 1999c. Confucian views on suicide and their implications for euthanasia. In R. Fan (ed.), *Confucian bioethics* (pp. 69-101). Dordrecht: Kluwer.

Lo, P. 1997. *Freedom and its moral boundary.* Hong Kong: Logos Publishers (in Chinese).

Lo, P. 1993. *Starry heaven and morality. Ethics and its applications.* Hong Kong: Joint Publishing (in Chinese).

Lo, P. 1994. *Ethical issues in birth, death and sex.* Hong Kong: Breakthrough (in Chinese).

Lo, P. 1996. Ethical reflections on artificial reproduction policies in Hong Kong. In G.K. Becker (ed.). *Ethics in business and society. Chinese and Western perspectives* (pp. 181-195). Berlin: Springer.

Lo, Chung-mao. 2001. Problems and practice with the development of liver transplantation at Queen Mary Hospital. *The Hong Kong Medical Diary* 6(4): 16-17.

Loewy, E.H. 1997. *Moral strangers, moral acquaintance, and moral friends. Connectedness and its conditions.* Albany: State University of New York Press.

Nie, J. 2000. The plurality of Chinese and American medical moralities: toward an interpretive cross-cultural bioethics. *Kennedy Institute of Ethics Journal* 10(3): 239-260.

Nie, J. 1999. Human drugs in Chinese medicine and the Confucian view: an interpretive study. In R. Fan (ed.), *Confucian bioethics* (pp. 167-206). Dordrecht: Kluwer.

Pang, S.M. 1999. Protective truthfulness: the Chinese way of safeguarding patients in informed treatment decisions. *Journal of Medical Ethics* 25(3): 247-253.

Pang, S.M. 1998. Information disclosure: the moral experience of nurses in China. *Nursing Ethics* 5(4): 347-361.

Pang, S.M. & Shae, W.C. 1998. The "code of professional conduct for nurses in Hong Kong": a critique and recommendation. *Asian Journal of Nursing Studies* 4(3): 46-55.

Postiglione, G.A. 1992. The decolonization of Hong Kong education. In G.A. Postiglione (ed.), *Education and society in Hong Kong* (pp. 3-38). Hong Kong: Hong Kong University Press.

Report of the Provisional Council on Reproductive Technology (2000). Hong Kong: Department of Health and Welfare.

Roetz, H. 1993. *Confucian ethics of the axial age*. Albany: State University of New York Press.

Shaw, S. 2000. Back to a culture of subservience. *The South China Morning Post*, 27 August.

Smith, A. 1997. Childless couple pay maid $40,000 to have their baby. *South China Morning Post*, 19 May.

Smith, D. 1996. The ethics of the physician patient relationship. *Critical Care Clinics* 12(1): 179-197.

Siu, H.F. 1996. Remade in Hong Kong: weaving into the Chinese cultural tapestry. In T.T. Liu & D. Faure (eds), *Unity and diversity: local cultures and identities in China* (pp. 177-198). Hong Kong: Hong Kong University Press.

Tao, J. 2000. Two perspectives of care: Confucian ren and feminist care. *Journal of Chinese Philosophy* 27(2): 215-240.

Tao, J. 1999. Does it really care? The Harvard report on health care reform for Hong Kong. *Journal of Medicine and Philosophy* 24(6): 571-590.

Tao, J. 1998. Confucianism. In R. Chadwick (ed.), *Encyclopedia of applied ethics* (pp. 597-608). San Diego: Academic Press.

Tao, J. 1996. The moral foundation of welfare in Chinese society: between virtues and rights. In G.K. Becker (ed.). *Ethics in business and society. Chinese and Western perspectives* (pp. 9-24). Berlin: Springer.

Tu, W. 1989. *Confucianism in an historical perspective*. Singapore: The Institute of East Asian Philosophies.

Weaver, S. 1998. A feminist perspective: gender and age as categories of analysis in biomedical ethics. *Ethics and Society* 6(2): 8-11.

Wong, T.W.P. & Ng, C.H. 1995. Education ethos and social change. In: S. Lau et al. (eds). *Indicators of social development: Hong Kong 1995* (pp. 233-254). Hong Kong: Hong Kong Institute of Asian Pacific Studies.

Yip, K. 1997. An overview of the development of psychiatric rehabilitation services in Hong Kong. *Hong Kong Journal of Mental Health* 26(1).

Zimbelman, J. 1996a. Technology assessment, ethics and public policy in biotechnology: the case of the human genome project. In G.K. Becker (ed.), *Changing nature's course: the ethical challenge of biotechnology* (pp. 85-108). Hong Kong: Hong Kong University Press.

Zimbelman, J. 1996b. Testing for HIV in Hong Kong: challenge to ethics and public policy. In G.K. Becker (ed.), *Ethics in business and society. Chinese and Western perspectives* (pp. 196-231). Berlin: Springer.

17 The Long History of Indian Medical Systems and Current Perspectives in Health Care Bioethics

Jayapaul Azariah

I. Introduction

The premise on which the Indian approach to ethical, social and legal issues with regard to the recent progress in modern science and technology is grounded in the following stanza from an ancient scripture:

> Right (*dharma*) and wrong (*adharma*) do not go about saying
> "Here we are!"
> Nor do gods, Centaurs and ancestors say
> "This is right and that is wrong"
>
> (*Apastamba Dharma Sutra*, 1.7.20.6).

The moral tradition which developed during the past four thousand years of Indian history is mainly due to intuitive knowledge combined with a rich blend of nature-based common sense ethics. Religion served as an effective base for implementation of these social, cultural, and religious practices. They defined the framework for understanding individual health as well as appropriate community conduct. The ancient Indian concept of ethics has many shades of understanding and meaning. The *Bodhisattva* (a Buddha in the making) ethics is that of refraining from or restraining selfishness. In Sanskrit, the word for "ethics" is *sila*, which, etymologically, means: "attainment of coolness". When a person possesses ethics, his mind has a peacefulness or coolness and is free from the heat of regretting what he has done (Chitkara, 2000, pp. 413-431).

II. General Background

A. Sexuality

Indian civilization is dominated by the Vedic period, which roughly extended from 2500 B.C. to 800 B.C. Altekar (1959) records that, in the land of the Ultarakurus and in the city of Mahismati, the institution of marriage did not exist (*The Mahabharata* XII, 102, 26 [B]). There was also an astounding degree of laxity in sexual morality. Sarmishtha reports "there is no difference between one's own husband and the husband of a friend" (*The Mahabharata* [Mbh.] I, 76, 28; Altekar, 1959, p. 380). The Cankam period of Tamil civilization (300 B.C. to 300 A.D.) records two time periods in the sexual life of a person: a) *kalavu* and b) *karpu*. The former indicates premarital promiscuous sexual experiences, which is to be learnt and forgotten (i.e., not to be practiced) after marriage. The latter word (*karpu*) indicates marital union, which is to be stable. Later, the word *karpu* was used to denote the important virtue of chastity in a woman. Given such social relationships and circumstances, it is to be expected that sexually transmitted diseases were rampant, as they continue to be today.

In Indian culture, elaborate external indications inform an approaching male that a woman is married. There are three such signs: (1) application of the red (*kungkum*) powder at the parting of the hair in the forehead region of a married woman, (2) a thick yellow thread around a woman's neck tied by her husband during the marriage ceremony (commonly called the *thali*), and (3) metal rings on her toes, sometimes on both legs as well. With these external caution indications, there is no chance that any approaching male will mistake a married woman for a permissible sexual partner. This cultural practice is being followed even today. Maybe, with such external symbols, promiscuous sexual relationships were minimized so as to avoid sexually transmitted diseases. It may be of interest, that even today sexual laxity still exists in certain pockets of Tamil Nadu (Salem and Dharmapuri Districts) and the concept of *karpu* ("chastity") in marriage is non-existent. As a result, the incidence of AIDS is also on the rise. By logical inference, diseases like AIDS very likely existed in the early period of Indian civilization. It is not known whether there was any incidence of AIDS-like disease, as there is no reference to it in the *Rig Veda*. Also, diseases like syphilis were unknown in the medical works of Charaka and Sushruta of the late Vedic period. However, "there are, no doubt, undoubted references in the earlier Sanskrit works to diseases of the genitals due to lewd or impure sexual connections" (Bhisagacarya, 1922, p. 134). A syphilis-like disease was described in the *Bhava Prakas*, a Sanskrit work written as early as 350 A.D.

B. The Quest for Good Health

Brhadavanyaka Upanisd 1.3.27 reads: "Lead me from unreal to the real, lead me from darkness to light, lead me from death to immortality". This quest was in the mind of every ancient Indian. Jainism, which is a non-vedic religion, took great interest in the alleviation of sickness and pain from the world, and its practitioners found the society of sick needing health care and medical attention. They were responsible for two great works in medicine, the *elati* (concoction of six or more medical substances) and *ciru-panca-mulam* (a medical concoction of five small roots).

Earlier than Hippocrates, King Darius, who ruled the kingdom of the Mediterranean region (600 B.C.), had contact with the Tamil kingdoms and imported medicinal items. In ancient Greece (circa 400 B.C.), the Hippocratic collections contain direct references to Indian drugs and other medical formulae (Kennedy, 1898). Later, around 300 B.C., in the Chaldean city of Ur, two types of wood, ornamental timber wood and fragrant wood, were found to possess medicinal properties (Wavmington, 1974, p. 14). Taxonomic identification of about 1008 plants with medicinal properties was carried out (Pillai, 1963, p. 175).

C. The Quest for Immortality

The *Rig Veda*, the oldest religious scriptures of the Vedic period (2500-800 B.C.), discloses that the Aryans used the Soma plant as a medical agent to heal human diseases and to reach immortality. It is not quite certain what the Soma plant was, but it may belong to the genus *Ephedra*. The common plant *Ephedra* has many alkaloids and ephedrine and had religious connotations as its juice was used as a medicinal agent. The Soma – The Divine Ambrosia – is the source of bodily pleasures, brilliancy, and extended life (*Rig Veda* 9.44.1); it removes the spirit of rivalry and enmity (Mandihassan, 1997, pp. 3936-3940). The Indo Aryans used the plant for sacrificial purposes and its juice is described in the ancient Aryan literature as a stimulating beverage. The word *oshadhi* literally means heat-producer. The Soma plant was used for some therapeutic purposes, and hence *oshadhi* applied to all herbs and medicinal plants. The Soma plant possessed intoxicating properties, and the Vedic Aryans recognized that it was capable of quickening the intellect. "Soma like the sea has poured forth songs and hymns and thoughts. The beverage [i.e., Soma juice] is divine; it purifies, it inspires joy, it is a water of life ... it gives health and immortality."

> We've quaffed the Soma bright,
> > And are immortal grown;
> We've entered into light
> > And all the gods have known
> What mortal now can harm,
> > Or for man vex us more?
> Through thee, beyond alarm,
> > Immortal god, we soar.
> "Thou Soma, fond of praise, the lord of plants, art life to us."
> "Be unto us Soma the bestower of wealth, the remover of disease."

Soma is supposed to preside over medicinal herbs and, therefore, the Rishi Medhatithi continues his hymn as: "Soma has declared to me 'all medicaments as well as Agni, the benefactor of the Universe, are in the waters; the waters contain all healing herbs. Waters take away whatever sin has been (found) in me, whether I have (knowingly) done wrong or have pronounced imprecations (against holy men) or have spoken untruth" (Kirtikar et al., 1933, p. 838).

D. Medicine through Food

Ancient Indian views on cosmology (study of cosmic elements) and cosmogony (application of cosmic wisdom to real life situations on earth) resulted in a close link between human well-being and human dietary food systems in their social, religious, and legal systems of life (Keith, 1998, p. 312). The Indian farmers identified a total of nine food grains and associated them with cosmic bodies. These grains were prescribed for their physiological influence on humans, such as stimulation of circulation and balance, control of the nervous system, and stimulation of intelligence, due to their cosmic connections (Azariah, 1999). A perusal of the ancient literature indicates that the health philosophy of the Indian forefathers was to incorporate plants, with pharmaceutical properties, into the food system of society. Such spices often possessed powerful antibiotic activity, which was needed in a geographical location where bacteria easily multiply, due to the prevalence of a warm to hot climate. As early as 600 B.C., the Chinese writer Sze Teu wrote: "some algae are a delicacy fit for the most honored guests, even for the king himself". The effectiveness of seaweed in human health is now known due to their bio-dynamic substances; they have curative properties for tuberculosis, arthritis, cold, influenza, and intestinal worm infection (Abdussalam, 1990).

E. Ancient Indian Medicine

The medical works of Charaka and Sushruta appear to have been composed in the pre-Buddhist period. The rise of Buddhism gave an impetus to the study of medicine in ancient India. Their knowledge of about 1008 medicinally important herbs and plants, together with their knowledge of 25 types of salts, 64 kinds of arsenic, 9 different metals, and about 120 varieties of metallic essences would have given them added advantage in medical practices to alleviate pain and cure diseases. The health of the community was a central focus. Sir William Jones, first President of Asiatic Society of Bengal in 1799, said:

> ... some hundreds of plants which are yet imperfectly known to European botanists and with the virtues of which they are wholly unacquainted, grow wild on the plains and in the forests of India. The Amarakosha, an excellent vocabulary of the Sanskrit language, contains in one chapter, the names of about 300 medicinal vegetables, the Medini may comprise many more and the *Dravyabhidhana* or Dictionary of natural productions includes, I believe a far greater number, the properties of which are distinctly related to medical tracts of approved authority (Kirtikar et al., 1933, p. 838).

There was a well-established health care system with well qualified surgeons and physicians like Charaka, who was the official physician of the kings Kanishka (1 A.D.), Sushruta (sometimes spelled as Sustuta) (4 A.D.), and Vak-Bhata. Medical facilities included features like lithotomy (operation for the removal of bladder stones), extraction of the fetus *ex uterus*, and repair of a damaged nose. They had about 127 surgical instruments. Since they knew the art of extracting the fetus, it is likely that the procedure was analogous to present-day abortion (whether elective or for medical reasons). Since such practices were common occurrences in society, killing a fetus was considered one of the five cardinal sins (Azariah, 1998a) Further, the Manu Smrti (1 A.D.) promulgated rules and regulations for [against?] abortion (4.208; 5.90; 8.317; and 11.88). There were also provisions for restoration for killing embryos (Doniger & Smith, 1992, p. 362; Prakash, 2000, p. 188). Such rules and regulations (equal to present day Acts or laws) attributed personhood to the fetus and embryo (Azariah, 1998a).

F. Ancient Indian Systems of Health Care

Indian experience developed many systems of health care, such as *Unani, Ayurvedic*, and *Siddha* medicines, which use a combination of medicinally active plant extracts and inorganic compounds. For instance, the *Siddha* system identified three humors that activate the body: *vatam* (wind pressure that maintains body equilibrium and equipoise), *pittam* (an aspect of human physiology that covers the area responsible for metabolism), and *kapam* (phlegm that is secreted on the wall of the respiratory tract). Disturbances in any one of these humors was believed to cause disease. It was an in-depth study of humoral pathology, as opposed to the modern approach of cellular pathology. If a woman suffered from headache during coition, then it was considered to be due to pressure in her uterus; if she felt pain in her chest, then it was due to the inflexibility of vaginal passage. A blood clot in the vagina can result in severe pain in the nape of the neck. *Sittars* (from *citti* meaning "perfection"), who were experts in medical, literary, social, devotional, magical, and religious matters, used plant extract of *Ocimum sactum* in combination with oxides of copper to treat peptic ulcer. They suggested a medicine prepared from pomegranate and seeds of castor plant (*Ricinus communis*) for promoting pregnancy, while strengthening the fetus may be done by taking long pepper powder along with a drink prepared out of a mixture of sesame oil, milk, sugar, curd (yohards), and ghee (Samuel, 1998, p. 450). *Sittars* have classified 20 kinds of venereal diseases and 18 kinds of leprosy.

III. Specific Issues

A. Beginning of Life and Reproduction

1. *The fetus as a human person and embryo cloning.* In the famous epic, the *Mahabharatha*, Krishna was engaged in conversation with his pregnant sister, Subhathtra, about the details of breaking a complex military formation. When the fetus, named Abhimanyu, responded to the narration, Krishna stopped his account abruptly without providing information on the method of escape once the complex military formation was broken. Abhimanyu, in his teens, broke the complex *Chakaravyha* formation but was killed, as he did not know how to escape it. This epic story implied that the fetus in the womb is capable of listening and understanding the essence of the conversation and implementing the same after birth. The fetus is understood as able to learn and reason (Azariah, 1998a). In the same epic, Queen Kandhari, the wife of the King Dhritrashtra, was pregnant. However, the early embryo in the womb was split into one hundred parts by a punch. Each bit was kept in a earthen vessel and one hundred sons were born (Minakshi & Azariah, 1998, p. 20). This story is an example of their knowledge on the potency of the human embryo and the possibility of multiple cloning. Hence the Vedic people have formulated laws governing fetal extraction and regulating abortion.

2. *Reproductive Health.* Modern India has taken an effective step to implement a reproductive health agenda. Many national agencies (like the Ministry of Health and Family Welfare, Government of India [GOI]) and non-governmental agencies (NGOs) (like the Indian Council of Medical Research [ICMR] and The Institute of Research in Reproduction in Mumbai) have taken action to promote reproductive health and rights. Due to the ethnic and cultural diversity in India, many sensitive areas, such as the gender-sensitive issues of sexuality, the role of men as responsible sexual partners, the empowerment of women, and reproductive choice have been addressed. The contribution of NGOs has been significant in bringing down the mortality and fertility rates among the poor, disadvantaged, and the vulnerable populations, including the sizable population living in urban slums and the adolescent. The fourth Five Year Plan of the GOI (1969-1974) set a target of reaching 60% contraceptive prevalence rate (CPR) and to achieve just 1% of net reproductive rate. During the 1960s, a demographic emphasis and a contraceptive method-specific target fixed on family planning was followed; however, it was abolished in 1996, as the approach did not yield the projected results. The new approach envisaged a

predictable monitoring system based on ground realities, unmet need, access to services, availability of resources, and overall improvement in reproductive health including a decline in maternal mortality rate (MMR) and infant mortality rate (IMR) rather than increase in CRP alone (Puri, 1999). The GOI launched an innovative "Reproductive and Child Health" (RCH) program in October 1997 to encourage parents to reduce family size, so as to provide better health care services and longevity for their children. The chief highlights of the program have been to allow the local state governments to set the target and the integration of the existing intervention techniques of fertility. Among the three states in which such a "target-free" approach has been implemented, variable results have been achieved. It is likely that the ethnic and cultural diversity of India may not yield a uniform result all over India. Moreover, Swaminathan (1997) points out that the RCH program approaches the problem more from the supply side with accent on quality of care, access to service, and coverage of the relevant population. She has rightly pointed out that:

> ... even assuming the program (RCH) is able to provide the best of services with the widest possible coverage, our contention is that we would still be tackling only 50 per cent of the problem of reproductive health. What the program does not address is the existing structural nature of women's work (domestic as well as non-domestic) which has severe built in hazards for women's health (reproductive and otherwise) which no amount of first rate quality of care and/or access to health services alone can deal with. Such supply side responses can only mitigate the adverse consequences of work; they can't address the fundamental causes of these health problems (pp. 1-25).

However, the significant current shift in the GOI's health policy has been to provide a broad range of health care to enable individuals to achieve sound reproductive health across the life span – a position which indicates that reproductive health is seen as a human right. A special program on safe motherhood – namely "Pregnancy is Special: Let Us Make it Safe" (7 April 1998) – was launched in accordance with the declaration of the year 1998 as the "Year of Safe Motherhood" by the World Health Organization. The gap between the developed world and the developing world is too wide in the area of reproductive health of women during pregnancy. Vital statistics of a woman's lifetime risk of dying from pregnancy is one in 1800 births in developed countries and one in 48 in developing countries. For Indian women, the risk is one in 37 (Azmi, 2000). The risk of maternal death is high due to a lack of skilled personnel to attend to the mother in labor. In India, over 50% of infant deaths occur during the neonatal period, nearly two-thirds of which occur with in the first week of birth, mostly due to perinatal causes. It has been suggested that MMR could be reduced by 50% or more by placing a skilled attendant, backed by a functioning referral system, at the service point (Koblinsky et al., 1999; Thapa, 2000).

Women are also employed in many work situations that do not provide an atmosphere conducive for promoting reproductive health, such as agriculture, (plantation), construction, hired manual labor, and domestic service. Even after 50 years of independence, about 80% of female workers in Tamil Nadu are still confined to the primary sector of the economy; of these, 56% are female agricultural laborers (Swaminathan, 1997). It is surprising to note that the number of female agricultural child laborers under 14 years-of-age, is rather high, with the highest number being 52,608 in the district of Madurai (rural and urban; rural alone: 47,218) (Swaminathan, 1997). She points out that

(1) The infant mortality indicators are uniformly high in the rural areas and more so in the districts where paddy cultivation dominates;
(2) infant mortality indicators are particularly high among agricultural laborers and among manual workers; and
(3) the mortality indicators are considerably higher for births to scheduled caste women (*dalit*, untouchables/deprived community) than for births to non-scheduled caste and scheduled tribe women.

Health problems among women child laborers and adults are many. Moreover, among the adult pregnant women who work as agricultural laborers, adverse pregnancy is a common occurrence. Woman usually weed and transplant the saplings in paddy cultivation, which requires squatting on their haunches, exerting physical strain and pressure on the uterus, resulting in premature labor in the last trimester of pregnancy and still births (Jayaraj, 1999). Since the male fetus is larger in size and less hardy than the female fetus, it aborts more often under these circumstances (Miller, 1981).

3. *Unplanned pregnancies and abortions.* The mean age at marriage has shown a dramatic change during the past century. During the early 1900s, it was below 13, but it has risen to 19.5 years in 1991 (Jayaraj, 1999). Census data show that in more than 13 states the median age at first birth is less than 20 years, which may contribute about 50% of first order birth in adolescent mothers. The incidence of abortions is higher if conception takes place at an early age; hence biological maturity is a crucial determinant of sex ratio at birth (Jayaraj, 1999). Rates of spontaneous abortion and still births are higher in adolescents than women in the age group of 20-29 years: 205% and 121% respectively (Pachuri & Jamshedji, 1983).

Unplanned pregnancies and the unmet needs of teenagers lead to higher incidence of induced abortions. Data on the percentage of people who use condoms is alarming. The current [CPR] is about 46%. Recent statistics show that:

> ... less than 10% of the married couples in the age group of 15-19 years use contraception in any form. There are at least 35 million people who are not currently using any form of contraception in spite of the fact that they would like to limit their family size. These alarming statistics imply not only an early start of reproduction, but also a large unmet need for contraception. Young people, in particular, face an excessive risk of unintended pregnancy because of their sexual behavior, lack of information and little or no access to sexual and reproductive health services (Puri, 1999).

It is reported that about 300 million Indian couples lack access to safe, effective, affordable, and acceptable contraception. "It is, therefore, the responsibility of the heath care providers to provide safe methods of termination of pregnancy when unwanted or un-timed pregnancies occur" (Mandlekar & Krinhna, 2000, p. 8).

Although abortion was legalized through the Medical Termination of Pregnancy Act (MTP) of 1971, an estimated 4.7 million abortions are performed annually in ill-equipped places (Jesani & Iyer, 1993). It is generally true nationwide that for every one case of reported induced abortion, there may be ten other unreported cases, mostly illegal. Performing such abortions under unhygienic conditions and by untrained persons increases the risk to the mother's life. Puri (1999) records the alarming state: It is estimated that annually 11 million abortions occur in India, of which approximately 6.5 million are induced and 4.5 million spontaneous. Analysis of India's 1992-93 National Family Health Survey data on 301,400 pregnancies collected from married women from urban and rural areas showed that 9.3% of the induced abortions were performed on females in 15-19 years age group and 31.9% in the age group of 15-24 years. The high incidence of induced abortions in the country indicates that pregnancy termination is being used as the primary method of family planning. However, precise data on spontaneous abortions in the early months of pregnancy are difficult to find in the records (Jayaraj, 1999). What happens to the aborted fetuses is not well documented. Whether they are used in any research studies, such as fetal stem cell research, is also not documented. The ICMR is in the process of preparing a "Consultative Document on Ethical Guidelines on Biomedical Research Involving Human Subjects (1997)". At this time the document is still in draft form.

4. *Contraceptive methods and reproductive health.* During the post-independence period, the common birth control methods were temporary methods, like the use of condom and intrauterine device (IUD), and permanent methods, such as tubal ligation and vasectomy. The "pill" was introduced during the 1980s. The National Family Planning Program, through the Primary Health Centres, has carried out sterilization, insertion of IUDs, and distribution of condoms. The present status of the Indian approach to contraceptive methods and reproductive health is aptly summarized in a recent issue of the ISSRF Newsletter (July 2000, No. 5). In accordance with the declarations at the International Conference on Population and Development in Cairo and the Fourth World Conference on Women held in Beijing, India has made significant advancements in the development of contraceptive technologies and has introduced new practices in reproductive health. Further policy changes have been made in the area of family planning and population control to the comprehensive concept of reproductive health and contraception. Research development in reproductive technology includes hormonal methods with the use of a non-steroidal antiestrogen centchroman, which has been tried on 377 women volunteers, androgens alone/anti-androgen in combination with progestins, antiprogestins, such as RU-486, ZK 98.299, and ZK 98.734, vasocclusion, immunological therapy, hCG vaccine, FSH vaccine, sperm antigens, inhibin, zona pellucida antigens, and riboflavin carrier proteins (Puri, 2000). Further, development of improved delivery systems for the male, such as nasal sprays, silastic implants, and injectable intravasal contraceptives are also in progress.

The Central Drug Research Institute in Locknow, in collaboration with the Indian Council of Medical Research and other international organizations, has identified about 67 plants which have bioactive compounds with antifertility activity. Indian Plants like *Hibiscus rosasinensis*, *Embelica ribes*, *Vicoa indica*, and *Montanoa tomentosa* of Mexico have antifertility activity in women. It is interesting to note that other plants, such as *Tripterygium wilfordii*, containing biodynamic and physiologically active substances like gossypol and glycosides, have antifertility effects in men (Lohiya, 2000). Extracts from the seeds of *Carica papaya* have been shown to have potent testicular/post-testicular contraceptive effects in rabbits and meet the essential criteria such as safety, efficacy, and reversibility. The following plants induce instant sperm immobilization: *Cyclamen persicum, Primula vulgaris, Gypsophyla panculate, Acicia concinna, Albizzia procera,* and *Anagallis arvensis.*

5. *Abortion and fetal tissue research.* Annually there are about 7 million abortions in India, of which 32% are on women below the age of 24 years (Puri, 2000). There has been an increase in female feticide in the country through the misuse of modern techniques of ultrasonography and amniocentesis, which help to identify the sex of the baby at very early stages of pregnancy. Female infanticide is a built-in socio-economic evil of the Indian society. Out of 8,000 abortions performed in one hospital in Mumbai (Bombay), 7,999 were female fetuses (Azariah, 1994). It is not known whether fetal tissue is being used in research work. However, judging from the intellectual climate of medical research, preparations are being made to formulate guidelines on research using fetal tissues or organs for transplantation in India.

B. Professionalism

1. *Physicians' code of ethics.* The Vedic people had their own moral code of ethical conduct of physicians (Pillai, 1963), which read as follows: A good physician must be a person of strict veracity and of the greatest sobriety and decorum, holding intercourse with no women but his own. He ought to be well versed in all commentaries of *Ayul Vedham* or the Science of Life and he otherwise be a man of sense and benevolence. His heart must be charitable, his temper calm and his constant study must be to do good to the people. He must be mild and courageous, frank, communicative, impartial and liberal, yet ever rigid in exacting an adherence to regimen or rules.

2. *Ethics committees.* Rules for the manufacture, use, import, export, and storage of hazardous microorganisms, and genetically engineered organisms or cells (New Delhi 5.12.89) recommend the formation of the following committees. They are (1) Recombinant DNA A.D.visory Committee (RDAC), (2) Review Committee on Genetic Manipulation (RCGM), (3) Institutional Biosafety Committee (IBSC), and (4) Genetic Engineering Approval Committee (GEAC) (CPCB, 1997). The ICMR's draft document "Consultative Document on Ethical Guidelines on Biomedical Research Involving Human Subjects, 1977" contemplates the formation of a number of bioethics committees in areas such as human genetics, organ transplantation (including fetal tissue transplantation), clinical evaluation of drugs/diagnostics/vaccines/herbal remedies, epidemiological research, and assisted reproductive technologies. The culture of forming bioethics committees as a necessity is becoming recognized in India. For example, some NGOs, like YRG Care in Chennai, an organization working among people living with HIV/AIDS, have a research advisory committee with a position for a bioethicist. Recently, the Government of India issued a government order in which the formation of bioethical committees to address animal research was made mandatory.

3. *Informed consent.* The practice of obtaining informed consent is also difficult in India because of illiteracy. Many rural people will not put their thumb impression on the informed consent forms. Such fears are aptly summarized by Majumder (2000): "many are unable to write and hence unable to sign the consent form. Asking for a thumb impression on the consent form is tantamount to packing up and going home, most rural Indians are extremely wary of placing a thumb impression on a piece of paper because their common experience has been that they have lost their property" (p. 20).

C. Social Issues
1. *Life expectancy, reproductive, and mortality rates.* Indicators like life expectancy at birth as well as mortality and morbidity rates reflect the health status of India. Post-independence India witnessed a tremendous advancement in these indicators. The life expectancy at birth was about 23 years in 1901 and increased to 60 years in 1992; at the beginning of the third millennium, it stands around 68 years. Similarly, infant mortality has declined from 215 per thousand live births in 1901 to 82 in 1992. The death rate has declined from 44 per thousand (1901) to 10 in 1992. Duraisamy (1998), using the National Sample Survey's individual level data for the year 1986-87, assessed the preva-lence of morbidity rate in Tamil Nadu. The study showed a U-shaped pattern indicating an age-related morbidity. The overall morbidity prevalence rate is 28 and 32 per thousand in rural and urban Tamil Nadu respectively. The prevalence rate of illness was higher among children aged between 0-4 and in adults above 60 years of age. There is a gender bias in the perception of illness, since the morbidity prevalence rate of boys was higher when compared to girls in the 0-4 age group in rural areas. Women in the age group of 15-44 years exhibited higher prevalence of illness, perhaps due to complications in preg-nancy and child birth (Duraisamy, 1998).

Approximately 33% of India's population and 40% of Tamil Nadu's population lives below the poverty line. With a higher literacy rate of 63%, Tamil Nadu registers a lower fertility and infant mortality rate (2.2 and 58 per 1000, respectively). However, there is significant variation among the different states of India. For instance, the Northern state of Uttar Pradesh has a lower literacy rate (42%), a higher total fertility rate (5.1 per thousand), and the highest infant mortality rate (98 per thousand) in the population (Jejeebhoy, 1998). The South Indian state of Kerala has a 100% female literacy rate. That women empowerment through literacy has a strong impact on mortality indicators is sup-ported by a comparison of data available for Kerala and Tamil Nadu. Estimated mortal-ity indicators for India, Kerala, and Tamil Nadu (1989) are summarized below:

Location	CDR	Mortality IMR	Indicators NMR	PNMR	PMR
INDIA					
Rural	11.1	98.0	62.1	36.4	50.9
Urban	7.2	58.0	31.4	26.3	31.0
Average	10.3	91.0	56.4	34.5	47.2
KERALA					
Rural	6.0	23.0	15.2	7.6	23.4
Urban	6.1	15.0	9.7	5.1	21.9
Average	6.1	21.0	14.2	7.2	23.1
TAMIL NADU					
Rural	9.7	80.0	60.4	19.6	58.7
Urban	6.8	43.0	29.9	13.5	43.8
Average	8.7	68.0	50.1	17.6	53.8

CDR: Child Death Rate; IMR: Infant Mortality Rate; NMR: Neonatal Mortality Rate; PNMR: Post-Neonatal Mortality Rate; PMR: Prenatal Mortality Rate
(Source: Office of the Register General, India. Vital Statistics Division. Sample Registration System [1989, 1992], New Delhi, India, pp. 73, 95-159.)

Adnan (1998) considers that a decline in fertility may be due to a complexity of other factors besides the use of contraceptive methods. These factors include a decline in demand for children among reproductive couples, urban growth, and changes in production and family organization, women's position, literacy rates, health conditions, and medical technology. However, literacy has its negative points in Kerala, since prenatal sex diagnostic techniques are abused, which has led to the selective abortion of female fetuses and the death of female infants. In this state alone, about 50,000 female infanticides occur per year (Verma, 2000). Such an onslaught on female babies has resulted in an adverse change in sex ratio. The national sex ratio in 1901 was 972 females for every 1000 males; in 1991, it declined to 927, which is an all-time low female to male ratio. Over the century, the decline in the sex ratio at birth has been steady. The present status in some of the Indian states like Delhi (810), Chandigarh (770), and Adaman and Nicobar (761) is alarming. Kerala is the only exceptional state, where the ratio was 1034 (1991 census), which is still a steep drop from 1056 in the 1961 census. Krishnaji (2000) predicts, "Some probing into what lies behind the long term trend and its reestablishment in 1991 suggests – as the studies here do – that a further decline in the ratio is quite probable when the first count is made in the next millennium" (February 2001).

2. *Childhood diseases and immunization programs.* There was a very important shift in the health policy of immunization in 1985 when the GOI introduced the Universal Immunization Program (UIP) targeting childhood diseases that are vaccine-preventable. Active immunization programs exist for diseases like childhood tuberculosis, diptheria, whooping cough, tetanus, polio, and measles. A campaign against the crippling disease of polio is being conducted by the State Government of Tamil Nadu and various NGO organizations. The first round of vaccines were administered during December 2000, covering about 72,000,000 children statewide and involving about 40,000 immunization posts manned by health staff and volunteers from NGOs. Remote areas in hill tracts were covered with the help of 592 mobile teams (Reporter, 2000). The second round of vaccine administration was covered a month later. Using demographic projections for estimating the target population for immunization, it is predicted that in the year 2006 the total number of children will steadily increase in all the states, including underachieving states, such as Uttar Pradesh, Rajesthan, Madhya Pradesh, Bihar, and Orissa, where children currently have no access to immunization (Das et al., 2000).

3. *Health care and gender issues.* Gender-based violence causes pain and ill health to women. The physically and psychologically painful condition of Indian women is aptly summarized by Nayar:

> True, partner violence occurs in all countries, and transcends social, economic, religious and cultural groups. It is generally part of a pattern of abusive behavior and often referred to as "wife beating", "battering", or "domestic quarrel" all over the world. But this is maximum in India. Very little comes to light except though occasional reports in the press. Women suffer silently and patiently. The courts entertain cases of bride burning; not wife beating. Of course, there are laws to ensure legal rights. But they are seldom enforced to punish abusers. Many beliefs, norms and social traditions legitimize and even perpetuate violence against women. Orthodox and perverse Hindus customs protect fundamentalists (2000, p. 12).

Fundamentalists in Kashmir valley have violated the basic human rights of women by killing women who visited beauty parlors. Even though about 700,000 elected women are in the village *panchayat* system of governance, their husbands make the major decisions, and their wives simply sign the papers. "In a patriarchal Indian society the attitude of men in treating women as subordinate commodities should change. Customs and traditions and religious mumbo-jumbo beliefs must be reformed to enforce and protect the basic and fundamental rights of women" (Nayar, 2000, p. 12).

4. *Female deficiency syndrome*. The practice of female infanticide and the neglect of female children are the cultural heredity of Indian civilization. Krishnaji (2000) cites a recent news item published in the *Times* of India (Mumbai) dated September 17, 1999: "in a village called Devra in Rajasthan ... a girl child not only survived – through a series of accidental circumstances – but also brought a *barat* – groom's marriage party – to the village for the first time after 110 years. Girl children were routinely killed in such villages. The early Indian census reported villages with no girls in some parts of the Northeast. Presumably such villages still exist in India (p. 1161). Such female deficiency has significant sociological impacts.

Think-tank discussions among the post-graduate students of the University of Madras for the past decade have indicated an alarming trend in the attitudes of students in the age group of 21-25 years. Assuming an extreme situation of 700 girls to 1000 boys, a challenging situation was posed to them. Under the Indian law of monogamy, it is only possible for seven boys to get married to seven girls. Three boys will be "left out", since the "market" for girls is closed with the notice "girls are out of stock". The question posed to them was: "If you are among the three who are left out, then what would you do?" The responses of the upcoming student generation can aptly be called the female deficiency syndrome, which may bring about serious changes in the social order. These responses varied from "I will kill the already married boy to release the bride", "divorce one's husband to satisfy the unmet needs of the unmarried close boyfriend/classmates", "I will become a *sanyasi* (unmarried sage)" and "sharing a wife/part time wife"! Polyandry was not favorable among girl students. Some south Indian states were more conservative in their responses.

5. *Health and the practice of inbreeding*. The Indian subcontinent is culturally diverse and linguistically pluralistic with a varied morphological, genetic and cultural singularity. Based on a recent study on the heterozygosity among the Indian population, Majumder (2000) has recognized three major morphological groups: caucasoids, mongoloids, and negroids. Moreover, the South Indians have a genetic identity of their own from the populations of North, West, East, and Central India. Inbreeding is one of the characteristic features of the southern population of India, which has a telling effect on health; i.e., it leads to an increase in the frequencies of recessive diseases. In four states of India, namely, Tamil Nadu, Andhra Pradesh, Karnatak, and Maharastra, 25% of all marriages are between relatives (Jayaraj, 1999). Jayaraj (1999) also reported that, since the sex ratio is high in the southern Indian states (where the incidence of consanguineous marriages is high), the sex ratio among births to women married to blood relatives will be higher than that for women who are married to non-blood relatives. Rao (1984), while studying the populations of Tamil Nadu in South India, found significant differences in fertility, sterility, fetal, perinatal, and infant mortality between consanguineous and non-consanguineous couples. Similarly, Bittles et al. (1991) also reported higher rates of postnatal mortality in children of consanguineous parents in the State of Karnataka. The variable of the age at

first childbirth may be a strong determinant of the incidence of postnatal mortality with consanguineous parents. The Department of Biotechnology, Government of India, has envisaged in its attempts to map the human genomic diversity to study the relationship between genomic variations and the incidence of disease-genetic epidemiology. The proposed study will identify gene loci responsible for the susceptibility of humans to common diseases, including infectious diseases (Majumder, 2000).

6. *Biomedical waste and health management.* The metropolitan city of Mumbai (Bombay) has about 1,200 public and private hospitals and nursing and maternity homes and about 13,000 private medical practitioners (including pathology labs), all of which generate about 0.5% of the total general municipal solid waste (4,500 tons a day). Street children, who are the rag pickers, salvage the discarded needles, syringes, and other medical wastes from the municipal garbage bins and solid waste dumping sites, and resell these items to make a living. These vulnerable para-health care related workers are at risk of exposure to injuries from contaminated needles and other sharp objects (Kewalramani, 2000). Furthermore, they are not trained in handling hospital wastes and are not aware of biomedical safety precautions. Infectious and non-infectious biomedical waste is not separated, which renders the entire 4,500 tons of municipal waste as infectious medical waste. When the salvaged needles are recycled by ill-equipped factories and resold, it has its own toll on consumer health.

D. Agricultural Issues

1. *Genetically modified food and reproductive health.* The field trials of genetically modified (GM) food plants has been tested in many parts of India. Recently, an objection has been raised to the field trials of a cotton plant with the Bt gene in India on the grounds that the area of land to carry out field trials is too small in India. Studies of genetically modified crop trials in the United States have shown that even 100 acre trials areas were being considered too small for safe extrapolation from field trials to large-scale cultivation. There have been attempts in India to do field trials of GM food crops without any adequate precautions and without any public consent. There have also been attempts by multinational companies to manage the processing of fruits. In these areas, no health guidelines exist for the cultivators as well as for the end users through the multinational processing companies.

Furthermore, genetically modified food may affect human reproductive health. The *Cangam* literature of South India (300 B.C. to 300 A.D.) recognized seven well-defined stages of womanhood based on the age and physiological status of body, namely (1) simple minded ignorant person (5-7 years), (2) age of accepting instruction and correction (8-11), (3) young girl but not attained puberty (12-13), (4) young girl (14-19), (5) a girl with wisdom (20-25), (6) a woman with knowledge, understanding, clarity, transparency and brightness (25-31), and (7) a young woman who is older (30-40/55). Two points emerge from these stages of life, namely, (a) the onset of puberty is well identified with the age of 14 and (b) female life expectancy was only about 40-55 years. The marriageable age of a woman was just under 12, which favored child marriages. The life expectancy of women was short, which may be due to hard domestic labor as well as to labor and delivery complications.

In modern India, the life expectancy has risen to around 68, and the average Hindu family size is much smaller than it used to be. However, it has been reported that 1 in 6 girls and 1 in 14 boys reach puberty at the alarmingly young age of 8. (One important question is what they think about sex, *Sunday Express*, 2000). One of the possible reasons may be due to the use of genetically modified food, which has built-in health risks. "Roundup Ready" plants can tolerate the Roundup herbicide. In the case of soya beans, isoflavonoids are produced as byproducts of metabolism, which has estrogenic activity. They are also called phytoestrogens, since they mimic human estrogen. Systematic accumulation of phtoestrogen may result in breast cancer, tumors, and vaginal adenocarcinoma, besides initiating the maturity status of women at an early age (Lappe & Bailey, 1998). In men, a female hormone may cause a reduction in sperm production, testicular retention in infants, and testicular cancer, besides initiating the process of feminization of males.

2. *Animal reproductive health.* Animal reproduction involves the enhancement of the reproductive rates of farm animals by increasing their fertility. It has been reported that India has about 196 million cattle and 80 million buffaloes (Kulkarni, 1999). Animal husbandry is an important source of food production in India, since any decline in their productivity affects the economy and the nutritional health of the people. Infection of the reproductive tract of animals with sexually transmitted diseases, causing pathogens such as *Brucellosis, Leptospirosis, Vibriosis, Trichomoniasis, Listerosis, Mycoplasmosis, and Salmonellosis,* have led to abortion, still birth, premature birth, infertility, and sterility in farm animals (Kulkarni, 1999); consumption of infected animals has led to health problems in human beings.

E. Organ Transplantation

In India, the medical art of organ transplantation is in its infancy. Economic conditions, the need to improve success rates, and the availability of organs are the main constraints. Moreover, potential organ donors also face many hurtles in convincing a hospital to accept organs as donations. Azariah (1998b) reported on a specific case in which two donors faced legal problems. With much difficulty, the donors succeeded in getting a court order directing the Chennai Medical College to accept their body after their death. The Transplantation of Human Organs Act of 1994 was amended as "Transplantation of Human Organs Rules, 1995" so as to include transplantation research, including transplantation of fetal tissues or organs in clinical practice. Both of these documents specify the criteria for brain death as "entire, permanent, irreversible cessation of functions of the brain stem – that is synonymous with brain-stem death, since the centers for the control of such essential body functions as consciousness, respiration and blood pressure are situated within the brain stem". It is significant that guidelines on live donor transplantation, cadaver donor transplantation, and on recipients of transplantation are being considered. Currently, xenotransplantation between animal species may also be permitted. However, transplantation involving an animal and a human being has not been allowed due to lack of technical expertise. There is also a deep concern, due to the current level of knowledge, about the possible transgenic infection of bacteria and virus and other microorganisms, such as fungi, hitherto not known to infect human beings.

IV. Conclusion

Compared to the Western world, India has a very different set of bioethical concerns, mostly due to its unique social and cultural history. The results of its history are a stratified social system, the poor treatment of women, and a large impoverished lower class. These in turn give rise to specifically bioethical problems, including the lack of quality medical care, high abortion rates for female fetuses, deficient vaccinations for children, and questionable food production. Whether these problems can be equately solved or lessened is difficult to see, since their sources are long-standing cultural issues.

Bibliography

Abdussalam, S. 1990. Drugs from seaweeds. *Medical Hypotheses,* 32: 33-35.

A.D.nan, S. 1998. Fertility decline under absolute poverty. *Economic and Political Weekly* 33: 1337-1348.

Altekar, A.S. 1959. *The position of women in Hindu civilization,* New Delhi: Motilal Banarsidass.

Azariah, J. 1994. Global bioethics and common hope: 1. Ecology and religion: spirituality Mode – a keystone in ecobalance. In D.J. Macer (ed.), *Bioethics for the people by the people* (pp. 98-104). Christchurch: Eubios Ethics Institute.

Azariah, J. 1998a. Status of human life in/and fetus in Hindu, Christian and Islamic Scriptures. In J. Azariah, H. Azariah, & D.J. Macer (eds), *Bioethics in India* (pp. 52-56). Christchurch: Eubios Ethics Institute.

Azariah, J. 1998b. Incomplete history of bioethics. *All India Bioethics Association Newslink* 1(6): 2-3.

Azariah, J. 1999. Biopiracy, environment and culture. Paper presented at the International Conference on Genetics, Law and Society: St. Paul, Minnesota, Oct. 11-14, 1999.

Azmi, S. 2000. Safe motherhood: Women's views and concerns. *Indian Society for the Study of Reproduction and Fertility Newsletter* 4: 7-9.

Bhisagacarya, G.M. (1922 [1994]) *History of Indian medicine, Vol. I.* New Delhi: Munshiram Manoharlal Publishers Pvt. Ltd.

Bittles, A.H., Mason, W.H., Greene, J. & Appaji Rao, N. 1991. Reproductive behavior and health in consanguineous marriages. *Science* 252: 789-794.

Central Pollution Control Board (1997). *Pollution control acts, rules and notifications issued thereunder, Vol. 1* (p. 502). New Delhi, Ministry of Environment and Forest, Government of India.

Chitkara, M.G. 2000. A world faith. Buddhist nirvana. In M.G. Chitkara (ed.), *Encyclopedia of Buddhism: A world faith* (chapter 47, pp. 413-431). New Delhi: A.P.H. Publishing.

Correspondent, Science. 2000. Genetically modified cotton outstanding. *Monsanto,* Sept. 11, p. 12.

Das, V., Das, R.K. & Coutinho, L. 2000. Disease control and immunization: A sociological enquiry. *Economic and Political Weekly* 35: 625-632.

Doniger, W. & Smith, B.K. 1991. *The laws of manu.* London; New York: Penguin Books.

Duraisamy, P. 1998. Morbidity in Tamil Nadu: Level, differentials and determinants. *Economic and Political Weekly* 33: 982-990.

Jayaraj, D. 1999. Sex ratio at birth: An exploratory analysis of its determinants. Working Paper No. 157, Madras Institute of Developmental Studies. Adyar, Chennai 600 020. pp. 1-26.

Jejeebhoy, S. 1998. Wife-beating in rural India: A husband's right? Evidence from survey data. *Economic and Political Weekly* 33: 855-862.

Jesani, A. & Iyer, A. 1993. Women and abortion. *Economic and Political Weekly* 28: 2591-2594.

Keith, A.B. 1998. *The religion and philosophy of the Veda and Upanishads. Part I.* Delhi: Motilal Banarsidass Publishers Ovt. Ltd.

Kennedy, J. 1898. The early commerce of India with Babylon. *Journal of Royal Asiatic Society,* 243.

Brihand Mumbai Municipal Corporation. 2000. Hospital waste management – Initiative. In N. Kewalramani (ed.), *National seminar on biomedical and solid waste management.* Mumbai: Veermata Jijabal Technological Institute.

Kirtikar, K.R., Basu, B.D. & I.C.S. 1933. *Indian medical plants*. Dehra Dun: Bishhen Singh Mahendra Pal Singh.

Koblinsky, M.A., Campbell, O. & Heichelheim, J. 1999. Organizing delivery care. What works for safe motherhood. *Bulletin of the World Health Organization* 77(5): 399-406.

Krishnaji, N. 2000. Trends in sex ratio. *Political and Economic Weekly* 35: 1161-1164.

Kulkarni, B.A. 1999. Reproductive problems of Indian dairy animals. *Indian Society for the Study of Reproduction and Fertility Newsletter* 1: 10-11.

Lappe, M. & Bailey, B. 1998. *Against the grain: biotechnology and the corporate takeover of your food*. Monroe: Common Curage Press.

Lohiya, N.K. 2000. Plant products for contraception: How to make it a reality? *Indian Society for the Study of Reproduction and Fertility Newsletter* 5: 9-12.

Mandihassan, S. 1997. Three important Vedic grasses. In N.K.R. Singh (ed.), *Encyclopedia of Hinduism* (Vol. 14, pp. 3936-3940). New Delhi: Anmol Publications Pvt. Ltd.

Majumder, P.P. 2000. Genes, diversities and peoples of India. In D.R.J. Macer (ed.), *Ethical challenges as we approach the end of the Human Genome Project* (pp. 20-33). Christchurch: Eubios Ethics Institute.

Mandlekar, A. & Krinhna, U. 2000. Surgical and non-surgical methods for termination of pregnancy. *Indian Society for the Study of Reproduction and Fertility Newsletter* 3: 8-11.

Minakshi, B. & Azariah, J. 1998. Does cloning mean new ethics? Paper presented at the International conference on "Ethics in Science and Medicine", VMKV Medical College, Salem. Abstract No. 2, p. 20.

Miller, B.D. 1981 *The endangered sex: neglect of female children in rural north india*. Reprinted (1997) New Delhi: Oxford University Press.

Nayar, K. 2000. Reforming Society – Human Rights Diary. *The Hindu*, Sept. 26: p. 12.

Pachuri, S. & Jamshedji, A. 1983. Risks of Teenage Pregnancy. *Journal of Obstetrics and Gynaecology* 37: 6-10.

Prakask, S. 2000. *Concise manu smrti*. Delhi: ISPCK.

Pillai, M.S.P. 1963. *Tamil India*. Madras: The South India Saiva Siddhandha Publishing Society.

Puri, C.P. 1999. From family planning to reproductive health: Role of ISSRF. *Indian Society for the Study of Reproduction and Fertility Newsletter* 1: 1-8.

Puri, C.P. 2000. Reproductive health: Research leads and needs. *Indian Society for the Study of Reproduction and Fertility Newsletter* 5: 1-6.

Rao, P.S.S. 1984. Inbreeding in India: Concepts and consequences. In J.R. Lukacs (ed.), *The people of South Asia* (pp. 239-268). New York: Plenum Press.

Reporter, Staff 2000. Pulse polio campaign covers 72 lakh children. *The Hindu*, December 11, p. 1.

Subramanian, P. (ed.)1998. *A descriptive catalogue of palm-leaf manuscripts in Tamil, Vol. 5, Part II*. Chennai: Institute of Asian Studies.

Sunday Express. 2000. Too Young to be Mothers, June 25, pp. 45-46.

Swaminathan, P. 1997. "Work and Reproductive Health: A Hobson's Choice for Indian Women?," Working Paper No. 147, Madras Institute of Developmental Studies (Adyar, Chennai 600 020), pp. 1-25.

Thapa, R 2000. Safe Motherhood: Issues and Perspectives. *Institute of Research in Reproduction Newsletter* 4(1): 3-7.

Verma, D. 2000. Fears over increasing female feticide. *The Hindu*, December 25, p. 6.

Warmington, E.H. 1974. *The commerce between the Roman Empire and India*. New York: Octagon Books.

18 Bioethics in the Philippines: An Overview of Developments, Issues, and Controversies

Leonardo de Castro

I. Introduction

This overview of bioethics in the Philippines covers developments, issues, and controversies that have arisen in the last 30 years. It deals with policies reflected in legislation as well as executive and administrative orders promulgated by the executive branch of government. It touches upon issues and controversies reported by media and written about in the published literature. It pays minimal attention to academic publications, guides and manuals dealing with various aspects of bioethics, since these have been very limited, both in terms of number and of influence upon popular awareness and sentiment.

A large part of this overview deals with legislation because bioethical issues in the country have tended to find resolution in the houses of Congress. Academic publications have had limited influence on government policy and public sentiment. The media and the pulpit have had greater impact, but, in these venues, there has been a tendency to appeal more to popular emotion or dogma rather than to secular arguments.

Hence, this overview makes extensive use of recently passed and pending legislation to focus on important issues and concerns. Indeed, for a long time in the country's schools, medical ethics was synonymous with medical jurisprudence. It dealt mainly with what the law said, and many in the medical community had the limited understanding that ethics pertained to whatever was considered legal. Another reason for this overview's approach is that lobbyists have been active in working for the passage of bills consistent with their ethical positions. Hence, many debates on issues of bioethics originated in the halls of congress even before they generated wide public attention.

Compared to other fields of study, bioethics is very young and it is certainly so in the Philippines. Although discussions of ethical issues pertaining to matters of medicine and biology have taken place for a long time, awareness of these issues as matters of bioethics started to develop only about 30 years ago. This development came largely as an offshoot of what was taking shape in North America and Western Europe, where the use of the term "bioethics" has served to provide a conceptual umbrella for related matters. Hence it is not surprising that bioethics in the Philippines has largely followed the examples set by Western countries in terms of theories and frameworks for analysis.

II. Characterizing Philippine Bioethics

A. *Tension Points*

The Philippines often is referred to as the only Catholic country in Asia. Over eighty percent (83%) of Filipinos declare affiliation with the Catholic Church. The rest belong to Muslim or other Christian groups.

The primarily Catholic orientation of the Filipino population has largely defined the focal points around which bioethics debates have revolved. This has been manifested in public debates regarding such issues as abortion, euthanasia, contraceptive use, and other reproductive health issues. Regarding these issues, public debate often has been drawn along lines defined mainly by Catholic partisans. Depending on the specific issues being considered, we could find Catholic groups often perched on one side of the debate, with government technocrats or feminist groups on the other. The positioning could be observed in symposia, position papers, academic publications, press statements, radio and television discussions, and other venues for public debate.

This kind of conflict in orientations surfaced in the jockeying for appointments to the Constitutional Commission of 1986 and subsequently became evident in the deliberations of that body. Appointments to government positions that exert considerable influence on pertinent policies have also come under scrutiny from religious sector lobbyists competing with influential traditional political power blocks.

Very recently, issues surrounding governmental population-related policies have surfaced once more because of religion-based initiatives. The newly-installed president, recognizing her mid-term assumption to power as a debt to the politically influential Catholic Church, has announced that programs dealing with the country's high population growth rate shall be guided by positions espoused by the local Catholic hierarchy. The announcement does not necessarily indicate a long-term commitment to religious fundamentals, but it does confirm the parameters around which public debates on issues of bioethics have had to be conducted. The public stance of government is certain to come under review, if not under attack, when funding sources for such projects remind policy-makers of the conditions under which support can be forthcoming.

Aside from bringing to the surface the pronounced influence of the Catholic Church on matters relating to bioethics, the bloodless Philippine revolt of 1986 brought along a different kind of power, which has had a strong impact on government policies. Non-governmental organizations have increased in number and in the magnitude of their capacity to influence public opinion, legislation, and policy-making. To the extent that they take on an advocate's role for consumers, they represent interests that conflict with those of producers and manufacturers, or with policies laid down by government.

An example is to be found in the government's efforts to accelerate food production through biotechnology and, more specifically, the use of genetically modified organisms. Early research in this area has been opposed aggressively by non-governmental organizations. Among these groups, the environment-oriented ones have lobbied strongly against field trials of genetically modified corn, citing consumer safety and environmental risks as reasons. The country's Supreme Court has so far denied petitions to stop field trials using these organisms. Notwithstanding their early setback, those opposed to the use of genetically modified organisms appear to be determined to pursue their cause. Their imposing presence will help to define the character of local bioethics in this century.

Socio-economic conditions constitute a third major factor that affects local bioethics. Many decisions on issues of bioethics have had to give way to considerations of economy and social status. This has been evident in cases of organ donation and transplantation, as well as in other critical care situations. The policies of the National Kidney and Transplant Institute in the recruitment of living non-related donors have digressed from established international guidelines because of the pressures brought about by economic and social considerations. Judging from recent media reports, the well-publicized controversy ignited by the recruitment of paid organ "donors" a few years ago has not eliminated the practice. The developments in this regard reflect the tension between theoretical ethical considerations, on the one hand, and socio-economic realities, on the other.

A fourth major factor that has started to influence local bioethics is to be found in feminist initiatives. Support groups for women have taken up the cudgels against positions espoused by Catholic groups on reproductive health issues. Some of these groups have endorsed the use of contraceptive methods frowned upon by the Catholic Church. A few have come out openly in favor of abortion and the use of RU-486. On the whole, feminist initiatives have focused on the interests of women, thus challenging what are perceived as traditionally masculine approaches to bioethics.

At this point, it seems proper to characterize Filipino bioethics in terms of the tensions created by these strong influences. In concrete terms, one can see tensions developing in the following instances:

(1) Between church-oriented positions and positions taken by support groups for women on population, and reproductive health issues;
(2) Between consumer and environment advocates, on the one hand, and bio-technocrats, on the other, regarding the use of genetically modified organisms to improve productivity; and
(3) Between socio-economic imperatives, on the one hand, and ethical concerns, on the other, as regards practices in organ donation and transplantation.

These tensions define the issues that have been raised in deliberations on public policy. It is important to observe how they are tending to be resolved.

Shortly after her assumption to power in January 2001, President Gloria Macapagal-Arroyo acknowledged her debt to the Catholic Church for its role in initiating the public demonstrations that toppled the government of President Joseph Estrada and installed her in the seat of power. On the matter of reproductive health issues, many people see that this debt has put her in the same position as President Corazon Aquino who, like her, was installed in office after church-instigated demonstrations led to the removal of the incumbent president.

The Catholic Church heavily influenced Corazon Aquino's administration insofar as choices of family planning methods were concerned. "Non-natural" contraceptive methods were taboo and the population growth rate remained at a high 2.3%. When a Protestant President replaced Aquino, things changed significantly with the appointment of a health secretary, who aggressively promoted artificial contraception. Before the changes could be firmly established, however, the health secretary left office to run for a senate seat. Notwithstanding the opposition of the Catholic Church, he won handily. His victory illustrated a growing gap between the official thinking of the Catholic Church and the attitude of its followers regarding issues of bioethics. It demonstrated, in a way, that while the people go to church, they do not necessarily think the same way that the Cardinal does regarding their family planning methods. It also showed that in the minds of the faithful, bioethical issues are not necessarily resolved by the edicts of their Church. Still, the Catholic influence is pre-eminent and the Church strives to maintain its impact on the political scene. It counts on the political hierarchy to enforce its morals and, judging by the record, politicians continue to oblige.

Notwithstanding the characterization in terms of religious tensions, it would be grossly inaccurate to picture Filipino bioethics as having Catholic theoretical foundations. There is no single dominant bioethical theory. Nevertheless, it is true that there is a strong Catholic influence on government policy.

B. Important Institutions

There are three national organizations that are primarily concerned with bioethics in the country: the Philippine Bioethics Network, the Reproductive Health, Rights, and Ethics Center for Training and Research, and the Bioethics Society of the Philippines. In addition, the Philippine Health Social Science Association has devoted many of its activities to the promotion of bioethics awareness.

Among the country's schools, the University of Santo Tomas has the oldest Department of Bioethics. The department offers an annual postgraduate course on bioethics. The University of the Philippines also offers courses in bioethics and has a program for bioethics education, which is integrated into the medical school curriculum.

Biomedical research involving human subjects has been the responsibility of the Philippine Council for Health Research and Development (PCHRD), which provides the secretariat for the National Ethics Committee. It also organizes training workshops for members of institutional ethics review committees. Similarly active in this regard is the Forum for Ethics Review Committees in Asia and the Pacific (FERCAP). Local members of FERCAP are collaborating with the pharmaceutical industry to upgrade research ethics review in a way that would complement the initiatives of the PCHRD.

The committee on the Code of Practice of the Philippine Association for Laboratory Animal Science has taken on the responsibility of regulating research involving laboratory animals. It has promulgated a Code of Practice for the Care and Use of Laboratory Animals in the Philippines.

C. Ethics Committees

Ethics committees have had a minimal impact on the country's bioethics. At the national level, one can identify three committees that have played a prominent and influential role in the recent past: the National Ethics Committee of the PCHRD, the National Committee on Biosafety of the Philippines, and the Ethics Committee of the National Kidney and Transplant Institute (NKTI).

The National Ethics Committee was organized by the PCHRD in accordance with its mandate to direct and coordinate all health research in the Philippines, in order to facilitate adherence to ethical principles and promote values, such as respect for the sanctity of life and the dignity of man. The Governing Council of the PCHRD initially laid down the basis for ethical review of research in the country with the adoption of the National Guidelines for Biomedical Research Involving Human Subjects, which was formulated by the National Ethics Committee for the first time in 1985.

The National Guidelines provide for the creation of institutional ethics review committees (IERCs), where there are biomedical research programs involving human subjects. The IERCs deal mainly with protocols generated by in-house researchers. In government hospitals, they also conduct an ethical evaluation of research proposals coming from other government agencies. Existing IERCs are mostly based in the large metropolitan centers. They are also called upon to review protocols for foreign drug companies or agencies when their institutions serve as the venues for research undertaken by their consultants.

The National Committee on Biosafety of the Philippines is a multi-sector body responsible for regulating field tests on biotechnology. Its role has come into public attention because of the controversy generated by ongoing field tests involving genetically modified organisms.

Although the direct responsibility of the Ethics Committee of the NKTI is limited to its own policies and activities, its decisions have had an impact on a broader scale. This is due mainly to the fact that the NKTI has been the center of ground-breaking activities in organ transplantation and other institutions in the country have looked to it for guidance and direction. Even when others have not agreed with its policies, it has nevertheless served as a basis of comparison.

At the institutional level, there have been very few fully functioning ethics committees, whether for medical research or for other purposes. In many cases, the committees have operated on an *ad hoc* basis, being called to a meeting only when there is an urgent need. There is very little opportunity for the members to build their capacity for review and assess their decisions.

D. Health Care Professionals

Health care professionals in the Philippines are generally very paternalistic in their relationships with patients. Patients often defer to doctors when important decisions have to be made. This holds true even in the case of biomedical research, thus making it relatively easy for medical practitioners to recruit subjects for experimentation.

The structure of relationships among health care professionals is very hierarchical, with doctors being firmly ensconced at the top. Although the hierarchy is to be expected (considering the well-defined responsibilities of members of health care teams), it is also important to note that the hierarchy exists even outside the health care environment. This is evident in the very limited participation of nurses in decision-making in clinics and hospitals. A study on the treatment of severely deformed neonates has shown that, in comparison with nurses from some developed Western countries, those from the Philippines are seldom consulted about decisions to withhold or withdraw life support from patients.

III. Reproductive Health

A. Abortion

The legal standards on abortion that are still in effect in the country are found in the provisions of the Revised Penal Code that was enacted into law on December 8, 1930. Articles 256-259 of Section 2 of the Code provide prison terms for:

(a) any person who intentionally or unintentionally causes an abortion with, or without the permission of the pregnant woman;

(b) a woman who practices abortion upon herself or gives another person consent to do so;

(c) a physician or midwife who takes advantage of scientific knowledge or skill to cause an abortion or assist in causing the same; and

(d) a pharmacist who dispenses an abortive.

It is interesting to note the socio-cultural context of the prohibition that is hinted at by the Code: "If this crime be committed by the parents of the pregnant woman or either of them, and they act with the consent of said woman *for the purpose of concealing her dishonor*, the offenders shall suffer the penalty of prison correctional in its medium and maximum periods" (Article 259, emphasis added).

These provisions of the *Penal Code* are echoed in the *Child and Youth Welfare Code* of 1974. Article 3 (1) of this Code says that "every child is endowed with the dignity and worth of a human being *from the moment of his conception*" (emphasis added). It also provides that "the civil personality of the child shall commence from the time of his conception" (Article 5).

In 1987, the above legal provisions were reinforced by the approval of the new Constitution, which declares that the State "shall equally protect the life of the mother and the life of the unborn from conception" (Section 12).

Although the law categorically prohibits abortion, social reality seems to point in the other direction. A study published in 1997 revealed that 20 to 30 women out of every 1000 undergo induced abortion in the Philippines every year (Perez, et al., 1987). In absolute figures, this translates to approximately 320,000 to 480,000 induced abortions every year. The medium level estimate of 25 induced abortions out of every 1000 is lower than figures reported in predominantly Catholic Latin American countries, but it has given the local Catholic hierarchy a reason to intensify its anti-abortion efforts. In the wake of talks that RU-486 could be allowed entry into the country, these efforts have found even stronger motivation.

Last year, the Bureau of Food and Drugs announced that it was likely to approve the entry into the country of the contraceptive RU-486. The head of the agency was reported by newspapers to have described the pill as "safe" and as "not an abortifacient." He explained that the drug works by preventing the implantation of the fertilized egg and does not work in the same way that a drug like misoprostal triggers uterine contractions.

In contrast, the Catholic Bishops' Conference of the Philippines (CBCP) said that women taking the RU-486 drug and similar pills will be considered automatically excommunicated from the Catholic Church. Speaking in behalf of the CBCP, Monsignor Pedro Quitorio said that RU-486 and other pills that induce abortion are prohibited under Church regulations. He said that *ipso facto* excommunication is automatic for those who take the pill.

When she was still Vice-President, Gloria Macapagal Arroyo announced her opposition to the entry of RU-486 into the country, saying that it was an abortifacient and its use was contrary to Philippine law. She warned that groups endorsing the use of the drug could be prosecuted for a criminal act. The Mayor of Manila warned that he was going to conduct a raid of any Department of Health warehouse or of any company that maintained stocks of this abortion pill. He noted that allowing the drug in the country would grossly violate the provisions of the Constitution proclaiming a pro-life policy. Congressman Leonardo Montemayor also cited the constitutional provision against abortion as he threatened to slash the budget of the Department of Health, if it allowed RU-486 to enter the country.

On the other hand, some women's organizations have argued that the pill should be made available locally to give women, especially rape victims, an effective option for asserting their reproductive rights. The study conducted by the University of the Philippines Population Institute partly provides the context for discussion concerning women's rights. Apart from the number of women who have undergone induced abortion, the study is noteworthy for establishing the type of women who are involved and the methods used. Due primarily to the illegal nature of abortions, many women have sought medical advice or assistance only when they were already suffering from infections or were directly threatened with serious harm.

In the Eleventh Congress, a bill was filed to allow abortion if the conception resulted from rape or was the offshoot of an incestuous relationship into which the mother was lured by force, intimidation, or fraud. The bill would also have legalized abortion when the conceiving mother was suffering from a disease that could prejudice the health of the unborn child, when the conception endangered the life of the expectant mother, or when the unborn child was found to be suffering from a terminal disease or an incorrigible abnormality. Up to this point, economic priorities have taken precedence over the abortion bill. However, we can expect it to be filed again in the next congress.

B. *In Vitro Fertilization and Assisted Insemination*

It was not until 1998 that a child was first reported to have been conceived in the Philippines through the use of either assisted insemination or *in vitro* fertilization (Macaso-Samson, 1998). However, the law has contained specific provisions dealing with such children since the Family Code of the Philippines was issued on July 6, 1987. The Code provides that "children conceived as a result of artificial insemination of the wife with the sperm of the husband or that of a donor or both are ... legitimate children of the husband and his wife, provided, that both of them authorized or ratified such insemination" (Article 164).

In the absence of public venues for the discussion of theoretical positions pertaining to this area of reproductive health, very little has been expressed on the related issues. Committee work leading up to the revision of the National Guidelines for Biomedical/Behavioral Research in 1995 brought out limited commentaries. After the consultations, the National Ethics Committee came out with guidelines relevant to the use of assisted reproductive techniques that included provisions:

(1) Prohibiting the intentional creation of human zygotes, embryos or fetuses for study, research and experimentation, or for commercial and industrial purposes;
(2) Limiting research on an embryo to procedures intended to improve its life and health;
(3) Prohibiting the sale of human gametes or zygotes;
(4) Limiting the application of the procedures to married couples;
(5) Ensuring the emotional stability and maturity of beneficiary couples;
(6) Upholding the dignity and anonymity of the couples involved; and
(7) Prohibiting the selective reduction of embryos.

In effect, the guidelines endorsed conservative Catholic values, including the inviolability of life from the moment of conception and the sanctity of marriage as an institution.

IV. Death and Dying

Bills regarding patients' rights and advance directives have been filed in Congress since the new Constitution came into effect in 1987. In 14 years, none has come close to approval. The most recent version is called "An Act Declaring the Rights of Patients and Prescribing Penalties for Violations Thereof."

House Bill No. 12406 attracted public attention mainly for its provision asserting a "right to refuse diagnostic and medical treatment." Section 6 of the bill lays the legal grounds for advance directives executed by "mentally competent patients" who are at least 18 years of age. The document would direct physicians not to put patients on prolonged life support in the event that their conditions develop "such that there is no hope of reasonable recovery." This is supplemented by a provision in Section 7 that "the patient has the right to refuse medical treatment which may be contrary to his religious beliefs."

The proposals sparked critical commentaries from representatives of the religious sector who see in the proposed bill a lack of respect for the value of human life. The Office on Bioethics of the Catholic Bishops' Conference of the Philippines manifested opposition saying that the bill is open to interpretations that could lead to the mercy killing of long-standing patients. Executive Director Tamerlane Lana expressed the fear that patients would refuse treatment if they can no longer afford the medical attention. There is also the argument that the bill fails to make the distinction between active and passive euthanasia. Although the local Catholic Church holds that patients could ask doctors to withhold treatment that would be futile in curing them or in prolonging life, it opposes the intentional killing of an incurable patient.

The reference in Section 8 of the bill to the right of a patient "to leave a hospital or any other health care institution regardless of his physical condition" has gone virtually unnoticed, but this provision may be seen to provide protection to physicians attending to patients covered by a Home-Against-Medical-Advice notice. Very few hospitals have clearly laid out policies and regulations relating to this practice. Passage of the bill could encourage hospitals to deal with the issues squarely by opening the pertinent issues to debate and coming out with their own implementing guidelines.

V. Access to Health Care

Government efforts to promote access to health care in the country are exercised mainly through a system of public hospitals that have mechanisms for accepting paying as well as charity patients. A nation-wide network of community health centers complements the public hospitals. The system is very inadequate, and many non-government as well as private individual efforts have needed to fill the gaps in the provision of health care access on an *ad hoc* basis. Some of these efforts generate peculiar ethical concerns (de Castro & Sy, 1998). For the purposes of this review, two government initiatives are worth discussing – the promotion of generic drug use and parallel drug importation.

The official commitment of the State to the promotion of health is embodied in the Declaration of Principles of the 1987 Constitution, which says that "the State shall protect and promote the right to health of the people and instill health consciousness among them" (Section 15). This commitment was initially manifested by the Congress of the Philippines when it sought to broaden access to health care through the passage of the Generics Act of 1988 in order "to ensure the adequate supply of drugs with generic names at the lowest possible cost and endeavor to make them available for free to indigent patients."

A. Generic Drugs Act

The Generics Act (Republic Act No. 6675) was passed to minimize the additional cost of drugs that come from expensive promotional and advertising activities. The law directed all government health agencies and their personnel to use generic terminology or generic names in all transactions related to the purchasing, prescribing, dispensing, and administering of drugs and medicines. It also required all medical, dental, and veterinary practitioners to write prescriptions using the generic name and ordered pharmaceutical companies to indicate prominently the generic names of their products. In addition, every drug manufacturing company operating in the Philippines was mandated to produce, distribute, and make available to the public the medicines it produces in the form of generic drugs.

The gains arising from the passage of the Generics Act have been minimal, and medicines in the Philippines are still quite costly compared to those in other developing countries. Medicinal products cater mostly to those who are financially well-off, and the local pharmaceuticals' pricing structure has had the effect of denying access to the poorer sectors of society. According to the Department of Health, prices pegged by multinational drug companies set the reference prices for domestic medicines produced in the Philippines or imported into the country. The effect is that when Filipinos get sick, they do not have options for low-cost drugs. Many patients purchase medicines on a day-to-day basis instead of having their prescriptions fully filled. In some cases, they must wait until money becomes available or until a charitable organization comes to their rescue. Thus, their treatments remain incomplete and their diseases are not cured. In its desire to address the issue of inequitable access to medicines, the government has decided to resort to parallel drug importation.

B. Parallel Drug Importation

The Department of Trade and Industry and the Department of Health (DOH) have collaborated on the importation of selected drugs from other countries even if these are already being made by multinational drug companies in the Philippines. Prior to parallel importation, these medicines were sold in the Philippines at five times their prices abroad. The scheme enables (for example) Filipinos suffering from hypertension to pay only P4.54 for a 20 mg tablet of Nifedipine (Adalat Retard) at one of the participating DOH hospitals instead of P25.25 at a drugstore for an identical product manufactured by locally-based multinational drug companies.

The exercise is not intended to be a permanent measure. It is meant primarily to emphasize to the multinational companies the defeasibility of their pricing structure. Its viability as a strategy to promote fair access to medicines rests on its ability to convince multinationals that, in the long run, it will be more economically feasible for them to adopt fairer pricing mechanisms. The hope is that a fair pricing structure can ensure access to essential medicines across poor and needy populations on a more equitable and permanent basis.

The initial reaction of local pharmaceutical companies has been negative and confrontational. The Pharmaceutical and Healthcare Association of the Philippines (PHAP) filed a petition with the Makati Regional Trial Court to prohibit the importation of high quality drug products of popular brands from foreign manufacturers.

A primary target of the objections is the authority granted to a government agency to compete with the private sector in an area that is supposed to be governed by free enterprise. The Philippine International Trading Corporation (PITC), a government owned and controlled corporation, has been responsible for the parallel importation of the products.

In reply, Health Secretary, Alberto Romualdez, Jr. emphasized that the PITC was subject to the same requirements set by the Bureau of Food and Drugs (BFAD) for any other company intending to engage in such a business. The medicines are subjected to the same tests as those carried out on products made by locally based pharmaceuticals. These are also labeled with prominent generic names to comply with the requirements of law. In addition, the government-controlled agency has been required to pay taxes for the importation, just like any other company.

Thus far, the exercise has shown that the PITC need not lose money when it brings in the products and sells them at such low prices. The PITC registered a net profit from the importation and distribution of these drugs, thus proving that the multinational companies can lower their prices considerably and make their products accessible to the poor as well as to the financially capable sectors of the population. Eventually, the Department of Health is hoping to persuade these companies to sell larger volumes of their products at lower prices to more Filipinos in need of medicines rather than to sell small amounts at high prices to the few who can afford them.

VI. Major Issues and Concerns

A. HIV/AIDS Regulations

The "Philippine AIDS Prevention and Control Act of 1998" was passed to protect the rights and civil liberties of all persons known to be infected with HIV/AIDS. Many of its provisions are illustrative of important issues and concerns that have come to the awareness of the Filipino public in matters of bioethics.

To protect infected individuals from discrimination and injustice, Section 16 of the Act specifically prohibits compulsory HIV testing as a precondition to a broad range of rights and services, including the following: (a) employment, (b) admission to educational institutions, (c) exercise of the freedom of abode, (d) entry to, or continued stay in the country, (e) travel, (f) the provision of medical or any other kind of service, or (g) the continued enjoyment of these undertakings.

In addition, specific measures to prevent injustices may be found in provisions that:

(1) Prohibit discrimination in matters of hiring, promotion, or assignment of employees (Section 34);
(2) Consider termination from work on the sole basis of actual, perceived or suspected HIV status as unlawful (Section 35);
(3) Bars educational institutions from expelling, disciplining, segregating, or denying participation, benefits or services to a student or prospective student on the basis of his/her actual, perceived or suspected HIV status (Section 36);

(4) Prevents quarantine, isolation, refusal of entry or deportation from Philippine terri-
    tory on account of perceived or suspected HIV status (Section 37);
(5) Protects the right to seek an elective or appointive public office (Section 38);
(6) Preserves the eligibility of HIV/AIDS patients for credit and insurance (Section 39);
(7) Preserves the right to receive health care services without additional cost (Section 40); and
(8) Entitles deceased patients to decent burial services (Section 41).

Patient-empowerment and the enhancement of informed consent are the aims of the provisions on counseling in Section 20, which directs all testing centers, clinics, or laboratories
to provide and conduct free pre-test counseling and post-test counseling for persons who
utilize their HIV/AIDS testing services.

    Access to insurance is promoted through the recognition that it is part of an individual's
right to health and is the responsibility of the State and of society as a whole. Section 26
directs the Secretary of Health and the Insurance Commission to implement a viable insurance coverage program for persons with HIV.

    As a guarantee of privacy, the AIDS law directs the State to provide a mechanism for
anonymous HIV testing and to ensure anonymity and medical confidentiality in the conduct
of HIV/AIDS tests (Section 18). Although the law provides for the mandatory reporting
of HIV/AIDS cases to authorities, it also directs all hospitals, clinics, laboratories, and
testing centers to ensure the "confidentiality of any medical record, personal data, file, including all data which may be accessed from various data banks or information systems" (Section
28). Moreover, it requires the offices concerned to protect client anonymity. It provides
that any information gathered in the process of contact tracing should remain confidential and classified. Such information can only be used for statistical and monitoring purposes and not as basis or qualification for any employment, school attendance, freedom
of abode, or travel.

    As a further indication of how seriously it takes the preservation of medical confiden-
tiality, the HIV/AIDS law contains detailed provisions dealing with the handling of all
medical information pertaining to the identity and status of persons with HIV, the limited
exceptions to the mandate of confidentiality, the giving of information to health workers
directly involved in the care of persons with HIV/AIDS, the conduct of judicial proceedings involving patients, and the release of HIV/AIDS test results.

B. Organ Transplantation

The provisions of the law on organ donation and transplantation are found in Republic
Act No. 7170 *Authorizing the Legacy or Donation of All or Part of a Human Body after
Death for Specified Purposes*. This Act, passed in 1991, defines death both in terms of the
absence of unaided cardiac and respiratory functions and in terms of brain criteria. It also
authorizes the retrieval of organs from brain dead patients whose relatives could not be
located within 48 hours. Section 2 of the Act defines death as "the irreversible cessation
of circulatory and respiratory functions or the irreversible cessation of all functions of the
entire brain, including the brain stem."

    These provisions were invoked by the doctor defendants in a landmark case filed
before the local ombudsman, alleging that a patient who was initially rendered comatose
by an accident was still alive at the time that a kidney, liver, and pancreas were taken out

of his body for the purpose of transplantation. In that particular case, the doctors were accused of murder after the relatives of the "donor" belatedly discovered that organs had been taken from him for transplant upon the authority of the director of the hospital in which he was confined.

C. Kidney Selling

In August 1999, a television program shook the medical community by exposing questionable practices relating to the solicitation of kidneys for organ transplantation. About 100 men from the seaside poverty-stricken district of Bagong Lupa were recruited as donors. The documentary highlighted the fact that those who sold their organs were very poor men who were convinced to give up one of their healthy kidneys for monetary gain. They were paid P70,000 to P100,000 (US$1400 to 2000) for their kidneys. The transaction was usually facilitated by an "agent" who received a fee of P12,000 (US$140) per "sale."

The program brought out the absence of adequate informed consent in the transactions, since it pointed out that poverty pressured many of the organ sources into giving up their kidneys due to a monetary offer that they could not refuse. Moreover, some sources claimed that they were not fully informed of the implications of the surgery for their long-term health. A few said they were forced to continue participation even when they wanted to drop out.

Many of the donors did not have the foresight to anticipate that the amount of money paid to them was not going to last very long and was, therefore, not proportionate to the harms and risks to which they were exposed. Having quickly spent the money received, they were left with nothing to show but the scars on their bodies. According to many of them, they were refused work as laborers because they were thought to be unhealthy by prospective employers.

The Philippine Medical Association (PMA) expressed opposition to the "commercialization" of organ procurement. It urged the government to set up an organ procurement program to encourage voluntary donation. The PMA President issued a statement that organs should not be sold as they are gifts of God to us, though they can be shared with others. Nevertheless, she added that the recipient could show appreciation or gratitude to the donor in whatever manner desired. She also called on the government to encourage donors by reminding them that sharing an organ is an act of love and solidarity for their neighbor.

Notwithstanding the public outcry generated by these controversial organ donations, the National Kidney and Transplant Institute issued guidelines in support of living non-related donor transplants under the following conditions:

(1) Absence of a blood related donor;
(2) Absence of a cadaver donor after a reasonable waiting period;
(3) No coercion;
(4) No profit-motivated broker or agent; and
(5) Recipients have technical and medical difficulties on dialysis.

The guidelines also provide for the grant of incentives other than the reimbursement of expenses incurred by the donor.

After the initial hysteria caused by the exposé died down, the debate tended to converge on the notion of incentives. Dr. Modesto Llamas, former president of the PMA, has said that his organization approves of the provision of incentives for organ donation.

D. Organ Donation for Commutation

The idea of providing incentives to organ donors also gave rise to a proposal to encourage death-row convicts to utilize an organ-for-commutation plan. Under the proposal, death-row convicts can have their sentence commuted by making a declaration before their execution that they are donating an organ as a gesture of atonement for their crime. The proposal was put forward by the Kidney Patients Association of the Philippines (KPAP), which has been searching for legislators to author and sponsor a corresponding bill. Bishop Teodoro Bacani, a ranking Catholic Church leader, expressed support for the proposal. Newspapers have reported him as saying that there is nothing morally objectionable about the idea, provided that the donation is voluntary. Bishop Bacani has also indicated that the proposal involves a very creative way of seeking reparation for a crime, as it involves the giving of life by one who has been convicted for being anti-life.

Prisoners serving jail terms of eight to 20 years have also been identified as prospective donors. Their penalties will be lightened in exchange for such goodwill, provided they spend some kind of "incubation period" in jail before their release.

Even before the current proposal was put forward, an editorial in the *Manila Bulletin* suggested a similar idea. The editorial came out in response to the public appeal of a blind woman for the eyes of a convict who was about to become the first person to die by lethal injection in the country after the return of capital punishment:

> It is marvelous if those who are sentenced to die by lethal injection can be given the chance to prove their generosity and nobility through organ donations ... Let us challenge them to let their inherent goodness bloom (Dimaculangan, 1999, p. 5).

Thus far, the Department of Health has rejected the organ-for-commutation proposal, taking the position that dangling the option to prisoners constitutes a coercive offer, which can be likened to compelling poor men to give up their organs in exchange for money.

E. Bioprospecting and Genetic Resources

The Philippines is protective of its biological and genetic resources. This attitude has been manifested in the government's effort to regulate access to such resources through the issuance of Executive Order No. 247. Among the Executive Order's features is a provision that the informed consent of local communities, including indigenous ones, should be sought before any prospecting of biological and genetic resources can be done within their territories, ancestral lands, or domains. Moreover, out of respect for customary laws, these were required to be the basis for obtaining consent. An Inter-Agency Committee on Biological and Genetic Resources has been given the responsibility of ensuring the protection of the rights of the indigenous and local communities.

To provide further safeguards against exploitation, research is subject to the following conditions:

(1) The type and quantity of samples obtained and exported requires approval by the Inter-Agency Committee.
(2) A complete set of all specimens collected is to be deposited in the country.
(3) Filipino researchers are to be allowed access to collected specimens and relevant data wherever these specimens are found in depositories abroad.
(4) The Philippine Government and affected cultural communities are to be informed of all discoveries and of commercial products derived from the activity.
(5) Royalties are to be paid to the National Government, local or indigenous cultural community, and individual person or designated beneficiary in case commercial use is derived from the biological and genetic resources.
(6) Filipino scientists are to be actively involved in the research and collection process as well as in the technological development of products derived; and
(7) Services of Philippines universities and academic institutions are to be used whenever appropriate, and equipment used in the process should be transferred to a Philippine institution or entity.

F. Genetically Modified Organisms

Many non-governmental organizations have consistently expressed opposition to using genetically modified organisms (GMO) for food. Their activities have had two main focal points: the testing of Bt-corn in Philippine farms, and the importation and sale of food items with GMO components.

The National Committee on Biosafety of the Philippines, a multi-sectoral body responsible for regulating field tests on biotechnology, initially approved the conduct of field tests in General Santos City in August 1999. Some groups went to the Supreme Court for a restraining order but were turned down. Hence, the tests have gone on and more sites are being prepared in other parts of the country.

In the meantime, non-governmental organizations (NGOs) have been holding demonstrations and circulating petitions asking the government to declare a moratorium on field testing in the country. The reasons that they have cited include the following:

(1) The side effects and illnesses arising from the consumption of products with GMOs may take years to manifest and could be fatal.
(2) The genetic engineering of crops is not focused on improving yield or nutritional quality but on increasing resistance of commercial crops to herbicides, thus giving rise to safety and environmental concerns.
(3) Most crops being developed are not staple food crops of poor countries but are export crops of developed countries. Even if the tests prove to be successful, there is no assurance that genetically modified food would redound to the benefit of the country, because control over the products is in the hands of multinational companies that have no clear obligations to the economic development of the country.
(4) The country's rich natural resources could be destroyed by the release of GMOs into the environment.

On the other hand, agriculture-based scientists argue that genetic engineering can be the answer to the problem of hunger as they increase the crops' resistance against pests, diseases, and even herbicides. Without GMOs, corn farmers have been incurring heavy losses due to corn borer infestations and have largely depended on the application of pesticides. The locally based International Rice Research Institute (IRRI) has pointed out the beneficial uses of genetic engineering in terms of greater productivity, vitamin- and nutrient-enriched grains, and a chemical pesticide and herbicide-free environment.

While the debates concerning the field testing of Bt-corn have continued, some food items already available in Philippine markets have been alleged to contain genetically modified organisms. According to Greenpeace, 11 out of 30 products chosen for examination because of their soy and corn ingredients have tested positive for GMO content. Of the 11, at least one infant formula being sold locally has been found to contain ingredients extracted from genetically altered soya beans. To deal with this development, environment-oriented NGOs have asked the government to implement a labeling system for ingredients of food products derived from GMOs. The suggestion has been heeded by the Department of Agriculture, which has said that it will ensure transparency by requiring manufacturers to inform consumers of the GMO contents of their products through the use of appropriate labels.

VII. The Future of Filipino Bioethics

There are two legislative items that are indicative of future directions for bioethics in the Philippines. The first of these items is a proposed *Magna Carta* of Patient Rights. The second is the Traditional and Alternative Medicine Act (TAMA) that was signed into law in 1997.

A. *A Magna Carta of Patient Rights*

The rights enumerated in a proposed *Magna Carta* reflect some of the present shortcomings in the system that must be addressed. They also constitute a statement of the aspirations of many people relating to the ethical delivery of health care.

Although the proposed *Magna Carta* provoked public reaction mainly on the issue of euthanasia, it has also served to encapsulate central issues of bioethics that are relevant to the health concerns of ordinary patients. The pending bill seeks to integrate the important concerns into a single document that could be the focus of public attention.

The proposed *Magna Carta* could also serve as a source of practical guidelines for physicians and other health care workers in dealing with patients because of the detail that it accommodates. It may not have the sophistication of well-established guidelines on similar subjects, but it seeks to go beyond the usual level of medical jargon. For instance, it explains voluntariness in terms of the patient's opportunity to ask questions, to consult relatives, and to seek another expert opinion. Elsewhere, it is not content to recognize a right to "information necessary and indispensable ... to intelligently give ... consent, ... which may include, but may not be limited to, the benefits, risks and side effects, and the probability of success or failure, as a possible consequence of ... proposed ... procedures." It goes on to say that: In the explanation of the proposed procedure or procedures, the comprehensive ability of the patient shall also be considered taking into account his level of education, the dialect or language that he speaks and understands, and if possible, the use of anatomic sketch, or otherwise the use of those materials or visual aids that may aid the patient or his legal surrogate, in fully understanding the proposed procedure or procedures (Section 4).

Regarding critical situations, the bill authorizes a physician to perform any emergency diagnostic or treatment procedure "as good practice of medicine" dictates when the patient is unconscious or otherwise incapable of giving consent and there is no one who can give proxy consent. If a legal surrogate refuses to give consent to a diagnostic, medical, or surgical procedure necessary to save life or limb, a court, upon petition of the physician or any person interested in the welfare of the patient, may issue an order allowing the emergency diagnostic, medical, or surgical procedure or procedures.

Among the other entitlements recognized in the proposed *Magna Carta* are the following:

(1) The right to privacy and confidentiality,
(2) The right to disclosure of and access to information,
(3) The right to choose one's physician,
(4) The right to leave,
(5) The right to refuse participation in medical research, and
(6) The right to be informed of one's rights and obligations as a patient.

In Section 4 (3), the bill explains the right to privacy and protection from unwarranted publicity in terms of the patients' not being subjected to exposure by photography, publication, video-taping, discussion or by any other means that would tend to reveal their identity and the circumstances under which they are under medical or surgical care or treatment. Confidentiality applies to information acquired by attending physicians and hospital staff in connection with the confinement of patients and the hospital care rendered to them.

The exceptions allowed under these provisions on privacy and confidentiality include considerations of public health, safety, and medical or scientific discussions for the benefit and advancement of science and medicine. Moreover, in recognition of the extended role of the Filipino family in matters of individual health and safety, there is the additional qualification that any information revealed to the spouse or a member of the family shall not be considered as a violation of the provisions of the proposed law but shall instead be treated with leniency and caution.

A mechanism to protect the patients' autonomy is to be found in the "right to disclosure of, and access to information" in Section 4 (4). This entitles patients to information about the nature and extent of their disease, the contemplated medical treatment and surgical procedures, and any possible complications, pertinent facts, statistics or studies regarding their condition. However, the bill allows exceptions on paternalistic grounds. It states that "if the disclosure of information to the patient will cause mental suffering and further impair ... health, or cause the patient not to submit to medically-necessary treatment, such disclosure may be withheld or deferred at some future opportune time upon due consultation with the patient's legal surrogates."

Also in Section 4 (4), the proposed *Magna Carta* gives importance to autonomy and the capacity of patients to understand and direct the course of their treatment by requiring that the attending physician provide the patient, at the end of confinement, a brief, written summary of the course of the illness, which shall include at least the history, physical examination, diagnosis, medications, surgical procedure, ancillary and laboratory procedures, and the plan for further treatment. In addition, the bill declares that patients are entitled to an explanation and viewing of the contents of the medical record of their confinement.

The "right to leave" was partially explained above in connection with the protection of doctors whose patients decide to go home against medical advice. It has additional relevance in the case of patients who are confined under emergency conditions but do not have the means to pay for hospital services. Section 4 (8) provides that "no patient shall be detained against his will in any health care institution on the sole basis of his failure to fully settle his financial obligations with the physician or the health care institution." This provision has caused private hospitals to lobby intensely against the passage of this bill and others with similar contents in the past. In the absence of a comprehensive health insurance system, a provision such as this protects indigent patients from unreasonable, unnecessary, and unjust periods of forcible confinement for which they cannot pay anyway. But lobbyists argue that the threat is necessary to protect them from huge operating losses. If this provision is approved, hospitals might find a way to pass the cost on to paying patients, thus giving way to another type of injustice.

The reservations of private hospitals about the proposed *Magna Carta* are addressed also to a related provision in Section 4 (1) that "patients in emergency who are in danger of dying and/or who may have suffered serious physical injuries shall be extended immediate medical care and treatment without any deposit, pledge, mortgage or any form of advance payment for confinement or treatment." Like the provision on the right to leave, this feature of the bill exacts a toll on the resources of private health institutions, which many of them are either unable or unwilling to shoulder. Although the broadening of access to critical health care is an important component of justice, there is a need to ascertain who should bear the costs of implementation.

Section 4 (9) of the proposed *Magna Carta* recognizes the "right to refuse participation in medical research." It acknowledges that patients have a right to be advised on how plans to involve them in medical research may affect their care or treatment and requires their written, informed consent for such purposes. Two major considerations make this provision important. The first is the prevalent attitude of respect and deference towards doctors, which makes it virtually impossible for any patient to refuse participation in medical research. This is magnified by a propensity on the part of pharmaceutical companies to recruit hospital-based consultants to carry out their research. By virtue of their influence, these consultants can obtain the consent of their patients almost at will and without adequate documentation.

The second factor is poverty and the reliance of charity patients on drug samples provided by the drug company representatives proliferating in the wards of public and private hospitals. Since the importance of the boundary between therapy and research in the minds of many doctors is underemphasized, patients could unknowingly be exposed to risks.

The "right to be informed of his rights and obligations as a patient" is perhaps the most important among those enumerated in the bill because, without such information, patients would not be in a position to assert their entitlements. Many patients become the victim of negligence, carelessness, or even gross malpractice without even being aware of it. Guilty parties get away with harmful practices because patients are ignorant of their rights. Thus, it is necessary to put the burden on health care institutions to provide the pertinent information.

B. Indigenization of Philippine Bioethics
One can quite safely predict that the discussion of bioethics issues in the near future will proceed along the tension points that have been mentioned above. The forces that have

given rise to those tensions can be expected to persist through the next 25 years. The religious influence is well entrenched, as it has been for centuries. The feminist movements, after having initially taken a cue from foreign developments, have adapted to local conditions and can be expected to grow stronger as they cater to the problems and needs of poor Filipino women. As an alternative to regular government agencies, non-government organizations have proven to be reliable and trustworthy providers of basic services. They are poised to play an active role in facilitating and processing public sentiment as regards issues of bioethics. These various sectors will continue to act on the basis of their own perceived responsibility to Filipino society, thus providing continuance to the tensions described above.

The social, economic, and cultural conditions that provide the context for those tensions can also be expected to remain. Although everyone is hoping that significant economic improvements will be experienced as soon as possible, the general conditions that define the parameters for bioethics issues will not disappear overnight.

One movement that should start to gain prominence is the indigenization of Filipino bioethics. By this is meant the application of indigenous Filipino concepts in the effort to understand and provide solutions to problems of bioethics. Already, some publications have surfaced that make use of Filipino concepts to define and clarify issues of bioethics (Miranda, 1994, 1998; de Castro, 1997, 1998, 1999, 2000).

The passage of the Traditional and Alternative Medicine Act (TAMA) of 1997 was also an important development. It was passed, among other reasons, to promote and advocate the use of traditional and alternative health care modalities, and to formulate standards, guidelines, and codes of ethical practice appropriate for the practice of traditional and alternative health care. As Filipinos come to terms with the homogenizing forces of globalization, the process of indigenization will be seen as an indispensable complement. It will be an invaluable asset as Philippine bioethics moves towards the future.

Bibliography

de Castro, L. 1997. Transplanting values by technology transfer. *Bioethics* 11(3-4): 193-205.

de Castro, L. 1998. *Teknolohiya at Pagkatao: Mga Isyu ng Etika sa Medisina.* Quezon City: Sentro ng Wikang Filipino.

de Castro, L. 1999. *Sakit* and *Karamdaman*: Filipino concepts of disease and illness. In *Global bioethics from Asian perspectives* (pp. 16-21). Tokyo: University Research Center, Nihon University.

de Castro, L. 2000. Kagandahang Loob: a Filipino concept of feminine bioethics. In R. Tong, G. Anderson & A. Santos (eds), *Globalizing feminist bioethics: women's health concerns worldwide* (pp. 51-61). Boulder: Westview Press.

de Castro, L. & Sy, P. 1998. Critical care in the Philippines: the "Robin Hood principle" vs. Kagandahang Loob. *Journal of Medicine and Philosophy* 23(6): 563-580.

Dimaculangan, J. 1999. Organ donation: a reparative option for lethal injection. *Manila Daily Bulletin* 10 February, 5.

Macaso-Samson, G., Almeda, L.A. & Vera, T.R. 1998. First test tube baby in the Philippines. *Philippine Journal of Obstetrics and Gynecology* (April-June): 67-69.

Miranda, D. 1994. *Pagkamakabuhay: on the side of life (prolegomena for bioethics from a Filipino-Christian perspective).* Manila: Logos Publications.

Miranda, D. 1998. Hindi Maatim: conscientious objection in health care. In F. Gomez, et al. (eds), *Conscience, cooperation, compassion* (pp. 33-52). Manila: University of Santo Tomas, Department of Bioethics.

Perez, A., Cabigon, J., Singh, S. & Wulf, D. 1997. *Clandestine abortion: a Philippine reality.* New York: The Alan Guttmacher Institute.

Philippine Council for Health Research and Development. 1996. *National guidelines for biomedical/behavioral research.* Metro Manila: Philippine Council for Health Research and Development.

19 Japanese Bioethics

Darryl Macer

I. Introduction

Japan emerged as one of the global economic superpowers in the twentieth century. It is a country of 125 million persons speaking a distinctive language, Japanese, with a history of at least three millennia. It has an illusive property for Europeans: it is an island at the Far East of Asia, which had an isolationist policy during the time when Europe was colonizing much of the world over the past four centuries. Since the Meiji restoration in the nineteenth century, the doors of Japan have been opened to all countries, and their ideas have been undergoing rapid change with globalization, which is itself driven by the communication devices which Japanese industry has exported around the world.

Japan has developed its own medical ethics, merging Buddhist and Confucian rules into a Shinto background, with a recent importation of Western values (Macer, 1999). Japanese ethics could be said to be rather pragmatic and authority centered. There is tax-payer financed universal health insurance, which supports the concept of social justice and access for all to health care. While the principle of justice is accepted socially, the increasing proportion of aged persons means sick people have recently been expected to pay a higher proportion of the medical costs themselves to lessen the tax burden. While the sick expect to be covered by this insurance, most do not want to be a burden on the state or their families. Informed consent is becoming accepted, and bioethics is part of a transition which is transforming Japanese society from a paternalistic society to an individualistic one.

II. History

Japanese medical ethics is a mixture of Buddhist and Confucian influences combined with Shinto influences, and more recently Hippocratic and Christian influences. From the fifth and sixth centuries A.D., the medical profession has been restricted to the privileged classes. With the centralization of government in the seventh and eighth centuries, a bureau of medicine was established, with the Yoro penal and civil codes creating an official physician class. After the Heian period (A.D. 800-1200), the government-sponsored health service was replaced by professional physicians. In the sixteenth century, a code of practice was drawn up that is very similar to the Hippocratic code, called the "Seventeen Rules of Enjuin". This code, developed by practitioners of the Ri-shu school, also emphasized a priestly role for a physician. The physicians "should always be kind to people. You should always be devoted to loving people." There is a very strong paternalistic attitude by doctors even today. The code also had a directive to keep the Art secret and to be concerned about quacks, as does the Hippocratic ethic. No abortions were allowed, nor poisons. A number of virtuous rules were included, such as: "You should rescue even such patients you dislike or hate" and "You should be delighted if, after treating a patient without success, the patient receives medicine from another physician and is cured."

Modern Western medicine took hold in Asia in the nineteenth century. The rapid progress of medical technology has led to changes in the way that medicine is practiced. The existing health care delivery systems and the relationships among patients, families, health care professionals, and society in general are changing. At the same time, as the technology is transferred, alien moral values are also being imported, beyond the general acceptance of the new technology as an improvement.

The black episode in Japanese medical ethics is the war-time experiments conducted on prisoners in Manchuria China, while China was under Japanese occupation in World War II. At least 3000 persons, mainly Chinese, were murdered by or after vivisection and other experiments in facilities under Unit 731 at several locations in China. The functions included vivisection practice for nearly qualified army surgeons, intentional infection of diseases, trials of non-standardized treatments, and discovering the tolerances of the human body (Tsuchiya, 2000). Unlike Nazi war crimes, the Japanese war criminals were only prosecuted in the Soviet Union, but the United States gave those in authority immunity from prosecution in exchange for all the records, so that the knowledge gained for biological warfare experiments could be kept secret (Harris, 1994). The United States actually tested some of the weapons in North Korea in 1952. Neither Japanese nor Chinese bioethics has analyzed these experiments and the ethical issues they raise (Morioka, 2000; Tsuchiya, 2000, 2003; Macer, 2001; Nie, 2001), which contrasts with the German preoccupation with the war crimes of their country's past. Because of the opportunity to have access to the best medical research facilities in Asia, many physicians went to the Unit, and after the war it was only in the mid 1990s that some members of the Unit started to confess and apologize for their actions, as they reached old age. However, the discussion of the issues in bioethics has only just begun.

Currently Japanese medical ethics is changing and a diversity of moral views similar to that experienced within Western ethics has been recognized. The hesitant introduction of bioethics is more related to the structure of Japanese society than to any real difference of attitudes between Japan and Western countries. This can be shown from the results of opinion surveys: for example, when individuals were asked to give their reasoning for their opinions over bioethical issues such as genetic manipulation or screening, there was at least as much variety in opinions expressed by members of the general public in Japan as there are in other countries (Macer, 1994a).

Since the 1970s, people have become more conscious of their rights to informed consent, which could be attributed to the importation of the civil rights debates that occurred in the United States and Japan in the 1960s (Kimura, 1995). However, the concept of human rights was recognized in the constitutions of the Meiji era and the post-Second World War. In the nineteenth century, some philosophers, such as Nakae Chomin, also introduced concepts of human rights (Hamano, 1997). He reinterpreted Confucianism by injecting concepts of popular sovereignty and democratic equality, and provided an internal tradition of human rights. Macer places the origin of informed choice with the older samurai tradition, which includes the control of when one will die and the choice of suicide (1999). In addition, the concept of informed consent is seen in the writings of Hanaoka Seishu on breast cancer from the nineteenth century.

With the introduction of Western medicine, there has also been an influx of Western religion, philosophy, and professional etiquette. As cultures evolve, it becomes impossible to separate which aspects were introduced from which sources at which time. Within a few decades, a culture may see something as unique to its own tradition, even though it was imported. Even the concept of a written text is seen as a cultural import in some Asian countries. Although ancient Japanese and Chinese books date back more than 1300 years, and legal systems were established at earlier times, the Westernization of Asia led to the introduction of European-style laws. This affects the types of laws and guidelines that govern medical practice.

The growth of international "bioethics" has had the effect of stimulating cultures around the world critically to assess the relationships between patient and practitioner, as well as between the public and the government (Macer, 1994b). A Japanese reaction during the 1990s, following the introduction of Western, particularly American, medical ethics in the 1980s, was a cultural backlash; the claim that Japanese are different from Westerners. This moral and cultural claim was used to defend existing practices, while also anchoring the rapid social changes. We have seen the development of the Asian Bioethics Association as one attempt to break with the domination of U.S. bioethics. At the 1997 UNESCO Asian Bioethics Conference (Fujiki & Macer, 1998), there was discussion by a number of Asian researchers on the need for recognizing traditional Asian bioethics, rather than importing bioethics from the United States. There has been discussion, for example, on whether the idea of fundamental human rights is compatible with the Asian *ethos* (Sakamoto, 1999).

III. Topics

A. Bioethics in General

1. *Important institutions.* Currently, professional responsibility is outlined by law and guidelines. In Japan, there are several basic laws, including the Doctor's Act. The Japanese Medical Association approved the concept of informed consent in 1991, superseding the Physician's Code of Ethics of 1951, which was more paternalistic (Kimura, 1995). There are professional guidelines issued for members of academic societies to follow, but physicians can still practice medicine outside of the professional society. Consensus is often more important than passing a law (Bai, et al., 1987; Shinagawa, 2000).

Physicians are required to obtain consent to medical treatment according to the Medical Practitioner's Act, Article 23. The obligation for treatment is based on assessing what can reasonably be expected in view of the knowledge and experience which ought to characterize the average physician. The obligation for consent means that the patient's will is to be respected when medical opinions are divided as to the necessity of the treatment.

The Council of Medical Ethics, established under the provisions of Article 25 of the Medical Act, is an advisory body supervised by the minister of public welfare and consists of the presidents of the Japan Medical Association, the Japanese Dental Association, and scholars and staffs from related administrative departments. Its function is to take administrative measures to eliminate physicians and dentists who commit malpractice or act unethically. Penal Code Article 211 states that if a physician injures a patient and the injuries cause death by mistreatment, he may be held liable for up to five years imprisonment and/or up to a 500,000 yen fine. According to Physicians Law, Article 7-2, if the doctor was sentenced to imprisonment or a fine, the Ministry of Health and Welfare can remove the license or stop the doctor's practice for a certain amount of time. This action follows the decision of the Medical Practice Council, according to Article 7-4. However, in practice, many Japanese are still reluctant to seek damages for malpractice (Feldman, 1985; Bai, 1983).

2. *Important personalities.* The Japan Association of Bioethics was established in 1990 and has had an annual meeting each year since then. There have been four Presidents of this Association to date: Hyakudai Sakamoto (philosopher), Kazumasa Hoshino (physician), Kinki Nakatani (lawyer) and Kiyoshi Aoki (biologist). The Association has over one thousand members; however, few persons in bioethics devote their full-time attention to the subject. Early pioneers of bioethics in Japan also include Koichi Bai at Kitasato Medical University, Norio Fujiki at Fukui Medical School, Rihito Kimura at Waseda University, and Shinryo Shinagawa at Hirosaki University, who have been introducing bioethics by public seminars and in newsletters and journals since the late 1980s.

Several university faculty positions have been established in bioethics, including Darryl Macer at University of Tsukuba (1990), Masahiro Morioka at Osaka Prefectural University (1997), Atsushi Asai (1998) and Akira Akabayashi (2000) at the University of Kyoto. Several centers of bioethics have existed for more than a decade, including the Eubios Ethics Institute. The Mitsubishi Kasei Institute of Life Sciences developed into a private bioethics institute in 2001. University degrees can be awarded in bioethics as part of other programs, but there is not a dedicated program in bioethics in Japan. A series of international conferences have also been held by the Eubios Ethics Institute: the Tsukuba International Bioethics Round tables (TRT1-8).

3. *Dominant bioethical theory.* Regarding the principles of bioethics in Japan, harmony has been discussed as a potential over-riding principle, but it is unclear if there really is any one principle that dominates (Macer, 1994a, 1998). Some commentators believe that autonomy is not seen in Japan; however, autonomy is applied to many life choices that are bioethical dilemmas. While privacy is regarded as a high virtue in some countries in law, such as Japan, there are common exceptions in practice. For example, while the Tokyo government issued guidance that employer tests for HIV may only be conducted with the informed consent of those tested, the Tokyo police department was found guilty of secretly testing potential recruits for HIV.

Significant family involvement in health care decision-making means that modern Western ideas on confidentiality have not yet been accepted in Asian medical practice. For example, families are often told medical news prior to the patient. Also, many patients, who are aware of their terminal diagnosis, play a "game of avoiding hurting others", in which they pretend that they do not know the seriousness of the disease, while family members pretend that the patient is not terminally ill. Modern Asia, however, is increasingly individualistic and patient rights are being promoted by many persons. So Japanese medical ethics is in a transitional phase which cannot be separated from broader socio-economic changes. The late twentieth century has seen rapid changes in family integration and the boundaries of the family (Maekawa & Macer, 1998).

The evolution of the concept of patient autonomy is seen as part of a trend that is reflected in all Asian cultures from paternalistic compassion and love towards individualistic informed decision-making. The situation is more complex, however, than the simple claim that in the past patients did not have autonomy and that physicians always acted paternalistically. The sick may prefer to leave decisions up to others or to use subtle linguistic expressions to convey their will. However, there is still a hierarchical social system which makes it difficult for patient and doctor to be truly at an equal level in their relationship. Even more so, the concept of informed choice, where patients are recast as medical consumers, is seen primarily in pharmacy stores rather than in medical consultation. Many sick persons are afraid to be a bother or burden to others, so they attempt to avoid any trouble which could occur if they clearly expressed their will and it differed from the decisions of others.

There are also theories of ethics in the West based on community, which argue that individuality, autonomy, and individual rights are not properly suited to preserve the community structure of society. Communitarians, for example, argue that societies need a commitment to general welfare and common purpose, and this that protects members against the abuses of individualism, which might be equated with the selfish pursuit of personal liberty.

B. *Professionalism*

There are separate laws outlining the activities of health professionals, including physicians, dentists, nurses, acupuncturists, masseurs, and other health care professionals. Non-registered professionals are not allowed to work. In 1990, there were 210,197 registered physicians at work in Japan, a ratio of 170 per 100,000 population. The Medical Practitioner's Law of 1971 contains guidelines on what the physicians should and should not do. There are some common exceptions to the law in practice. For example, Article 17 of the Act forbids non-registered persons from performing an action which may present harm to another person's body if not done by a sufficiently capable medical technique. This law technically outlaws non-registered practitioners from taking blood pressures or performing ear piercing. However, such actions are commonly performed everywhere. The curriculum for training is set by the Ministry of Education, but physicians are licensed after passing a national exam by the Ministry of Health and Welfare.

The Medical Service Law and the Health Center Law were two important laws in a series that control the operation of medical facilities. In 1991, there were 10,066 hospitals in Japan, with 1,685,589 beds. No physician introduction is required for admission to a hospital. About 81% of Japan's hospitals are privately operated. They tend to be smaller than public sector hospitals; many were developed from physician-owned family practices. The chief executive must be a physician. Of the 1048 mental hospitals in 1988, 90% were private (Koizumi & Harris, 1992).

In 1991, there were 82,118 general clinics in Japan. "Clinic" is the usual name for physician offices and about 94% are privately operated. A clinic cannot keep a patient for more than 48 hours and is legally defined as having less than 20 beds, whereas a hospital has 20 or more beds. About 60% of clinics have no patient accommodations, but they are usually well equipped. Physicians in clinics do not have access to hospital facilities and must refer patients to hospitals if they cannot provide the necessary services on site. The clinics compete with hospitals for patients, who can choose the facility they prefer. Under the Occupational Safety and Health Law of 1972, an occupational health physician was a designated physician for any workplace with more than fifty workers.

The number of physicians who had disciplinary action taken upon them between 1971 and 1988 included fourteen who lost their license for various reasons, including two for violations against the Physician's Act, three for patient abuse, two for pharmaceutical law abuses, and three for other reasons; 196 other physicians lost their license for some amount of time for other legal reasons. Licenses may be taken for actions against the medical laws and pharmaceutical and drug laws, as decided by the Medical Practice Council.

In 1990, there were 745,301 registered nurses and assistant nurses at work in Japan, a ratio of 602.9 per 100,000 population. There were 25,303 registered public health nurses, a ratio of 20.5 per 100,000 population. There were 22,918 registered midwives, a ratio of 18.5 per 100,000 population. The Medical Act of 1948 included guidelines on the activities of medical professionals including nurses. The specific guidelines are outlined in a special law: Law No. 86 of 26 June 1992 aimed at promoting and assuring the professional competence of nursing staff. In 1990, there were approximately 8700 psychiatrists, 53,000 nurses, 14,000 nurses aides, 2000 clinical psychologists, 469 occupational therapists, and 3000-4000 psychiatric social workers working with psychiatric patients. The number of psychiatrists per 100,000 population is 7.08. Attempts by the Ministry of Health and Welfare to introduce a licensing system for clinical psychologists and psychiatric social workers have been unsuccessful. Since the 1920s, the primary treatment for mentally ill patients in Japan has been long-term institutionalization. The Law of Mental Health of 1950 abolished private confinement of mentally ill persons. In 1989, the average length of stay in a Japanese mental hospital was 496 days, 41 times the average length of stay of patients in the United States. The Mental Health Law of 1988 encouraged community integration, but progress has been slow. The major goal of the law in mental health has been to avoid human rights abuses, through a series of periodic reports, requests for discharge, and notification of patients of their legal rights to have their case heard by a patient review board.

There are very few social workers in Japan, with an average of 0.2 per 100 beds in general hospitals and 0.5 per 100 beds in mental hospitals in 1991. However, there have been efforts to increase this ratio.

Insurance programs do not recognize counseling and psychotherapy as methods of medical treatment which need to be reimbursed. This means that counselors are encouraged to see as many people as possible a day and have many short visits, which is a general problem of dental and medical care in Japan. In 1998, the government altered the law to allow physicians some compensation for obtaining informed consent (Akabayashi, et al., 2000). The obligation for consent means that the patient's will is to be respected when medical opinions are divided as to the necessity of the treatment (Tokyo District Court, 1971, 5.19). The patient must be competent, and generally a person older than 15 years is considered competent in most cases. The consent of the person exercising parental authority is required in cases involving infants, children, and the mentally ill. A Tokyo District court in 1992 upheld a case brought against Tokyo University Medical School involving informed consent. The operation was a medical success, but the patient was not informed of the chances of failure and brought a case against the hospital. However, in other more recent cases, the courts have upheld informed consent (Swinbanks, 1989; Tanida, 1991). In practice the concept of fully informed consent is still being introduced into Japanese medical practice.

Privacy of communication is guaranteed in the constitution. Article 21 of the constitution guarantees freedom of assembly and association as well as speech, press, and all other forms of expression. There is the Law on the Protection of Computer Information on Individuals, which provides for the handling of information on individuals for processed and stored in computers by government agencies. The law states that government agencies are prohibited from using the information on individuals for any purpose other than the original purpose for which the files were compiled. Any person may require a government agency to disclose the information on himself which is stored in the computer system and, if necessary, demand its alteration. This could be interpreted as meaning that the truth of any health information entered into the system must be verified following the individual's request.

If someone informs others of personal medical data (for example, the result of a genetic screening test to an employer), section 134-1 of the penal code could apply. If the person who leaked the information is a national employee, they could be punished by the Law on Government Employees. The Occupational Health and Safety Law obligates the health care staff to keep secrets. Under Article 14 and 15 of the AIDS law, divulging this diagnosis will be punished beyond the measures of the penal code. Article 15 sets penalties of up to six months imprisonment or up to a 200,000 yen fine.

C. Reproduction

About two thirds of Japanese couples use contraceptives. However, despite the emphasis of the Eugenic Protection Law on control of the population, the Ministry of Health and Welfare only approved use of low dose birth control pills in September 1999. They were introduced at an estimated annual cost of over 50,000 yen, which is very expensive. Some claim that the pill may encourage promiscuity, and more recently that it may lead to an increase in cases of AIDS, if it alters condom usage habits. Governmental concern about the falling birth rate among Japanese, an image among women that the pill is not safe, and belief that it interferes with natural hormonal cycles, slowed wide-spread use of oral contraceptives.

The 1948 Eugenic Protection Act was designed to permit the sterilization of mentally incompetent patients. Sterilization is not generally performed for reasons of birth control. In 1948, Japan was one of the first industrialized countries to pass a liberal abortion law, because it was related to post-war population control. The Law of 1948 governed the use of abortion services in Japan, until it was replaced by the Mother's Body Protection Law in 1996. The number of abortions conducted is declining, but it is still high among developed countries. The viability limit of fetuses as defined in the Eugenic Protection Law was amended from twenty-four completed weeks of gestation to twenty-two completed weeks in 1991. Abortion is restricted to the period in which the fetus is not viable outside of the uterus, as determined by the Ministry of Health and Welfare.

Among some pressure groups, there is more acceptance of social abortion than selective abortion for handicapped fetuses because of concerns that this selection will lead to bad attitudes towards handicapped people (Morioka, 2002). The law does not specifically permit selective termination of fetuses with a disease, so some doctors will interpret the law loosely and others strictly, especially in some national university hospitals which want to be more careful to follow the letter of the law. The number of multiple pregnancies has increased following the wide use of assisted reproductive technology, and there is still debate inside the medical association on whether to condone the practice or not.

Examples of voluntary guidelines from other professional societies include one on *in vitro* fertilization (IVF) and assisted reproductive technology by the Japan Society of Obstetrics and Gynecology (JSOG) (Shinagawa, 2000). There were about 11,000 babies born from IVF in Japan in 1999, so the technique has been widely used. IVF is restricted to married couples and eggs are not donated. The Japanese Society of Obstetrics and Gynecology approved the procedure of oocyte drilling for treatment of infertility in 1993.

Surrogacy is not permitted, though foreign surrogacy agencies have been used by Japanese clients, and at least two agencies operate for the United States surrogacy businesses in Japan. Through these agencies, babies are born by means of surrogate motherhood or "womb leasing" surrogacy, since 1993. These surrogacy arrangements involve sperm from Japanese men inseminated into American women. On 5 November 1992, the Japan Society of Fertility and Sterility publicized their statement that they do not support the clinical practice of surrogate reproduction and they have shelved the production of any guidelines on the matter. According to their statement, they recognized serious gaps between the capability of technology and its ethical, legal, and social acceptability in Japanese society.

Donor insemination is conducted largely through the Obstetrics and Gynecology Department of Keio University, Tokyo, and there are no laws that regulate the practice. There are about 500 attempts a year at Keio University and over 250 births per year. Each sperm donor is used for up to fifteen pregnancies, and only married women are accepted. Keio University is the most public about its program. Other institutes do not admit to having such a program. The guidelines used are those of Keio University and the Japan Society of Obstetrics and Gynecology. Children conceived through donated sperm or eggs are still legally considered illegitimate; however, in February 2001, the Ministry of Justice announced it may change the law to recognize these children as legally the children of the birth parents rather than the current situation which recognizes the genetic parents. For several centuries, however, there has been a well-established tradition of recognizing adoption in Japan. Every year there are about 90,000 adoptions.

Preconception sex selection has been investigated in Japan, but in a 1993 survey, 76% said that if they had only one child they would want a girl, which suggests many do not consider traditional ideas of family inheritance important. The reason why more people wish to have a girl than a boy, which is in contrast to many other Asian countries, may be because girls are considered more cute or better care-givers for elderly parents. The Japan Society of Obstetrics and Gynecology and the Japan Medical Association committees both reached similar guidelines in September 1986. They decided that sex selection by Y-chromosome containing sperm concentration should only be adopted to help prevent the conception of a conceptus with severe sex-linked genetic disorders, such as progressive muscular dystrophy or hemophilia. However, there is no law against marketing methods for sex selection.

On 30 November 2000, the Human Cloning Regulation Act was enacted. It prohibits transfer of human or animal–human embryos made by somatic nuclear transfer to an animal or human uterus. The initial ban is for three years, at which time it will be reviewed. A breach of the prohibition can be punished by a fine of ten million yen and ten years imprisonment. It does not prohibit transfer of human-human chimeric embryos or embryos made by embryo splitting (Nudeshima, 2001). Embryonic stem cell research is not covered by law but by administrative guidelines, which the Ministries enforce.

D. Death and Dying

1. Issues in euthanasia and physician-assisted suicide.
Medical treatment to reduce or remove pain which may also cause premature death is considered lawful under several conditions (Nagoya High Court, 1962, 12.22):

(1) The patient suffers from an incurable disease as judged from contemporary medical knowledge and technology, and death is impending;
(2) Physical pain is unbearably extreme and without any other means of relief;
(3) There is consent or a contract based on the true will of the suffering person. In the case where the consciousness of the patient is not clear enough to express his wishes and there is no hope of recovery, the consent or earnest request of the immediate family is sufficient; and
(4) A generally practiced medical act is to be employed to this end.

The Japanese Medical Association (JMA) recommended that there be general legislation allowing doctors to withdraw life-sustaining treatment if patients wish to do so in cases of terminal illness. They want the law to recognize living wills, but they oppose legalizing euthanasia. The report by the JMA Bioethics Committee also suggested that cancer patients be informed of their disease "in principle".

A Japanese court decided that a man who helped his terminally ill female partner die in response to her requests in 1991 did so out of deep love, so he was only sentenced to one year with a two year stay of execution. In a 1993 case of physician-assisted active euthanasia in Japan, a doctor at a Tokai University injected KCl into an incompetent patient at the pleading of relatives. The University Committee judged it unethical. There are mixed opinions among physicians on the issue (Macer, et al., 1996).

Handicapped neonates are usually treated aggressively, with physicians paternalistically making treatment decisions. The general view is that parents are distraught and unable to decide. Even hopeless cases may be more aggressively treated with therapy than in most Western countries. This is in contrast to the traditional custom of *mabiki* which was to leave handicapped newborns to die. There have been no legal suits regarding the withdrawal of treatment for handicapped neonates. A survey of consultant pediatricians found that 90% would intensively treat a Down's syndrome baby even if the parents refused treatment, but that 90% of the public would not consider a doctor who did not treat a handicapped infant as a murderer.

2. Hospice care and care of the dying.
The Ministry of Health and Welfare and the JMA have published manuals to help practitioners resolve other difficult dilemmas (JMA, 1989; Akabayashi, et al., 1999). The latest manual lists four factors which should be taken into account when considering whether to disclose a cancer diagnosis: (1) the purpose of disclosure should be clear; (2) the patient and family members need to be able to accept the diagnosis; (3) the nature of the relationship between the practitioner and the family and patient should be considered; and (4) psychological support should be provided to the patient after disclosure. There exists a general reluctance to tell the truth about terminal illness in Japan, but a growing percentage of doctors support revealing such a diagnosis and a growing percentage of the public claim that they would want to know. Even in 1980, 61% of people said that they would like to be told the truth and, in 1981, only 27% of doctors said that they would never tell patients the truth. In 1989, a Government Task Force concluded that the truth should be told and this view is, in principle, official.

Japan has relatively few nursing homes, compared to Western countries. One of the reasons for the relatively low number is that bed-ridden elderly persons over sixty-five years of age can receive free medical treatment including hospitalization, and anyone over seventy years of age is eligible for free care. Government supported Health Services Facilities for the Elderly were established by "The Amendment of the Act for the Health and Medical Service for the Elderly". The facilities must be staffed with medical doctors, nurses, nursing care staff, physiotherapists or occupational therapists, health consultants, and nutritionists. The municipalities pay the medical expenses, while the elderly bear the cost of personal items such as meals, diapers, haircuts, and daily necessities.

3. *Ethics of pain management.* Japanese physicians have been reluctant to administer morphine because of tough laws on related drugs. The Narcotics and Psychotropics Law was amended in 1990 to improve the accessibility of morphine preparations to cancer patients with significant pain. The Ministry of Health and Welfare produced four volumes on palliative care with guidelines on cancer pain relief and legislative management of narcotics use in hospital, clinics, and pharmacies (Takeda, 1991). Morphine use in pain management increased seventeen-fold between 1979 and 1989 due to attitude changes in physicians for management of pain, and this further increased after the law changed in 1990 as more physicians accepted the need to alleviate pain in terminal care. Morphine has changed from an illegal drug to an accepted pain treatment, following the WHO Cancer Relief Programme in 1980. In 1989, the Ministry legalized the use of 10 mg tablets of slow release morphine (MS Contin) and 30 mg tablets in 1990. The amount of morphine consumed is still about one-fourth of the levels consumed in the United States and one-eighth of that consumed in the United Kingdom; notably, the reverse relationship exists for most other pharmaceutical products.

Public surveys in the 1990s found that 80% do not want continued treatment if they are in a vegetative state, and 75% said that they do not want treatment if they are in pain and close to death. Those who are over seventy years of age were more willing to have treatment continued. However, the euthanasia cases expose the inadequacies of Japanese terminal care, where many patients who have pain remain in pain because pain killers are not completely covered by the national health insurance. This creates the desire to die, and when combined with the inadequate medical communication and trust between patient and doctor, there will remain relatively high (about 50%) public support for informed and consensual active euthanasia of competent patients, despite its illegality.

E. *Access to Health Care*
1. *Right to health care.* The modern Japanese constitution, drafted by the occupation forces after the Second World War, was reviewed by the Japanese government, and voted into force by the Japanese Diet (Parliament) in 1948. It includes thirty-one Articles on the rights and duties of the people. Article 25 reads: "All people shall have the right to maintain the minimum standards of wholesome and cultured living. In all spheres of life, the State shall use its endeavors for the promotion and extension of social welfare and security, and of public health." Article 25 assumes a welfare state but does not have much legal meaning. It does not vest in each individual person a concrete right which can be enforced by the judicial process, since such type of right comes into force only through implementing legislation. The obligation for treatment is based on assessing what can reasonably be

expected in view of the knowledge and experience which ought to characterize the average physician (Supreme Court, 1949, 3.1).

2. *The national health care system.* The basic philosophy of the Japanese health care system is universally mandated, government provided health insurance coverage. There is little choice over which insurance scheme a person must join: either employees must join the one statutory plan offered by their employers, or the self-employed plan administered by local governments or trade associations. The government health insurance plans cover every Japanese person, and two thirds have employee-based systems and one third self-employed/pensioner schemes. The proportion of the population covered by each scheme in 1991 was: (1) Government Managed Health Insurance (28.9%), (2) Society Managed Health Insurance (25.5%), (3) Day Laborer's Health Insurance (0.1%), (4) Seaman's Insurance (0.4%), (5) Mutual Aid Associations Insurance (9.7%), (6) National Health Insurance (32.1%), and (7) NHI associations (3.3%).

The government is the insurer for all of the population, with very few persons taking out additional private medical insurance. The ratio of gross domestic product devoted to health care in 1990 was 6.8%, which is a small percentage relative to other countries. There is unlimited coverage to all persons, and even foreigners who have failed to join the legally mandated medical insurance schemes and lack a foreign medical insurance policy are treated. The part of the bill which cannot be paid by the person or their family is paid by local or Prefectural government contributions.

The government-based health insurance schemes pay for the services rendered. This is a system of insured diagnosis and treatment, with several basic assumptions:

(1) Freedom to set up a practice and to choose a place of treatment;
(2) Fee-for-Service Payment System; and
(3) Universal Medical Care Insurance.

Any qualified person can register a new clinic in any location, allowing competition, which should improve the quality of care. Full medical attention can be given as the patient's conditions require, and compensation is given based on the quantity and quality of service.

All the statutory plans cover medication, long-term care, dental care, and some preventive care. The Employee's Health Insurance provides various medical and dental care, hospitalization, medicines, transportation, and special nursing for non-occupational injuries and sickness of the insured and their dependents. There are cash benefits including an injury and sickness allowance, delivery expenses, maternity allowance, nursing allowance, and funeral expenses. To help offset increased spending by an aging population, in January 2001, the maximum cost a person may pay in one month doubled from 63,600 yen (for anyone) to 121,800 yen (for high income earners). Expenses beyond this level will be reimbursed. The sickness benefit is 60% of one's wages for up to six months. The maternity benefit includes 60% of one's wages for 42 days before delivery and 56 days after delivery. The guaranteed minimum delivery expenses include 240,000 yen. A nursing allowance of 2000 yen per child is paid when a mother continues to nurse a child. Pregnant women can receive assistance and health checks at their local health center, following registration of the pregnancy.

Ambulance and emergency care is covered under the universal health insurance scheme, and a network is organized at the local governmental level. Physically, most ambulances are in the same building as the fire service vehicles. The general principle is that every person living in urban areas should be within five minutes of ambulance services.

There are several special schemes for payments to persons who are unable to avoid health care, about 0.6% of the population as described below. Additionally, there are special schemes for diseases, such as the "Guidelines for Counter-measures Against Incurable Diseases" of 1972, which includes relief of the burden of medical expenses on those concerned. The number of recipients of certificates of medical services for different intractable diseases was 245,195 persons in 1992.

The Health Services System for the Elderly, established in August 1982, provides a comprehensive system for health and medical services and equitable sharing of the medical care cost for the aged in the entire nation. The Maternal and Child Health Law provides for municipalities to offer health education, counseling, examination, and home visitation services for three year-old children and their mothers. The original Law of School Health was established in 1925 to prevent infectious diseases in schools. The current system includes mass screening for many conditions, including heart disease, renal disease, and tuberculosis. There are lists made of persons according to the Law for the Welfare of the Physically Disabled and a quota system for employment.

3. *Lack of a two-tiered system?* Very few Japanese take out additional private medical insurance, and it has a very minor role. This is because everyone must join one of the government health insurance schemes, which provide universal access, so there is little need to take out any other insurance. The private insurance is mainly concerned with cash compensations to cover incidental expenses and reimbursement to the families of injured persons. Although providers are officially prohibited from charging more than the fee schedule allows, the prices which patients pay for treatment under private medical insurance depend upon the decision of the health care provider and are less regulated than the government system. Foreign persons under foreign health insurance can basically be charged any price the health care provider decides, within the principle of competition. Motor vehicle accident insurance for "damages" to third-parties is common, but the payments are not for medical expenses, but are much greater for loss of expected lifetime earnings and misery. Causing the death of a person usually involves the transfer of over 100-million yen via such insurance, and is pursued through legal suits which may be settled out of court.

This having been said, although anyone can access any physician directly, a recommendation letter or introduction is required to get treatment at a prestigious hospital. Thus those who can get introduction letters by contacts, which could also involve money, can access the best facilities. Although bribery is illegal, imminent specialists may be illegally paid monetary gifts in the range 100,00 to 300,000 yen. These practices are seen more among patients hospitalized in the private rooms of universities and prestigious hospitals (Ikegami, 1992). There are also reports of illegal payments in geriatrics hospitals for nonprofessional nursing care (diapers, and so forth), which hospitals claim are inadequately covered by health insurance (Niki, 1992).

F. *Other Issues*

1. *Organ transplants from brain dead donors.* One of the technologies which has been the most controversial in Asian countries is organ transplantation. In some ways, organ transplantation was a "flagship" for the introduction of bioethics debate into Japan (Macer, 1992), and thus this specific technology may have led to consideration of the need for the

public to be involved in the debate on medical ethics. The issue of consent was closely linked to this question, and it raised questions of trust in doctors. Rather than religious views, the fundamental doubt in people's minds may have been, and may still be, trust in the medical profession (Macer, 1992). This issue of trust has also been cited as a reason why African-Americans are reluctant to donate organs (Siminoff and Saunders Sturm, 2000).

The most controversial issue involving the use of modern scientific technology is organ transplantation from brain dead donors. On this issue, there has been more debate in Japan than in any other country in the world. The first heart transplant was performed in 1968, and the second was delayed by this debate until 1998. The brain death law was passed in 1997, and by February 2002, there had been 18 transplants approved under the new law (Masahiro & Sugimoto, 2001; Bagheri et al., 2003). For a country of 125 million people, that is almost nothing. There are still critics of the law permitting organ transplants from brain dead donors (Becker, 1999). One of the motivating arguments used to support organ donation is love of others. The organ donor cards in Japan feature four little angels (actually a Western concept) giving organs to save others.

A law enabling cornea transplantation was passed in 1958. This law, allowing physicians in general to transplant corneas from cadavers, requires prior written consent of the family of the dead donor, and does not require consent when there is no surviving family. In 1979, the Act Concerning the Transplantation of Cornea and Kidney was passed. The level of kidney donation (at least the reported level) has dropped in the last few years with the high profile of the brain death issue and fear of litigation. Reported by a survey from Japan's Women's hospitals, from 1980-85, ninety-six of 314 kidneys were donated from brain dead donors, and, in 1984-1988, 152 of 429 kidneys were from brain dead donors.

The Prime Minister's *ad hoc* Committee on Brain Death and Organ Transplantation report of January 1992 recommended unanimously that organ transplants from brain dead donors who have positively expressed a desire to donate organs should be permitted. They also say that no organ transplants should be performed from patients who have said they do not want to give organs. The committee also says that organs can be donated if family members agree that the deceased expressed a wish to donate organs, and that there has been no pressure on the relatives to make this decision. They recommended that a third-party should look at these cases to ensure there is no undue pressure to consent. In addition to these unanimous findings, there was a majority agreeing that brain death is real human death. A minority of four members said that brain death is close to human death.

Actually, since the mid 1985s, the level of public agreement is the same as the range as general opinion across Western countries, with about 25% rejecting organ transplants from brain dead donors. It was argued that Japanese have special cultural barriers to such donations, which has been dismissed by Japanese sociologists and religious groups (Nudeshima, 1997). In every culture, some people reject removing organs from bodies and their views should be respected. As mentioned, the more serious doubt in the minds of some people is whether they can trust doctors (Macer, 1992) and, among ten countries in Asia-Pacific area surveyed in 1993, Japan had the lowest trust in doctors (Macer, 1994a).

2. *AIDS.* Although there have been many infectious diseases throughout history, AIDS has been associated with much ethical debate in Asia. Confidentiality should be maintained for medical information, and in some countries there are laws against those who break confidentiality (as in Japan). In the case of a fatal infectious disease like HIV, there is a possible harm to others, so it could fail as a legitimate exception if that harm is a real

threat. The early years of the AIDS epidemic saw hospitals refusing persons infected with HIV and disclosures of HIV status to third parties beyond government reporting (Feldman & Yonemoto, 1992). The exceptions to confidentiality have revealed its real weaknesses.

In Japan, the Physician's Law Article 19-1 says that a physician must see a patient to cure unless sufficient reason exists. This is used to argue against refusals of HIV infected persons. In a court case, if a patient was hurt as a result of doctor's refusal, the doctor has responsibility to pay. On 30 June 1992, a Kobe District Court awarded damages to a patient based on a refusal of emergency medical treatment. The judge said the physician has the responsibility to compensate the damage the patient incurred as a result of the refusal of care.

Also, there is a quota system for employment for HIV infected persons, and it is against civil code Article 709 and 715 for a company under the quota to refuse to hire an HIV infected person. Breaking this law means that the company must pay consolation money to the person.

The contamination of blood with HIV in Japan eventually lead to prosecution of some of the responsible persons who failed to stop non-heat-treated blood products being sold. This also helped erode the trust people had in physicians and the Ministry of Health and Welfare.

3. *Gene therapy.* In 1994, the Ministry of Health and Welfare in Japan announced that members of their Ethics Committee were assessing applications for gene therapy. The Ministry of Education released their guidelines in 1995, and both sets were revised in 1999. Each Ministry has a separate committee (with overlapping members). In university hospitals, drugs already need the approval of both ministries, and so will gene therapy. By August 1994, one gene therapy protocol had been approved for Niigata University and one for Hokkaido University. The guidelines are basically those of the National Institutes of Health in the U.S. The guidelines rule out germ-line therapy and limit cases to terminal illnesses without effective therapy. However, they only require verbal informed consent, not written consent, which may be determined by local hospitals' policies. Japanese scientists and public strongly support the use of gene therapy (Ng, et al., 2000; Inaba & Macer, 2003).

4. *Support for the japanese pharmaceutical industry.* A 1993 scandal revealed that the Japanese Ministry of Health and Welfare was attempting to encourage Japanese industry not to use a foreign MMR (mumps, measles, rubella) vaccine, while risking public health with a vaccine with 100-200 times more frequent side effects. A controversy erupted in 1993 over the high incidence (1 in 400) of side effects from a MMR vaccine made and used in Japan. It was withdrawn after the media released unpublicized government risk data. The Preventive Vaccination Law was weakened in 1987 by removing its obligatory nature and was further weakened in 1993 with the broadening of exceptions and the removal of provisions which penalized parents who failed to have their children vaccinated.

One of the embarrassments of the Japanese health care system is the corruption which is implicit in the way drug prices are set and reimbursement is made, as well as the contributions from pharmaceutical companies to doctors who use their drugs. The Japanese are the world's highest spenders on prescription drugs. Almost all general practitioners and hospitals have their own pharmacies for outpatients. Every two years the Ministry of Health and Welfare sets the "official" prices for all drugs. These prices are used to determine the charges to patients and the national health insurance systems. However, pharmaceutical companies offer drugs to hospitals at a discount. The permitted discount is 10%,

which means that there is even official sanction of the scheme to have financial reimbursement for dispensing prescription drugs. In practice, the current discounts are 20-30%,
or more in competitive markets. This means that hospitals and doctors benefit from prescribing drugs, and this explains why the consumption of drugs is so high. For example,
antibiotic prescriptions around 1990 were about fifteen times greater per person than in
the United Kingdom. There are also financial incentives to use newer, more expensive broad-
spectrum antibiotics, because the profit for the hospital is greater than dispensing older
and cheaper antibiotics. This source of income is regarded as essential for private hospitals
and clinics, in the absence of government subsidies, to maintain the current wage system.

IV. Conclusions: The Future of Japanese Bioethics

The key issue for bioethics in Japan was the unprecedented social debate over the law to
allow organ transplants from brain dead donors. It is rare to see a debate between the public
and the policy makers over any issue, but this issue led to the introduction of informed consent and the need for medical policy to be more sensitive to public concerns. The future could
expect a further transition from paternalism to informed consent to informed choice.

There have been calls in academia for laws to control reproductive technology, but a
limited law on cloning is the only legal instrument specifically made to regulate reproductive technology, despite similar public disagreement with that technology, as for
declaring brain death. There is also discussion of amending the abortion law implicitly to
include abortion for reasons of fetal handicap, but it is likely that genetic counseling programs will continue to expand without such a legal change.

The Japanese health care system provides an equitable level of health care coverage for
a low proportion of the gross domestic product. In a national survey in 1985 of those persons who had experienced an illness but not seen a physician, only 0.4% gave economic
reasons. This suggests that almost no one is prevented from seeking medical care for economic reasons. There are a complex mesh of insurance systems to cover all persons, and
the major critic has been the JMA which has suggested one universal system. Other critics suggest it may be too rigid to allow proper competition. However, it is based on the ethical presumption of universal coverage for equivalent services. It is being challenged by the
aging population, and the gradual introduction of more "user" fees (Watts, 2000).

The bioethics debate may be the catalyst required to transform Japan from a "paternalistic democracy". People of any country may resist the rapid change and globalization of ethics,
ideals, and paradigms as ethnic and national identities may be changed, or lost, especially
countries with such a long history of culture. How countries approach globalization is a fundamental question, but many individuals in countries with access to common news media
have already answered the question by their converging lifestyles and values. To the extent
that human rights and the environment are more respected, this trend is to be encouraged.

When Japan opened its doors to Western society in the last century, it led to the introduction of a newly emerging science and scientific paradigm, only part of the fabric of
Western society. Meanwhile, Western society has continued to evolve and bioethics has
emerged. It is now time for bioethics to also be developed in Japan. Part of this development includes importing and developing ethical approaches which can be debated, but
a more important part is the involvement of the public in discussion and development of

the indigenous diversity of ethical traditions. However, it must be noted that, in terms of equity of access to health care systems, Japan has achieved this at a low cost, and the principle of universal coverage is unlikely to be challenged for the foreseeable future.[1]

Note

1. Further updated references on bioethics in Japan can be found at the Eubios Ethics Institute world-wide web site: <http://www.biol.tsukuba.ac.jp/~macer/index.html>.

Bibliography

Akibayashi, A., Fetters, M.D. & Elwyn, T.S. 1999. Family consent, communication, and advance directives for cancer disclosure: a Japanese case and discussion. *Journal of Medical Ethics* 25(4): 296-301.

Bagheri, A. et al. 2003. Death and organ transplantation: knowledge, attitudes, and practice among Japanese students. *Eubios Journal of Asian and International Bioethics* 13: 3-6.

Bai, K., Shirai, Y. & Ishii, M. 1987. In Japan, consensus has limits. *Hastings Center Report* (June) Special Supplement: 18-20.

Becker, C. 1999. Money talks, money kills – the economics of transplantation in Japan and China. *Bioethics* 13(3): 236-243.

Feldman, E. 1985. Medical ethics the Japanese way. *Hastings Center Report* (October): 21-24.

Feldman, E.A. & Yonemoto, S. 1992. Japan: AIDS as a "non-issue". In D.L. Kirp and R. Bayer (eds), *AIDS in the industrialized democracies: passions, politics and policies* (pp. 339-360). New Brunswick: Rutgers University Press.

Fujiki, N. & Macer, D. (eds) 1992. *Human genome research and society*. Christchurch: Eubios Ethics Institute.

Fujiki, N. & Macer, D. (eds) 1994. *Intractable neurological disorders, human genome research and society*. Christchurch: Eubios Ethics Institute.

Fujiki, N. & Macer, D. (eds) 1998. *Bioethics in Asia*. Christchurch: Eubios Ethics Institute.

Fukushima, M. 1989. The overdose of drugs in Japan. *Nature* 342: 850-851.

Hoshino, K. 1993. Legal status of brain death in Japan: why many Japanese do not accept "brain death" as a definition of death. *Bioethics* 7: 234-238.

Ikegami, N. 1992. The economics of health care in Japan. *Science* 258: 614-618.

Inaba, M. & Macer, D. 2003. Attitudes to biotechnology in Japan in 2003. *Eubios Journal of Asian and International Bioethics* 13: 78-90.

Japanese Medical Association and the Ministry of Health and Welfare 1989. Manual for terminal care of cancer patients. *Journal of the Japanese Medical Association* 102 (supplement) (in Japanese).

Kimura, R. 1995. History of medical ethics: contemporary Japan. In W.T. Reich (ed.), *Encyclopedia of bioethics* (pp. 1496-1505). New York: Simon and Schuster MacMillan.

Kitagawa, J.M. 1995. History of medical ethics: Japan through the nineteenth century. In W. T. Reich (ed.), *Encyclopedia of bioethics* (pp. 1491-1496). New York: Simon and Schuster MacMillan.

Macer, D. 1992. The "far east" of biological ethics. *Nature* 359: 770.

Macer, D. 1994a. *Bioethics for the people by the people*. Christchurch: Eubios Ethics Institute.

Macer, D. 1994b. Bioethics may transform public policy in Japan. *Politics & Life Sciences* 13: 89-90.

Macer, D., Hosaka, T., Niimura, Y. & Umeno, T. 1996. Attitudes of university doctors to the use of advance directives and euthanasia in Japan. *Eubios Journal of Asian and International Bioethics* 6(3): 62-69.

Macer, D. 1998. *Bioethics is love of life*. Christchurch: Eubios Ethics Institute.

Macer, D. 1999. Bioethics in and from Asia. *Journal of Medical Ethics* 25: 293-295.

Macer, D. 2001. What is our bioethics? *Eubios Journal of Asian and International Bioethics* 11(1): 1-2.

Masahiro, M. & Sugimoto, T. 2001. A proposal for revision of the organ transplantation law based on a child donor's prior declaration. *Eubios Journal of Asian and International Bioethics* 11: 108-110.

Morioka, M. 2000. Commentary on Tsuchiya. *Eubios Journal of Asian and International Bioethics* 6(6): 180-181.

Morioka, M. 2002. Disability movement and inner eugenic thought: A philosophical aspect of independent living and bioethics. *Eubios Journal of Asian and International Bioethics* 12: 94-97.

Ng, M.C., Takeda, C., Watanabe, T. & Macer, D. 2000. Attitudes of the public and scientists to biotechnology in Japan at the start of 2000. *Eubios Journal of Asian and International Bioethics* 106(4): 106-113.

Nie, J. 2001. Challenges of Japanese doctor's human experimentation in China for east Asian and Chinese bioethics. *Eubios Journal of Asian and International Bioethics* 11(1): 3-7.

Niki, R. 1992. *Shakaihoken Jyunpou* 1768-1770 (in Japanese).

Nudeshima, J. 1991. Obstacles to brain death and organ transplantation in Japan. *Lancet* 338(8774) 1063-1064.

Nudeshima, J. 2001. Human cloning legislation in Japan. *Eubios Journal of Asian and International Bioethics* 11(1): 2.

Sakai, A. 1991. Psychoactive drug prescribing in Japan: epistemological and bioethics considerations. *Journal of Medicine and Philosophy* 16: 139-153.

Salzberg, S.M. 1991. Japan's new mental health law: more light shed on dark places? *International Journal of Psychiatry* 14: 137-168.

Shinagawa, S. 2000. *Tradition, ethics and medicine in Japan*. Berlin: Humanitas Verlag.

Siminoff, L.A. & Saunders-Sturm, C.M. 2000. African-American reluctance to donate: beliefs and attitudes about organ donation and implications for policy. *Kennedy Institute of Ethics Journal* 10(1): 59-74.

Swinbanks, D. 1989. Japanese doctors keep quiet. *Nature* 339, 409.

Takeda, F. 1991. Changing attitudes towards narcotic use in cancer pain management in Japan. *Postgraduate Medical Journal* 67 (Supplement 2): S31-S34.

Tanida, N. 1991. Patient's rights in Japan. *Lancet* 337(8735): 242-243.

Tanida, N. 2000. Japanese religious organizations' view on terminal care. *Eubios Journal of Asian and International Bioethics* 10(2): 34-37.

Tsuchiya, T. 2000. Why Japanese doctors performed human experiments in China 1933-1945. *Eubios Journal of Asian and International Bioethics* 6(6): 179-180.

Tsuchiya, T. 2003. In the shadow of the past atrocities: research ethics with human subjects in contempory Japan. *Eubios Journal of Asian and International Bioethics* 13: 100-102.

Watts, J. 2000. Japan makes older people contribute towards their health care. *Lancet* 356: 2075.

Part V: New Zealand

20 Bioethics in New Zealand: A Historical and Sociological Review

Jing-Bao Nie and Lynley Anderson

New Zealand ("*Aotearoa*", "the land of the long white cloud", in the Maori language) is a small country far away from the rest of the world. Located in the Southern Pacific Ocean, New Zealand remains even a long distance (three hours flying time) from Australia, its closest neighbor. Its total land mass is about the same as that of Britain, with a population of almost 4 million, about 7% of that of the United Kingdom or that of a mid-sized city in Mainland China. New Zealanders (often self-called "Kiwis") include the indigenous Maori inhabitants and latecomers from Europe, the Pacific Islands, Asia, and other parts of the world.

Despite their geographical isolation, people in this country have not been able to avoid the perennial human problems of illness, suffering, and death, as well as the new ethical challenges brought about by developments in medical technology and the life sciences. In general, New Zealanders have been very sensitive to the moral issues related to abortion, euthanasia, allocation of health care resources, patient-physician relationships, biotechnological advances, and so forth. As in many other countries, bioethics in New Zealand explores the interface between health and illness, medicine, law, philosophy, politics, economics, and the mass media. Bioethics as an academic and intellectual discipline has become well established and institutionalized. As a public discourse or social movement, bioethics plays an important role in the critical evaluation of health care delivery, health policy, medical research, and patient rights. Internationally speaking, bioethics in New Zealand is, in some respects at least, rather advanced and progressive in spite of its small land size and population.

Although the development of bioethics in Aotearoa has kept pace with development overseas, New Zealand also has a unique voice shaped by particular historical events and its distinctive socio-cultural heritage. As in the United States (Jonsen, 1998), bioethics in New Zealand is both an academic discipline as well as a public discourse or a social-cultural movement. This review is historical because it outlines the birth, growth, and present state of bioethics in this country. It is also sociological because it identifies the socio-cultural forces that have shaped the features of "Kiwi" bioethics and the ways in which bioethics has contributed to New Zealand society.

I. Bioethics as a Social-Cultural Movement

A. The Socio-Cultural Context

Bioethics in New Zealand has not developed in a social vacuum, nor is it solely an academic discipline developed and discussed within the university context; rather, it is influenced by and in turn influences the ideologies and discourses surrounding health care issues in New Zealand. Health issues and public health policy are matters of great public interest and debate. Few remain unmoved when medical scandals are uncovered, new technological breakthroughs are made, or health budget cuts are suggested. Changes to health practices and health policy impacts on a deeply personal and highly political level within our community and, because of this, there is always much to be heard on these matters. This gives the field of academic bioethics a rich base from which to draw. People could be said to be "doing" bioethics in their homes and in the media, whether or not they are aware of it. This is obviously not unique to New Zealand; however, there are certain political and cultural features that are unique to these shores that invariably shape the kind of bioethical conversations that New Zealanders have and the conclusions they reach.

One of the seminal events influencing bioethics in New Zealand was the 1987-1988 Cartwright Inquiry (an investigation into a 1966 research trial on cervical cancer, to which we will return to in greater detail later). The Inquiry was an important catalyst for the development of bioethics in New Zealand and a pivotal event in New Zealand's social history. Of course, concern for patients' rights, allocation of scarce resources in health care, the delivery of medicine, and research ethics had emerged prior to the Inquiry. These concerns created the environment in which such an inquiry could occur and bioethics could flourish. Like all social movements, it was influenced by the nature of the society from which it developed. And so, it is to the salient historical, social, and political features of New Zealand that we will turn next.

New Zealand is a typical liberal democracy. It is peaceful, the rule of law operates, and it is economically and constitutionally stable. There is a strong commitment to the preservation of individual rights and freedoms. Historically, New Zealand has been known for having a robust social welfare system, featuring high quality public health and education systems. A move to the right in the 1980s saw an erosion of the welfare system, but a reasonable level of access to fully or partially publicly funded social goods, including health care, still exists.

The size and remoteness of New Zealand, the shadow of colonialism, and the well-honed national myth of egalitarianism, as well as a parliamentary system that easily allows for broad policy change also influence the values that New Zealanders embody. One such value that historically New Zealand has fostered is that of progress. From the "social laboratory" of the 1890s to the enthusiastic welfarism of the 1950s-60s to the wholesale adoption of the new right ethos of the 1980s, New Zealand has readily embraced new ideas that might provide social improvement. This concern for social improvement has not been limited to national boundaries. New Zealand has played a large role in the South Pacific and has taken active and controversial stands on highly contentious international issues. One such example is New Zealand's strong anti-nuclear stance. A commitment to fairness, progress, new ideas, and radicalism, if the issue is right, combined with belief in individual responsibility, shapes much of the public policy discourse in New Zealand. Bioethical conversations are not excluded from this influence (Gallop, 2001).

One other particularly important feature of New Zealand society is that of race relations. New Zealand was colonized mainly by European peoples. The process of colonization was significantly different to that of the United States or Australia. A partnership between the colonials and the indigenous people, Maori, was fostered from the outset. And although the "partnership" was not always upheld, a discussion about the rights of

Maori and the role of the crown has always been evident. The debate on biculturalism in New Zealand and reparations for land confiscation are two of the most important areas of focus for race relations (Gallop, 2001).

Biculturalism constitutes one of the most striking characteristics of New Zealand's values and thereby its bioethics. Biculturalism takes its roots in the Treaty of Waitangi, the fundamental document for New Zealand as a nation representing the partnership between Maori and the British Crown. Like Australian Aborigines and native North Americans, Maori suffered greatly due to Western colonization. In 1840, more than 500 Maori chiefs and representatives of the British Crown signed a landmark agreement, the Treaty of Waitangi. In the Treaty, Maori were imbued with authority over the resources of Aotearoa New Zealand. The key concept of the Treaty is the partnership between Maori and Pakeha (European settlers). Unfortunately, the Treaty of Waitangi was not acknowledged and honored as the founding document until two or three decades ago. Recently, government and other public institutions have made great efforts to recognize the distinctive place of Maori within this country and to acknowledge the spirit of the Treaty of Waitangi. For instance, a discussion document on Maori health issued by the Ministry of Health in April 2001 stressed that a Maori Health Strategy must be guided by the principles of the Treaty: partnership, participation and protection. Partnership means: "Working together with iwi, hapu, whanau and Maori communities to develop strategies for Maori health gain and appropriate health and disability services." Participation means: "Involving Maori at all levels of the sector in planning, development and delivery of health and disability services." Protection means: "Ensuring Maori enjoy at least the same level of health as non-Maori and safeguarding Maori cultural concepts, values and practices" (New Zealand Ministry of Health, 2001, p. 1).

B. Women's Movement, Women's Health, and Abortion

The birth and growth of bioethics in New Zealand emerges from several socio-cultural movements such as the women's movement, the patients' rights movement, and the consumer movement. Bioethics is not only a fruit of these movements but part of them. While the women's health movement was certainly not the only social force that helped create bioethics, it was significant. The character of the Cartwright Inquiry was strongly influenced by the women's movement and national attention to women's health.

In 1893, New Zealand became the first country in the world to grant women the right to vote. The move to enfranchise women was a major step toward gender equality and gave women the opportunity to influence society. This change came about following extensive nationwide campaigns, lobbying, and political maneuverings that continued for many years. However, the time was right for a move like this to succeed. In the latter part of the nineteenth century, New Zealand had become more prosperous and increasingly stable, and women's increasing community involvement indicated a growing shift in attitude toward their participation in the public sphere (Page, 2001).

Women's groups continued to be a strong lobbying force throughout the 20th century to improve women's health. These consumer-based movements incorporated action on at least four different aspects of women's health. These included the establishment of the Family Planning Association in the 1930s to improve access to sex education and contraceptives in the face of fears of New Zealand's declining population and entrenched moral views regarding women's procreative choice. The Parent's Centre was established to educate women about childbirth and to demand choices for women in childbirth that differed from the standard medically orientated birth, in which women were sedated and subject to the arbitrary rules, which were part of obstetrics at the time. Political lobbying by the above groups, joined by the Homebirth Association, led to the 1990 Amendment to the Nurses Act of 1961, allowing midwives to attend normal births without a doctor being present. Concurrent changes made to five other Acts supported midwives' new-found role, allowing limited prescription rights, access to laboratory testing, the ability independently to deliver babies in public hospitals, and to receive payment for this care from public maternity funds. Resistance to these changes came from obstetricians, but midwives and women's health groups were well prepared, having previously garnered political support (Pairman, 2001).

Abortion is a topic that has engendered much debate overseas, and this has also been true in New Zealand. Prior to 1977, abortion was covered under the Crimes Act of 1961, which allowed abortion so long as it was "supported by medical opinion given in good faith," yet only one clinic was established for this purpose. A Royal Commission was set up in the 1970s to examine issues surrounding contraception, sterilization, and abortion. Legislative changes in 1977 meant that women could access abortion under limited circumstances. The grounds for termination of a pregnancy in New Zealand are as follows: that the continuance of the pregnancy would result in serious danger to the life or to the physical or mental health of the woman; if it would lead to serious disability in the child; or if the pregnancy was the result of incest. Under the new legislation, women seeking an abortion, usually after an appointment with their general practitioner, must gain the approval of two authorized certifying consultants. The abortion must be carried out in a hospital or authorized clinic by a registered medical practitioner. In general, prior to 20 weeks gestation, New Zealand's abortion law could be characterized as being prescriptive in design, but in practice it is interpreted far more liberally. After 20 weeks gestation, the law becomes significantly more restrictive, allowing abortion only when the life of the mother is threatened. Since 1977, New Zealand's abortion rate has continued to rise from 5945 in 1980, to 15,208 in 1997, to 16,103 in 2000. This is a rate of approximately 19 per thousand women aged 15-44 years; this rate is slightly lower than the abortion rates in Australia and the United States which are both above 22 per thousand (Statistics New Zealand, 2002). Rising statistics have led some anti-abortion groups to claim that New Zealand's abortion law has been interpreted too liberally; that it has been interpreted as providing for abortion on demand. However, there is little to suggest that the majority of people in New Zealand society want any further restrictions (Abortion Supervisory Committee Report, 1998).

The women's health issues discussed above provided a background for events to unfold in the Cartwright Inquiry. Although having roots in the women's movement and women's health movement, what followed from the Inquiry would impact upon the delivery of health care for all in New Zealand.

C. The Cartwright Inquiry into the "Unfortunate Experiment": The Birth of New Zealand Bioethics

The birth of New Zealand's bioethics was a response partly to issues and problems created from the political, social, cultural, scientific, and technological changes of the 1980s within the country, and partly to events overseas, especially to events in the United Kingdom and the United States. Such events eventually led to the establishment of the first bioethics center and the development of research ethics committees. However, historically, the birth of bioethics as a public discourse in New Zealand was directly associated with what was officially titled "Inquiry into Allegations Concerning the Treatment of Cervical Cancer at National Women's Hospital" in 1987 and 1988 ("The Cartwright Inquiry").

The well-known inquiry started as a response to a cover story published in the Auckland (the largest New Zealand city) monthly magazine *Metro* in May 1987. The article, "An 'Unfortunate Experiment' at National Women's", was written by Sandra Coney (a freelance journalist and women's health activist) and Phillida Bunkle (then an academic and women's health advocate). Based on their careful examination of related papers in medical journals, letters, interviews with medical professionals and administrators, and a detailed description of a particular patient, the authors alleged that Professor Herbert Green, a consultant obstetrician and gynecologist at National Women's Hospital, conducted a medical experiment in which conventional treatment was withheld without the patient's knowledge or consent over a period of nearly twenty years. The *Metro* article attracted immediate and intense public attention. In June 1987, the Minister of Health appointed a Committee of Inquiry led by Silvia Cartwright, then an Auckland District Court Judge. The terms of reference for the Inquiry included whether there was an on-going research project, whether any women had received or were receiving inadequate treatment, and if so, the reasons for such a failure, and if any women involved required further treatment. Moreover, it considered the ways in which patients in medical research and practice could be better protected and properly informed as well as methods to improve the training of medical students (Appointment letter, Minister of Health, Cartwright Report, p. 19). While initially the Minister wanted a "short, sharp" inquiry completed in a couple of months, the deadline for reporting was extended on three occasions, until it lasted almost a year. In July 1988, Judge Cartwright submitted her final report of nearly three hundred pages: *The Report of the Committee of Inquiry into Allegations Concerning the Treatment of Cervical Cancer at National Women's Hospital and into Other Related Matters* ("The Cartwright Report").

The Inquiry validated the allegation of the *Metro* article that the physician had failed to provide sufficient treatment. The "unfortunate experiment" originated with Dr. Green's unconventional belief that "carcinoma in situ" (CIS, abnormalities in the cells in the neck of the womb) did not progress to invasive cancer and that no medical treatment was therefore required. This belief was unconventional because, in 1966 and onwards, when Green's research program was proposed and commenced, the internationally accepted view was that CIS is a pre-malignant disease and must be treated with the aim of eradication. The claimed goal of Green's research was to attempt to prove that CIS was not always harmful and, therefore, to reduce the need for aggressive surgery. Judge Cartwright concluded that failure to treat existed during the entire period of research, reaching a peak in the late 1960s and early 1970s. While a significant number were not managed by generally accepted medical standards, "the outcome of treatment for the majority of women has been adequate." Unfortunately, "for a minority of women, their management resulted in persisting disease, the development of invasive cancer and, in some cases, death" (The Cartwright Report, p. 210).

The primary goal of the Cartwright Inquiry was to investigate Dr. Green's unethical research project. However, it did not limit itself to medical misconduct by a particular physician or colleagues, or to activities at a particular hospital, or even solely to the issue of women's health. Rather, the Inquiry also examined many other related issues, such as patients' rights, medical power and hierarchy, and the institutional barriers that prevent effective and efficient problem solving in medical institutions. The Cartwright Inquiry can be seen as public scrutiny of medical practice, research, education, and institutions in New Zealand. The depth and breadth of this scrutiny was unprecedented in New Zealand. From an historical and sociological perspective, the secondary and more general aspect of the inquiry, regarding medical practice and systems, is equally if not more significant to the development of bioethics than the original basis for the Inquiry.

D. From Medical Ethics to Bioethics: The Importance of
Informing Patients and Obtaining Consent

The Cartwright Inquiry represents the most profound turning point in the history of New Zealand medical ethics. It signaled the shift from an era of traditional medical ethics (focusing primarily on the professional etiquette of physicians) to a new era of bioethics (encompassing a broader and more patient-centered perspective). Historically medical ethics in New Zealand, as in many other places in the world, has by and large been paternalistic and authoritarian, as well as physician- and medical profession-oriented. A good example is the 1887 Code of Medical Ethics of the New Zealand Medical Association (formerly the British Medical Association New Zealand Branch), adopted from the Code of the American Medical Association. On the one hand, the code emphasizes the greatness and nobleness of the medical profession to such a degree that it requires that "when pestilence prevails, it is their [physicians'] duty to face the danger, and to continue their labours for the alleviation of the suffering, even at the jeopardy of their own lives (p. 25)." On the other hand, it stressed that "Physicians should minister to the sick with due impressions of the importance of their office; reflecting that the ease, the health, and the lives of those committed to their charge depend on their skill, attention, and fidelity. They should study, also, in their deportment, so to unite *tenderness* with *firmness*, and *condescension* with *authority*, as to inspire the minds of their patients with gratitude, respect, and confidence" (p. 25 original italics).

The code puts forward a series of obligations of patients to their physicians. These include: a patient "should faithfully and unreservedly communicate" to the physician the "supposed cause of their disease", should "never weary his physicians with tedious detail of events or matters", and "should, if possible, avoid even the friendly visits of a physician". Also, the patient "should, after his recovery, entertain a just and endearing sense of the value of the services rendered him by his physician" and "should be prompt and implicit" in obeying the physician's prescriptions (p. 25).

Informed consent, the benchmark moral doctrine and principle in contemporary medical practice, did not formally enter into New Zealand medical ethics until the 1960s. In 1964, for the first time, the term "consent" appeared in the yearly manual issued by the British Medical Association New Zealand Branch. While there was always a section on medical ethics in the Annual Handbook, two paragraphs, one on consent and the other on medical information, were new. The subsection on consent to examination or treatment acknowledged that "The law touching this question is extensive and practitioners should make themselves familiar with their obligations" (1964, p. 23). It stated that, while it can be generally accepted that the patient's visit to the physician is "indicative of consent", it is "necessary to have a clear prior consent before embarking on treatment, except in an emergency" (British Medical Association New Zealand Branch, 1964, p. 23).

Telling the truth to patients about their medical condition is currently considered to be a fundamental element of informed consent and good medical practice in most Western countries, including New Zealand. However, this is a relatively new phenomenon. The 1887 Code of the New Zealand Medical Association required that a physician should not reveal gloomy prognostications to their patients if "not absolutely necessary". Since the physician "should be the minister of hope and comfort of the sick", it is regarded as a "a sacred duty" for a physician "to avoid all things which have a tendency to discourage the patient and to depress his spirits" (p. 25). The 1963-64 Handbook of the New Zealand Medical Association stated in the subsection on information to the patient: even though "the patient has a right to know the facts and the opinion about his case", "What to tell a patient about his illness calls for discretion on the part of the doctor in attendance. ... In the face of serious illness or where there is little or no chance of recovery, it calls for particular discretion as to what is said and how it is said." It went on: "In any circumstances the doctor must act in what he believes to be the best interests of the patient" (British Medical Association New Zealand Branch, 1964, p. 23). Even in the Cartwright Inquiry, several doctors expressed their concern about the possibility that a patient might be "frightened" by bluntly truthful medical information. Dr. Graeme Duncan, the then-president of the Royal New Zealand College of Obstetricians and Gynaecologists, testified that telling patients of all complications "would frighten a very large number of people from having necessary treatment, and it would also be beyond the intellectual comprehension of a considerable proportion of population." He challenged the notion of informed consent in general because it lacks a "clear" and "consistent" definition (Coney, 1988, p. 143).

The Cartwright Inquiry identified and highlighted the failure to inform patients and obtain their consent as the salient unethical feature of Dr. Green's experiment. During the entire research period, lasting two decades, many patients did not know they were in a research trial, nor had they always been properly informed of the treatment options available to them. In her report, Judge Cartwright pointed out that, while the doctrine of "informed consent" was far from developed in New Zealand in 1966, morally and professionally, the requirement to obtain consent to inclusion in a non-therapeutic trial had been clearly stated in the Nuremberg Code of 1947 and the World Medical Association's Helsinki Declaration of 1964 (pp. 132-135).

Informed consent is one of if not *the* central issue in the Cartwright Inquiry and the subsequent report. The Cartwright Report is such a remarkable document that it can be seen as the manifesto for bioethics in New Zealand. It concluded that "The lack of systematic seeking of consent to inclusion in research or treatment (except for operative procedures) and the inadequate procedures for approval and surveillance of research and treatment, pose a serious risk to patients' rights" (Cartwright Report, p. 212). It emphasizes that "Except in cases of serious emergency, the patient's autonomy and the right to participate in decisions concerning her treatment or management must be honored" (Cartwright Report, p. 215). The Report has a particular chapter on issues of ethics and patient rights. In general, Judge Cartwright advocated "a system which will encourage better communication between patient and doctor, allow for structural negotiation and mediation, and raise awareness of patients' medical, cultural and family needs. *The focus of attention must shift from the doctor to the patient"* (Cartwright Report, p. 176; italics added). The call for and promotion of patient-centered health care is a predominant concern for her inquiry and report. Cartwright lamented that too many consent forms for surgical or medical treatment "tend to offer protection to the doctor rather than information for the patient" and recommended this be redressed. Informed consent was widely misunderstood – and continues to be misunderstood – as a measure to protect medical professionals from being sued. For Judge Cartwright, informed consent is "a principle designed to protect and preserve the patient's rights, not to protect the doctor from liability" (p. 176).

Judge Cartwright articulated three crucial points about valid consent. First, the patient's consent is "a pre-condition to all treatment or research." The requirement "starts with the premise of the right of a person to his or her autonomy or self determination." Second, consent must be "freely given", i.e., the patient "must not feel obliged to be compliant because of a cultural, lingual or social gulf between her and the doctor". "As a corollary, the doctor has an obligation to know her [the patient's] cultural perspective and to ensure, if necessary by seeking the assistance of a respected member of her community, that 'yes' means 'yes' and is not just a desire to please." Third, the patient must have "adequate information on which to base her decision." This means that the information, as expected from and offered by a reasonable doctor to a reasonable patient, must not only be accurate but that the patient must also understand. "The amount of detail in the information will be determined by the degree of risk or the magnitude of possible harm" (Cartwright Report, pp. 137-139).

E. The Legacy of Cartwright: Patient's Rights, Codes and Legislation

The Cartwright Report concludes with a number of recommendations. Some pertain directly to the women affected by Dr. Green's research, ensuring that they receive adequate and immediate follow-up and care. Other recommendations, such as to improve medical ethics education and to establish a patient advocacy service, have been far-reaching and have had a strong and lasting impact on New Zealand medicine and bioethics. These recommendations, although originally referring specifically to National Women's Hospital and the University of Auckland, have been interpreted and applied generally within New Zealand. A few other recommendations, such as amending the Human Rights Commission Act of 1977 to include a statement of patients' rights, are directly concerned with national institutional change to protect patients. According to Cartwright, because the then current system for protecting patients involved in research and/or treatment failed in significant areas, a system focusing on the protection of patients and independent of the medical establishment needed to be created.

As an aftermath, in 1994 the Health and Disability Commissioner Act was enacted to allow for the appointment of a Health and Disability Commissioner, whose role was to define, monitor, and protect patients' rights. One of the initial tasks of the first commissioner (Robyn Stent) was to draw up a Code of Health and Disability Service Consumers' Rights following extensive consultation.

A lot of legislation, reports, codes, and statements have appeared since the Cartwright Inquiry. Among the most significant are the Health Information Privacy Code of 1994 and the Code of Health and Disability Services Consumer Rights of 1996. The Health

Information Privacy Code established rules regarding the collection, use, storage, correction and disclosure of health information of individual patients. As the title indicates, the Code of Health and Disability Services Consumer Rights defines patients as "consumers". This Code is unique internationally, as New Zealand is, so far as we know, the only country that has a code of patient rights enshrined in legislation. The Code established a series of rights for all patients and accordingly defined a series of health service provider duties. A health care provider includes anyone (people and organizations) providing any sort of public or private health or disability service. The Code articulates the following ten rights every consumer possesses and which every health professional must take reasonable steps to respect:

(1) The right to be treated with respect, including the right to be provided with services that take into account the needs, values, and beliefs of different cultural, religious, social, and ethnic groups;
(2) The right to freedom from discrimination, coercion, harassment, and exploitation;
(3) The right to dignity and independence;
(4) The right to services of an appropriate standard;
(5) The right to effective communication;
(6) The right to be fully informed;
(7) The right to make an informed choice and give informed consent;
(8) The right to support;
(9) The rights in respect of teaching and research;
(10) The right to complain.

On attending the launch of the Code on the 1st of July 1996, Judge Cartwright (now Governor General) stated, "the Code of Rights closes the book on the cervical cancer inquiry." Nevertheless, the Cartwright Inquiry continues significantly to influence medicine and bioethics in New Zealand.

The establishment of a nationwide independent advocacy service was seen as an important element of the Health and Disability Commissioner's office. The role of advocates is to assist patients to ensure that their rights are respected, working independently of government agencies, health providers, and even the Commissioner. For example, one of their major functions is to try to help patients resolve disputes that may arise between themselves and their health care providers. Resolution is often completed without the need for intervention from the Commissioner's office, although advocates will refer cases on to the Commissioner and the Commissioner can also refer cases to advocates.

Partly due to the influence of the Cartwright Inquiry and partly due to the changing international ethos of medical ethics, ethical codes of medical professions experienced a revolutionary change. The New Zealand Medical Association issued a Code of Ethics in 1989 whose spirit emphasizes the partnership between patients and physicians more than any earlier code. It acknowledges and endorses such World Medical Association's ethical codes as the Declaration of Geneva (1948), the Declaration of Helsinki on biomedical research (1964, 1975 and 1983), and the Declaration of Lisbon on patients' rights (1981) as general guides having worldwide application. One of the articles of the 1989 Code requires that doctors "Accept the right of all patients to know the nature of any illness from which they are known to suffer, its probable cause, and the available treatments together with their likely benefits and risks" (p. 8). Since 1989 the New Zealand Medical Council has issued several reports and statements on informed consent, confidentiality and public safety, etc.

The research program at National Women's Hospital was sad and tragic for those women who lost their lives or were harmed, and unfortunate and unethical in nature; however, the outcomes of the Cartwright Inquiry have been positive. In his report in an international journal, Alastair Campbell commented in these words: "the news from New Zealand is good news, manifesting two striking national qualities – openness and honesty about past mistakes and a real willingness to create a future out of the lessons learnt from such honest self appraisal" (1989, p. 166). Campbell also pointed out that nationwide changes brought about after the Cartwright Report "give medical ethics in New Zealand a distinctive character, and indeed it could be argued that a side effect of the Cartwright report has been a serious attention to ethical theory and practice well in advance of that in many other countries" (1991, p. 36). The Cartwright Inquiry left a legacy that, in the words of Robyn Stent, involved "transforming individual tragedy into systematic change to ensure mistakes are not repeated and the lessons benefit all" (Stent, 1998, p. 8).

The general approach taken by the Cartwright Inquiry, understandably, is to emphasize external regulations and even external control as the solution to ethical problems related to health care and medical research. As Charlotte Paul (medical advisor to Judge Cartwright in the Inquiry) has pointed out, the Inquiry and its legacy have been "shaped by a concentration on external morality – the view from the outside [of the medical profession], reflecting the ethos of the wider society and of bioethics" (2000, p. 114). But overemphasis on external morality meant that the internal morality of medical profession – "those values, norms, and rules that are intrinsic to the practice of medicine – was ignored or even denigrated" (Paul, 2000, p. 114). In this age of external regulation of medical research and practice there is a need to avoid alienating medical professionals and to restore the moral tradition of medicine itself.

F. Ethics Committees

New Zealand has a system of ethics committees covering regions, some institutions, and some specialist national committees. Institutional ethics committees, generally based in universities, limit their role to non-patient based research. Regional ethics committees generally assess research protocols that involve the use of personal health information and the use of patients in research.

Hospital ethics committees were already established before the Inquiry and, following the Inquiry, were involved in drafting guidelines with the Director General of Health leading to the establishment of regional ethics committees. The aim of the guidelines was to put in place mechanisms to protect participants in research or those consenting to participate in health care involving new, untried or unorthodox treatments. The objectives of the regional ethics committees were primarily to protect research participants, although the objectives were broad enough to allow a committee to consider any matter of ethics relevant to health care delivery. This meant that ethics committees could look at clinical issues including innovative treatment as well as research concerns. Health care ethics committees were distinctive in their constitution: half of the committee members were to be lay, with a requirement for the chairperson also to be a lay member, and to have two Maori representatives.

Setting national standards and overseeing the regional ethics committees has been the role of the Health Research Council Ethics Committee. A new National Ethics Committee has recently taken over this role (with Dr. Andrew Moore, a philosopher from Otago University, as chair). The Health Research Council Ethics Committee will continue the business of the Health Research Council, the grant funding body for human subjects research. Two other national ethics committees also exist. The first of these is the National Ethics Committee for Assisted Human Reproduction, which examines individual proposals for research and clinical treatment using assisted reproduction. The second is the Animal Ethics Committee that oversees the use of animals in research.

G. Responses to Biotechnology

Recent advances in the science of genetics have led to growing worldwide concerns about the manipulation of genes. New Zealand, with an important agricultural base and research, faces a myriad of issues regarding the development of genetically altered organisms. A Royal Commission was initiated in May 2000 to look critically at genetic modification. The Commission is made up of four people with backgrounds in science, law, medicine, and ethics/theology. These four have been asked to receive representations on, inquire and investigate into, and report upon all matters regarding genetic modification and genetically modified organisms in New Zealand. This brief includes examining the legal, cultural, ethical, and environmental issues that surround genetic modification of animals and food, as well as for medical purposes. The Commission's report was published in 2001. This topic is likely to continue to be a challenging ethical issue for New Zealand, as it is worldwide, as developments in technology and their application expands.

The use of biotechnology for addressing health concerns, making products and modifying living organisms is also becoming increasingly common in New Zealand society. To address and examine concerns raised by this practice, the Minister of Research, Science and Technology established the Independent Biotechnology Advisory Council, in May 1999. The objectives of this group were to enhance and stimulate public discussion and to advise and assist the Government in the consideration of environmental, economic, social, and health aspects of biotechnology. This group includes people with knowledge of ethics, Maori culture, law, science, business, agriculture, education, social and health issues regarding biotechnology. Two recent issues included stem cell technology and genetic screening. The Royal Commission on Genetic Modification took over the role of IBAC pertaining to genetic manipulation. The Royal Commission established the terms of reference for a new committee: the Bioethics Council, which is set to take over from IBAC at the end of 2002 with Sir Paul Reeves (a Maori who has been a past Governor General of New Zealand, and an ordained clergyman) as chair. The Bioethics Council has recently been established. Their task is to examine the ethical, cultural and spiritual dimensions of emerging biotechnologies. A central aim is to initiate public conversation about such techonology.

H. The Role of Media and Other Publicized Cases and Events

Like any modern socio-cultural movement, bioethics as a public discourse in New Zealand would be impossible without the media. The Cartwright Inquiry started with an article published in a popular magazine, and the inquiry itself was an extremely publicized event with heavy media coverage from beginning to end. In fact, it is probably the most publicized medical and bioethical event in New Zealand history. Since the inquiry, many other cases or events directly related to bioethics have occurred with heavy media coverage. The following are some notable cases.

1. *Resource allocation.* The rising cost of health care has been a worldwide problem and New Zealand has been forced to ration health care resources. As a result, since the early 1980s, the New Zealand health care system has undergone what have been called "incessant reforms and changes" or "revolving doors" (Gauld, 2001). Two cases highlighted the need for access to treatment that is fair and equitable. In 1997, Rau Williams, a sixty-four-year-old Maori man with diabetes, mild dementia, and other co-morbidities, was denied in-hospital dialysis treatment for end-stage renal failure. The hospital stated that this was solely a clinical decision; however, questions were asked by the media about the role that financial considerations played in the decision. The family of the patient took the case to the High Court, the Court of Appeal, and the Human Rights Commission, but they were not successful. Mr. Williams died a few months later. This case provoked heavy media coverage and street protests about such issues as rationing health care, resource allocation, and the right to health care. This public debate illustrated the danger of conflating clinical decisions with resource allocation.

The second case involved the death of Colin Morrison, a Southland farmer, while waiting for triple heart bypass surgery. Morrison's death in 1998 became a symbol for critics of the health reforms, illustrating regional inequity in funding that limited access to surgery. In 1998, a new booking system for referrals for elective services was launched, called the National Waiting Times Project. Under this system, patients requiring surgery are prioritized according to medical need using a points system. Once patients meet a clinically acceptable threshold (i.e., enough points) and there exists sufficient funds to meet the financial threshold, then they are booked for surgery. This system was designed to inject equity and increase transparency in waiting lists, and to make a clear distinction between clinical and financial barriers to treatment, something that was never clear in the Williams case.

2. *The case of Baby L.* This is the first New Zealand case of withdrawing life-support treatment from a severely impaired newborn decided in court. In 1998, Baby L, a girl, was born seven weeks prematurely with severe Mobius Syndrome, a brain stem abnormality. Since her neurological abnormalities were extensive and permanent, the prognosis was very poor, including not being able to breathe by herself, or to hear, see, swallow, smile, or cry. Medical staff and Auckland Healthcare's ethics committee concluded that putting Baby L on life-support – a ventilator – was not only futile but also inhumane, because treatment meant merely prolonging dying and suffering. Baby L's parents, especially her mother, wanted the life-support to be continued. Auckland Healthcare went to the High Court for permission to disconnect Baby L from the ventilator. Baby L was taken home by her parents and died in her mother's arms. The brief life of Baby L and her sad story raised the public's attention to and awareness of withdrawal of treatment, the limits of medicine and advanced technologies, the issue about what decisions should be made for severely impaired newborns, and who should decide when disagreements occur.

3. *The case of Liam Williams-Holloway.* In 1999 and 2000, the whole country was captivated by the case of Liam Williams-Holloway, an underage boy suffering from a life-threatening brain/bone cancer called "neuroblastoma". According to Liam's oncologist, chemotherapy, the standard biomedical intervention, was the best option, claiming a success rate of over 50 percent internationally. However, Liam's parents had a different opinion about their child's treatment, and they opted for a kind of alternative therapy

including the use of a "quantum booster" – an electrical oscillator. When the parents did not take Liam for scheduled chemotherapy, the hospital and the oncologist gained an order from the Family Court placing Liam in the custody of the Children, Young Persons and Their Families Agency. This required that Liam be located and delivered to the hospital for chemotherapy. On 11 February 1999, the Agency appealed to the public, and a nationwide search for Liam (four years old then) and his parents began. Yet, partly because of the popular support for the parents, the family successfully hid from authorities. Four months later (on 6 May 1999), the Family Court lifted the previous court guardianship. Liam and his parents came out of hiding and his parents took Liam overseas to receive treatment. In October 2000, Liam died in Germany. The sad case of Liam Williams-Holloway has resulted in enormous public debate on the issue about who should have the final say regarding medical treatment of children, children's rights to standard medical treatment, the state's interest in protecting the child, parental rights to decide for their children, the use of alternative and complementary medicine, the problem of "quackery", and even the role of the media in covering medical cases.

4. *The Gisborne inquiry.* In 1990, in direct response to the Cartwright Report, New Zealand developed a cervical cancer screening program designed to screen all women to detect the few with early signs of cervical cancer so that they could benefit from early medical interventions. Unfortunately, no formal evaluation of the program was put in place at the time, and so little was known about the program's effectiveness and whether women found to have cervical cancer were followed up successfully. A 1999 proposal to evaluate the program raised some interesting and fraught ethical, legal and policy challenges for New Zealand in 2000. Debate has centered over whether individual privacy concerns could or should be outweighed by societal interests. In the study proposed in 1999, researchers planned to carry out an audit examining the screening history and management of women who had subsequently been diagnosed with cervical cancer. The researchers wanted to gain access to the names of women on the national Cancer Registry, the National Cervical Screening Register, and then contact women directly following discussion with the women's general practitioner, all without the women's prior consent. When this research was taken to regional ethics committees for approval, some committees raised privacy and consent concerns suggesting amendments to the proposed study. The amendments were not acceptable to the researchers, who were concerned that by meeting these conditions, the scientific validity of the study would be undermined (Davidson, Dawson, & Moore, 2001). For researchers to obtain access, there would need to be a change in the legislation. The Minister of Health has proposed changes to legislation in June of 2001 that would allow auditors access to identifiable health information held by the screening program, the cancer registry, and the woman's doctor, hospital, and specialist without the prior consent of the women. What impact this may have on the cervical screening program is unknown. Women who are offended by the proposal to have their health information accessed may well remove themselves from the Register. There is a lot of public debate yet to go on, and no resolution is likely any time soon.

I. Significance of Tikanga Maori

The Cartwright Report mentioned the importance of respecting distinctive Maori cultural norms related to the body, illness, diagnosis, and treatment in any good medical practice.

It especially pointed out that Maori women have three times greater risk of suffering invasive cancer than other New Zealand women and recommended "developing a programme in consultation with Maori Women, which is sensitive to their needs, which will inform them of the nature of the disease and ensure that adequate screening, treatment and advice is readily available" (p. 217). All this reflects the spirit of the Treaty of Waitangi and the idea of biculturalism.

Actually, the spirit of the Treaty of Waitangi and biculturalism has given New Zealand bioethics some unique features. An example of the impact of biculturalism on New Zealand bioethics is the role of Maori values in social policy development regarding assisted reproductive technologies (ART). Early in the public debate, the Ministry of Maori Affairs formulated some fundamental and influential guidelines for dealing with ART and related issues within the framework of the Treaty. They include:

- "[T]he embodiment of the Treaty of Waitangi at all levels and in all processes associated with ART ensures that the role and status of Maori in the development of New Zealand society is advanced and recognized."
- "In the national interest and as Treaty partners, government has a responsibility to ensure that those who administer all the admissions of ART, inclusive of such things as research and the storage of gametes and embryos are not absolved from their Treaty obligations."
- "ART has implications for valuing human life and the sustenance of past, present and future family relationships. Therefore it is from the perspective of valuing human life and protecting family relationship that this working group choose to approach ART and the implications for Maori" (Cited in Nicholas, 1996, p. 215).

As a result, such values as the extended family relationship, ancestors and descendants, and cultural identity, rather than merely informed consent and individual choice, are very visible in New Zealand regulations on ART. Moreover, Maori culture and values continue to inform New Zealand public debate and policy formation in other areas of biotechnology – the human genome project, genetic research, genetic therapy and counseling (Nicholas, 1996).

Maori have their own cultural traditions, with significant differences from and similarities to Western and other cultures. Here, it is impossible to present Maori views on human body, health, illness and disease, life, death and dying, healing, and so forth, in any detail. The differences between Maori and dominant Western perspectives on bioethical issues are highlighted in the following sad incident regarding the human body. According to Maori custom, the *tangi* or funeral rites should be held when someone dies. A central part of the *tangi* is for family members, relatives, tribe members, and friends to talk to the dead person. This may last three or four days to make sure that all people involved have their opportunity to say what has been unsaid in the lifetime of the dead and to bid farewell to the dead. The dead will not be buried until this ceremony has been performed. In the Western rational and scientific discourse, if someone dies in an accident, he or she is subject to a coroner's post-mortem examination to determine the cause of death. When a young Maori man died in a car accident from severe head injury, his brain was removed for this standard post-mortem examination. The extended family of the young Maori man was outraged when they discovered that the body they talked to had an empty head and that the dead young man was buried without his brain (Gillett, 1998, p. 62).

Ancestors are of great moral significance in Maori culture. "Maori regard the past as intertwined with the present, and feel a spiritual link to their ancestors, who are accorded much higher value than in those cultures where they merely signify part of an historical record" (Jones, 2000, p. 130). This raises moral dilemmas since scientific interests, such as archaeological and anthropological interests, may conflict with indigenous concerns regarding human skeletal remains. Following a worldwide trend, indigenous people in New Zealand are becoming increasingly active in deciding how to treat the skeletal remains of their ancestors and other items of cultural significance (Jones, 2000, pp. 119-150).

II. Bioethics as an Academic Discipline and Ethics Education

Bioethics in New Zealand is not only a significant socio-cultural movement but also a well-established academic discipline. Bioethics is now taught in all medical schools, most universities, some polytechnics, and even in some high schools. Many non-medical health professional schools throughout the country now have a strong ethics component within their curricula. There are bioethics centers throughout the country and a peer-reviewed journal of bioethics. Currently, many scholars, medical professionals, and scientists are engaged in teaching and research directly related to bioethics.

One of the recommendations of the Cartwright Report was for formal ethics teaching to be included in the curriculum for medical students. In the Report, Judge Cartwright argued that "formal teaching throughout the undergraduate and postgraduate courses should include ethical concepts and improved communication skills." She went on to state: "The public does not see medicine purely as a scientific pursuit. Increasingly, it is demanding evidence that doctors think through the many dilemmas which surround its practice and that they involve the public in ethical decisions" (p. 288).

A systematic approach to ethics education commenced a few years prior to the Cartwright Inquiry at the University of Otago Medical School, with the appointment of philosopher and neurosurgeon Dr. Grant Gillett. This ethics program was developed further with the establishment of the Bioethics Research Centre in 1988 with Professor Gareth Jones as the interim Director while awaiting the appointment of Alastair Campbell as the first Professor of Bioethics in 1990. Professor Donald Evans is the current Director of the Bioethics Centre, having taken up the position in 1997. Since the Bioethics Centre was established, ethics education has flourished within the medical curriculum at the University of Otago with five academic staff now employed. Courses in bioethics are available at the University of Otago at the undergraduate and postgraduate level and in the health professional schools. Graduate programs include Masters degrees in Bioethics and Health Law, Health Science (Bioethics), and Medical Science, as well as Doctoral level studies. The bioethics graduate program of the University of Otago enrolls students from around the world and enjoys visiting scholars from Canada, the United States, Britain, Germany, China and Australia.

The implementation of a new curriculum in 1997 resulted in immense changes to all teaching within the University of Otago Medical School. Its model is unique. For example, ethics has been integrated into every year of medical education, from first to sixth, in contrast to a single course. Students' first contact with ethics begins in the pre-clinical years with a focus on understanding and applying bioethical frameworks and discussing issues raised by topical events presented in the media. The systems integration module, which runs through years two and three, integrates pre-clinical sciences and specializations into some 18 paper cases. Each of the paper cases demonstrates a particular bioethical dimension such as truth-telling, patient rights, etc., alongside the clinical and pre-clinical subjects. This gives students an opportunity to apply ethical frameworks to paper cases while also utilizing the pre-clinical sciences. Students respond well to ethics taught using these methods as they get to observe the direct relevance of bioethics to clinical practice in the early years. In the clinical years, ethics education is directly related to the clinical experience that the student is currently undergoing. Professional development is a thread with a strong ethics component that also runs throughout the clinical years, focusing on professional responsibilities and the ethical challenges faced by clinicians. The objective of the ethics program at the University of Otago Medical School is to raise the ethical consciousness of students and to help them develop skills in competently addressing ethical challenges in medical practice.

Auckland Medical School first introduced a formal and coordinated ethics teaching program in 1983, initiated by Dr. Val Grant. Ethics teaching was conducted in each of five years of medical study, provided primarily by Dr. Grant but also with the support of staff from the Philosophy Department and various clinicians. At the time of publication of the Pond Report in 1987, confirming the new status of medical ethics teaching, the ethics curricula at Auckland Medical School complied with all recommendations in the report. It is compulsory at all levels, and is tested by examination. In 1991, Dr. David Seedhouse took up a position as a full-time senior lecturer in Medical Ethics. In addition to teaching commitments, Dr Seedhouse edited the journal *Health Care Analysis*. Dr. Vanya Kovach now holds the teaching position at the Medical School, while Dr. Seedhouse has become Professor at the Centre for Health and Social Ethics at Auckland University of Technology. This Centre was established in 2000 and has both an undergraduate and postgraduate curriculum.

At the Auckland Medical School, Dr. Vanya Kovach formally taught ethics with the involvement of staff from the Philosophy Department of Auckland University. Dr. Matin Wilkison has recently been appointed to take over this role. The program, developed by Dr. Kovach, begins in the second year with a focus on cases that raise ethical issues for medical students in training rather than for doctors. The "basics" of ethical theories and principles are introduced alongside a rich conception of professional roles and obligations. The relationship between ethics, religion, and culture prepares students for their first encounter with patients at the end of their third year. Ethics in the third year encourages student inquiry into a range of traditional topics such as consent and confidentiality. In these two pre-clinical years, the emphasis is on values, principles and the sometimes-perplexing questions inherent in the practice of medicine. In addition to this, the acquisition and explicit use of higher-order critical thinking skills contributes to the development of abilities essential for good ethical decision-making. During these two years, a connection between ethics and communication skills is highlighted. Fourth year students are invited to reflect upon their clinical experience in relation to a number of different models of the patient–physician relationship. In the fifth year, students take part in formal case discussions with clinicians and philosophers and are required to present their own ethical analysis of cases or situations previously encountered. The overall aim is to create ethically informed student doctors, who are reflective and collaborative thinkers, able to deliberate thoroughly and effectively, and thereby to meet the requirement of public accountability for their decisions (Kovach, 2001).

The influence of religion over the birth and development of bioethics in New Zealand is not as visible or strong as in some other Western countries. Yet, it would be inaccurate to ignore the role of religion. The Presbyterian Synod of Otago and Southland was a major sponsor of the first professorship in bioethics in New Zealand, supporting Professor Alastair Campbell, a theologian, at the Bioethics Centre of the University of Otago, and the Centre itself. Barbara Nicholas, a feminist theologian, was one of the early staff members at the Centre. The current head of the Centre, Professor Donald Evans, is a former philosophy professor from Wales and minister of religion. The establishment of the Nathaniel Centre in Wellington in 2000 acknowledges and facilitates the role of the Catholic Church in New Zealand to debate bioethics. This Centre (headed by the Rev. Michael McCabe) provides the Catholic community in New Zealand with opinions on bioethical issues.

The *New Zealand Bioethics Journal* is a peer-reviewed journal published by the Bioethics Centre at the University of Otago. Although the Journal in its current form was first published in June 2000, it has a twelve-year history starting with the establishment of the Bioethics Research Centre at the University of Otago in 1988. The publication from the newly established Centre was initially called the *Bioethics Research Centre Newsletter*. In 1994, the newsletter was renamed the *Otago Bioethics Report* and continued to be published in this form until 2000. Editorship of the newsletter and then the *Otago Bioethics Report* was first held by Dr. Barbara Nicholas then later by Dr. John McMillan. Lynley Anderson edited the *Otago Bioethics Report* from 1998 and remains the editor of the *New Zealand Bioethics Journal*, having taken the publication into its new state. The aim of the journal is to provide a voice for the uniquely New Zealand perspective on bioethics and health law and to reflect on overseas influences which impact national health care practice, health law and policy. The journal is published three times a year.

The multidisciplinary nature of bioethics has meant that a great number of scholars, scientists, and medical professionals from many academic areas have contributed to the development of bioethics as a socio-cultural movement and as a discipline. Many bioethics works have appeared. Campbell, Gillett, and Jones co-authored *Medical Ethics*, an influential textbook focused on New Zealand context, which is currently in its third edition (Max Charlesworth joined the team in the later two editions). Campbell (now in Bristol), writes from the perspective of theology and philosophy; his manuscript *Health as Liberation* (1995) was written in New Zealand. The major works of Professor Grant Gillett include *Reasonable Care* (1989), *Medicine and Moral Reasoning* (as a co-editor, 1994), *The Mind and its Discontents* (1999), and *Consciousness and Intentionality*, co-authored with John McMillan (2001). Gareth Jones, professor and head of the Anatomy and Structural Biology Department at the University of Otago, writes from the angle of an anatomist and Christian bioethicist. His many publications in the field of bioethics include such books as *Brave New People: Ethical Issues at the Commencement of Life* (1984, revised edition 1985), *Manufacturing Humans: The Challenges of the New Reproductive Technologies* (1987), *Coping with Controversy: Helping Christians Handle their Differences* (1994, revised edition 1996), *Valuing People: Human Value in a World of Medical Technology* (1999), and *Speaking for the Dead: Cadavers in Biology and Medicine* (2000).

In 1990, the Eubios Ethics Institute was established by biologist and bioethicist Darryl Macer, creating a unique link between New Zealand and Asia, especially Japan. The

Eubios Ethics Institute publishes the *Eubios Journal of Asian and International Bioethics*, the official journal of the Asian Bioethics Association and the International Union of Biological Sciences Bioethics Program, available in hard copy and on the Internet. Actually, this journal was the first on-line bioethics journal in the world. The Institute also has published many volumes on bioethics.

Historically, bioethics as a discipline in New Zealand is mainly informed by medicine, law, philosophy, and theology. As an academic discipline, bioethics in New Zealand is facing two primary challenges: (1) to continue to inform the public about bioethical issues and contribute to bioethics as a socio-cultural movement, and (2) to move toward a more multidisciplinary and interdisciplinary environment, integrating into bioethics the perspectives, theories and methods of such subjects of learning as economy, anthropology and other social sciences, history, Maori studies, and so forth.

III. Concluding Remarks

The central event surrounding the birth of "Kiwi" bioethics was the Cartwright Inquiry into the unethical research program on cervical cancer at National Women's Hospital. Since then, bioethics has come a long way and is rapidly changing. Central features of New Zealand's bioethics include biculturalism, wide public awareness, active participation of the media, keeping pace with international developments, serious commitment to ethical medicine (practice, research and education), co-operation and commitment of medical professionals and establishments, efforts of government, devoted intellectuals and scholars, openness and honesty to ethical misconduct, and institutional mechanism designed to protect patients and research participants.

On the one hand, as the health system reforms, New Zealanders are troubled by "classic" bioethical dilemmas in medicine, such as sustaining an equitable health care system, decision making for minors, and the balancing of conflicts between protection of individual privacy and promotion of the public good. On the other hand, New Zealanders, together with people in many other countries, face many new challenges brought about by changing socio-cultural and medical environments, including recent advances in genetics and biotechnologies, and the wider use and more public acceptance of various kinds of alternative and complementary medicine and multi-cultural development. From this historical and sociological review of Kiwi bioethics, we have reason to believe that bioethics as a socio-cultural movement and an academic discipline in this country will continue to grow in New Zealanders' constant search for ethically sound answers to old dilemmas and new challenges.

Acknowledgements

This chapter is based on research which was financially supported by a grant from the Bequest Fund of the Dean's Research Advisory Committee, Dunedin Medical School, University of Otago. The authors would like to thank the research assistant Rebecca Keown and acknowledge the generous help of the following people: Professor Donald Evans, Claire Gallop, Dr. Neil Pickering, Professor Grant Gillett, Professor Gareth Jones,

Dr. Vanya Kovach, Professor Darryl Macer, Dr. Barbara Nicholas, Sally Pairman, Professor David Seedhouse, and Professor Peter Skegg.

Bibliography

_____. 1946-1949. Nuremberg code. In *Trials of war criminals before the Nuremberg military tribunals under control council law no. 10*. Washington, DC: United States Government Printing Office.

_____. 1998. Southern operation delay under fire after death. *Otago Daily Times*. Dunedin, New Zealand, (6 April): 3.

Abortion Supervisory Committee. 1998. *Report of the abortion supervisory committee*. Wellington.

Alexander, M. 1998. Tears in heaven. *Sunday Star Times* (4 October): C3.

American Medical Association. 1887. *Code of medical ethics for New Zealand*. Wellington: Lyndon and Blair.

Ansley, B. 1999. Mind that child. *Listener* (22 May) 18-20.

Auckland Healthcare Services Ltd. v. L. 1998. High Court, Auckland, NZFLR 998.

Brown, P. 1999. Back off state agencies – stop chasing young Liam and his parents. *The Dominion* (15 February).

Campbell, A.V. 1989. A report from New Zealand: an "unfortunate experiment". *Bioethics* 3(1): 59-66.

Campbell, A.V. 1991. Ethics after Cartwright. *New Zealand Medical Journal* 104: 36-37.

Campbell, A.V. 1995. *Health as liberation: medicine, theology and the quest for justice*. Cleveland: Pilgrim Press.

Chowka, P.B. 1999. New Zealand freedom of choice case resolved on a positive note [On-line]. Available: <http://www.naturalhealthvillage.com/newsletter/990515/liam.htm>.

Chowka, P.B. 1999. Underground in New Zealand: the search for medical freedom [On-line]. Available: <http://www.naturalhealthvillage.com/newsletter/990401/liam.htm>.

Committee of Inquiry into Allegations concerning the Treatment of Cervical Cancer at National Women's Hospital and into Other Related Matters, Judge Silvia Cartwright. 1988. *The report of the committee of inquiry into allegations concerning the treatment of cervical cancer at National Women's Hospital and into other related matters*. Auckland.

Coney, S. 1999. Chemotherapy in children – Where to draw the line? *The Lancet* 353: 819.

Coney, S. 1988. *The unfortunate experiment: the full story behind the inquiry into cervical cancer treatment*. Melbourne: Penguin.

Coney, S. & Bunkle, P. 1987. An "unfortunate experiment" at National Women's. *Metro*, (June), 46-65.

Danish Council of Ethics. 2002. *Genetic investigation of health subjects: report on presymptomatic genetic testing*. Copenhagen: Danish Council of Ethics.

Davidson, H., Dawson, J. & Moore, A. 2001. Law, ethics and epidemiology: the case of the cervical screening audit. *New Zealand Bioethics Journal* 2(2): 8-26.

Duffy, A.P., Barrett, D.K. & Duggan, M.A. 2001. *Report of the ministerial inquiry into the under-reporting of cervical smear abnormalities in the Gisborne region*. Wellington: Ministry of Health.

Fleming, D. 1999. A life in the balance. *New Zealand Woman's Weekly* (1 March): 14-15.

Fulford, K.W.M., Gillett, G.R. & Martin, J. (eds). 1994. *Medicine and moral reasoning*. Cambridge: University Press.

Gallop, C. 2001. Personal communication. Interview by Lynley Anderson. Dunedin, New Zealand, August 15.

Gauld, R. 1999. Policy disaster, public policy and the booking system. *Otago Bioethics Report* (June): 13-15.

Gauld, R. 2001. *Revolving doors: New Zealand's health reforms*. Wellington: Institute of Policy Studies and Health Services Research Centre.

Gauld, R. 2001. Restructuring, reform and more change: recent developments in New Zealand health policy. *New Zealand Bioethics Journal* 2(2): 3-7.

Gillett, G. 1989. *Reasonable care.* Bristol: Bristol Press.

Gillett, G. 1998. The case of the empty head: crossing cultures and preserving values. In: P. Komesaroff (ed.), *Expand the horizons of bioethics: proceedings of the Australian Bioethics Association fifth national conference* (pp. 62-67). Melbourne: Australian Bioethics Association.

Gillett, G. 1999. *The mind and its discontents: an essay in discursive psychiatry.* Oxford: Oxford University Press.

Gillett, G. & McMillan, J. 2001. *Consciousness and intentionality.* Philadelphia: John Benjamins Publishing Company.

Hartley, S. & Smith, D. 1999. Hawea cancer boy missing. *Otago Daily Times* (12 February): 1.

Healthcare Otago Limited v. Williams-Holloway. 1999. Family Court, Dunedin, NZFLR, 812.

Hills, B. 1999 *Fake healers* [On-line]. Available: <http://www.smh.com.au/news/spectrum/9909/11/spectrum1.html>.

Independent Biotechnology Advisory Council. 1999. *The biotechnology question.* Wellington: Ministry for the Environment.

Jefferson, S. 1999. Little Liam and civilisation as we know it. *Butterworths Family Law Journal* 3(2): 29-32.

Jones, D.G. 1985. *Brave new people: ethical issues at the commencement of life.* Grand Rapids: Eerdmans.

Jones, D.G. 1996. *Coping with controversy: helping Christians handle their differences.* Dunedin: Visjon Publications.

Jones, D.G. 1987. *Manufacturing humans: the challenges of the new reproductive technologies.* Leichester: Inter-Varsity Press.

Jones, D.G. 2000. *Speaking for the dead: cadavers in biology and medicine.* Brookfield: Ashgate.

Jones, D.G. 1999. *Valuing people: human value in a world of medical technology.* Carlisle: Paternoster Press.

Jonson, A. 1998. *The birth of bioethics.* New York: Oxford University Press.

King, A. 2001. *He Korowai Oranga: Maori health strategy discussion document.* Wellington: Ministry of Health.

Kovach, V. 2001. Personal Communication. Interview by Lynley Anderson. July 12.

Macer, D. 1994. Bioethical reasoning in New Zealand & Australia. In D.R.J. Macer (ed.), *Bioethics for the people by the people* (pp.139-145). Ibaraki: Eubios Ethics Institute.

Macer, D. 1998. *Bioethics is love of life: an alternative textbook.* Christchurch: Eubios Ethics Institute.

Macer, D. 1991. Letters of explanation and invitation. *Eubios Ethics Institute Newsletter* 1(1): 1.

Macer, D. 1990. *Shaping genes: ethics, law and science of using new genetic technology in medicine and agriculture.* Christchurch: Eubios Ethics Institute.

Macer, D., Asada, Y., Akiyama, S. & Tsuzuki, M. 1994. Bioethics in high schools in New Zealand, Australia & Japan. In D.R.J. Macer (ed.), *Bioethics for the people by the people* (pp. 177-185). Ibaraki: Eubios Ethics Institute.

Macer, D., Asada, Y., Akiyama, S., Tsuzuki, M. & Macer, N. 1996. *Bioethics in high schools in Australia, Japan & New Zealand.* Christchurch: Eubios Ethics Institute.

Macer, D. 1997. A big-hearted man who made the city his life. *New Zealand Herald* (13 October): A14.

Martin, Y. 1998. Soft side of harder. *Dominion,* (3 October): 14.

McCabe, M. 2000. Bioethics – challenges for the church. *The Nathaniel Report: A Publication of the Nathaniel Centre – the New Zealand Catholic Bioethics Centre,* 1 (August), 3-4.

McLoughlin, D. 2000. Liam Williams-Holloway and the triumph of quackery. *North & South* 167 (February): 72-81.

McMullen, J. 1999. Live Q&A with Brendan Holloway, father of Liam Williams-Holloway. *60 Minutes.* Sydney, Australia (23 May).

Ministry for the Environment. 2001. *Report of the royal commission on genetic modification*. Wellington: Ministry for the Environment.

Ministry of Health. 1990. *Amendment to the nurses act 1961*. Wellington: Ministry of Health.

Ministry of Health. 1996. *Code of health and disability service consumers' rights*. Wellington: Ministry of Health.

Ministry of Health. 1994. *Health and disability commissioner act*. Wellington: Ministry of Health.

Ministry of Health. 1994. *Health information privacy code*. Wellington: Ministry of Health.

Moore, C. 1999. How well do we look after our sick children. *The Press* (20 February), 4.

Morris, B. 1999. Child has a right to receive effective, modern therapy. *New Zealand Herald*, (16 February), A13.

Naylor, S. 1999. When parents and doctors disagree. *Otago Daily Times* (23 February), 19.

New Zealand Crimes Act. 1961. Wellington: New Zealand.

New Zealand Human Rights Act. 1993. Wellington: New Zealand.

New Zealand Medical Association. 1989. *Code of Ethics*. Wellington: New Zealand Medical Association.

Nicholas, B. 1996. Community and justice: the challenges of bicultural partnership to policy on assisted reproductive technology. *Bioethics* 10(3): 212-221.

Page, D. 2001. Not a privilege but a right: a brief history of the women's suffrage movement in New Zealand [On-line]. Available: <http://www.nzhistory.net.nz/gallery/suffragists/ suffintro.htm>.

Pairman, S. 2001. Personal Communication. Interview by Lynley Anderson. Dunedin, New Zealand. 15 February.

Paul, C. 2000. Internal and external morality of medicine: lessons from New Zealand. *British Journal of Medicine* 320: 114-118.

Price, N. 1999. Prioritisation and maximisation: drawing the ethical line. *Otago Bioethics Report* 8(2): 11-12.

Price, S. 1999. Parents won but Liam may have lost. *New Zealand Herald* (14 May), A11.

Rankin, K. 2001. Science, medicine and Liam Williams-Holloway [On-line]. Available: <http://pl.net/~keithr/rf99MedicalScience.html>.

Rankin, J. 2001. Authoritarian versus alternative thinking in godzone [On-line]. Available: <http://pl.net/~keithr/rf_shorts_1999_04apra.html#may16b>.

Revington, M. 1997. Blood money: after Rau Williams, how many more cases are waiting to pass the "clinical" test? *Listener* 161: 24.

Shortland v. Northland Health Limited. 1998. 1 NZLR, 433.

Statistics New Zealand. 2002 [On-line]. Available: <http://www.stats.govt.nz>.

Stent, R.K. 1998. Fulfilling the legacy of Cartwright. *Otago Bioethics Report* 7(3): 6-8.

Stirling, P. 1999. The cure. *Listener* (29 May): 21-23.

Taylor, R. 1999. Court on rare ground in smothering media fire it ignited. *New Zealand Herald* (1 March), A11.

The Treaty of Waitangi. 1840. New Zealand.

Wallace, N. 1998. Died waiting for by-pass. *Otago Daily Times* (6 April), 1, 3.

Warnock, M. 1984. *A question of life: the Warnock report on human fertilisation and embryology*. Oxford: Basil Blackwell.

White, M. 1998. The brief life of Baby L. *Listener* 165: 22-23.

World Medical Association Declaration of Helsinki. 1964. *Ethical principles for medical research involving human subjects*. Helsinki: World Medical Association.

World Medical Association. 1948. *Declaration of Geneva: physician's oath*. Adopted by the General Assembly of the World Medical Association, Geneva, Switzerland, September 1948 and amended by the 22nd World Medical Assembly, Sydney, Australia, August 1968.

World Medical Association. 1981. *Declaration on the rights of the patient*. Adopted by the 34th World Medical Assembly Lisbon, Portugal, September/October 1981 and amended by the 47th General Assembly Bali, Indonesia, September 1995.

Notes on Contributors

Sahin Aksoy, *Professor, Department of Medical Ethics and History of Medicine, Harran University, Dekanlik Binasi, Sanliurfa, Turkey.*

Lynley Anderson, *Lecturer, Bioethics Centre, University of Otago, Dunedin, New Zealand.*

Jayapaul Azariah, *Founder and President, All India Bioethics Association, Indira Nagar, Chennai, India.*

Gerhold K. Becker, *Chair of Religion & Philosophy, Founding Director of the Center for Applied Ethics, Hong Kong Baptist University, Kowloon Tong, Hong Kong.*

Hasna Begum, *Professor, Department of Philosophy, University of Dhaka, Dhaka, Bangladesh.*

Anne Bernard, *Professor, Centre de documentation en éthique de l'Insern, Paris, France.*

Leonardo de Castro, *Professor, Department of Philosophy, College of Social Sciences and Philosophy, The University of the Philippines, Diliman, Quezon City, Philippines.*

Ruth Chadwick, *Professor and Director, Institute of Environment, Philosophy, and Public Policy, Lancaster University Furness College, Lancaster, UK.*

Mark J. Cherry, *Assistant Professor, Department of Philosophy, Saint Edward's University, Austin, Texas.*

Ya-Li Cong, *Professor, Department of Medical Ethics, Beijing University Health Science Center, Beijing, Peoples Republic of China.*

H. Tristram Engelhardt, Jr., *Professor, Department of Philosophy, Rice University, Houston, Texas and Professor Emeritus, Baylor College of Medicine, Houston, Texas.*

Fabrice Jotterand, *Department of Religious Studies, Rice University, Houston, Texas.*

Anne Fagot-Largeault, *Professor and Chair of Philosophy of Biological and Medical Sciences, Collège de France, Paris, France.*

T. Garanis-Papadatos, *Department of Public and Administrative Health, National School of Public Health, Athens, Greece.*

Nuala Kenny, *Professor and Chair, Department of Bioethics, Dalhousie University, Halifax, Nova Scotia, Canada.*

B. Andrew Lustig, *Director, Joint Program on Biotechnology, Religion, and Ethics, Rice University and Baylor College of Medicine, Houston, Texas.*

Darryl Macer, *Professor at the Institute of Biological Sciences, University of Tsukuba, Tsukuba Science City, Japan.*

José Alberto Mainetti, *Director, Instituto de Bioetica y Humanidades Medicas, Buenos Aires, Argentina.*

Mirta Matinez, *Instituto de Bioetica y Humanidades Medicas, Fundacion Jose Maria Mainetti Centro de Referencia en Bioetica, Buenos Aires, Argentina.*

Brendan Minogue, *Professor, Center for Bioethics, Youngstown State University, Youngstown, Ohio.*

Guillermo C. Morello, *Instituto de Bioetica y Humanidades Medicas, Fundacion Jose Maria Mainetti Centro de Referencia en Bioetica, Buenos Aires, Argentina.*

Maurizio Mori, *Professor, Politeia and Consulta di Bioetica Via Cosimo del Fante, Milano, Italy.*

Jing-Bao Nie, *Senior Lecturer, Bioethics Centre, University of Otago, Dunedin, New Zealand.*

Michael Parker, *Professor, The Ethox Center, Institute of Health Sciences, Oxford University, Oxford, UK.*

Hécto H. Pinedo, *Instituto de Bioetica y Humanidades Medicas, Fundacion Jose Maria Mainetti Centro de Referencia en Bioetica, Buenos Aires, Argentina.*

Scott B. Rae, *Professor, Talbot School of Theology, Biola University, La Mirada, California.*

Jacob Dahl Rendtorff, *Professor, Social Sciences Department, Institut for Samfundsvidenskab og Erhvervsøkonomi VIII, Roskilde University, Roskilde, Denmark.*

Kurt Schmidt, *Professor, Center for Medical Ethics, Markus-Hospital, Frankfurt, Germany.*

José M. Tau, *Instituto de Bioetica y Humanidades Medicas, Fundacion Jose Maria Mainetti Centro de Referencia en Bioetica, Buenos Aires, Argentina.*

P. Dalla-Vorgia, *Department of Public and Administrative Health, National School of Public Health, Athens, Greece.*

Index